Register Now for Online Access to Your Book!

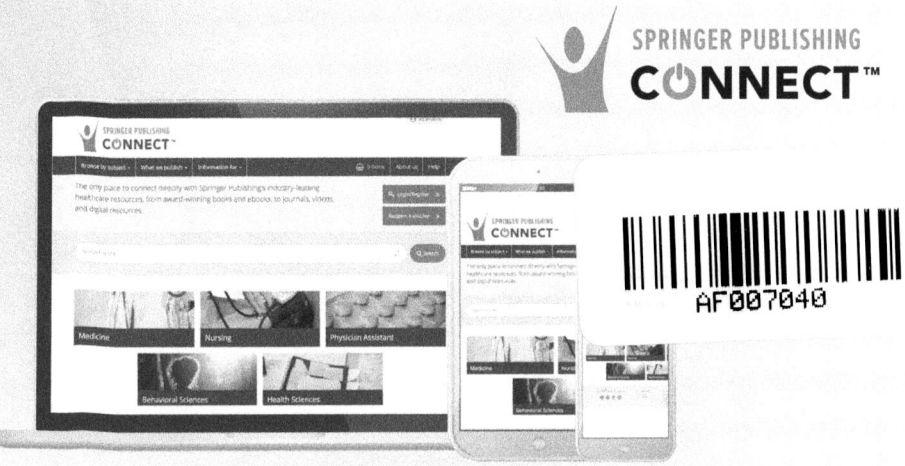

Your print purchase of *EMDR With Children in the Play Therapy Room* **includes online access to the contents of your book**—increasing accessibility, portability, and searchability!

Access today at:
http://connect.springerpub.com/content/book/978-0-8261-7593-9
or scan the QR code at the right with your smartphone
and enter the access code below.

5H86FA89

Scan here for quick access.

If you are experiencing problems accessing the digital component of this product, please contact our customer service department at cs@springerpub.com

The online access with your print purchase is available at the publisher's discretion and may be removed at any time without notice.

Publisher's Note: New and used products purchased from third-party sellers are not guaranteed for quality, authenticity, or access to any included digital components.

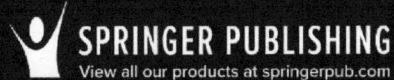
View all our products at springerpub.com

EMDR With Children in the Play Therapy Room

Ann Beckley-Forest, LCSW, RPT-S, is a licensed clinical social worker in private practice in Buffalo, New York. Her specialties include attachment and child and adolescent trauma; she also works with adult survivors. She is a registered play therapist and supervisor and an approved provider of play therapy continuing education through the Association for Play Therapy. She is also an EMDR International Association (EMDRIA)-approved consultant and a faculty member of the Child Trauma Institute, in addition to serving as the training chair of the EMDRIA Special Interest Group for children and adolescents. She provides clinical consultation in person and remotely and gives trainings locally and around the United States and Asia. Her primary interest is in the intersection of play therapy and eye movement desensitization and reprocessing (EMDR), and she has previously published on this topic in the *Play Therapy* magazine and the EMDRIA magazine, *Go With That*.

Annie Monaco, LCSW, RPT, is a licensed clinical social worker, a registered play therapist, and a faculty member of both the Child Trauma Institute and University at Buffalo School of Social Work. Annie travels throughout the United States and internationally providing trauma-informed trainings and agency and therapist consultation. She is a trainer of eye movement desensitization and reprocessing (EMDR) and Progressive Counting (PC) and attachment and dissociation and is the chair of the EMDR International Association (EMDRIA) Child and Adolescent Special Interest Group. She has extensive training in complex trauma, family therapy, play therapy, and restorative justice, and over 25 years of experience serving children, teens, families, and adults. Her private practice in Amherst, New York, includes complex issues such as foster care, out-of-country adoptions, juvenile justice, and dissociation.

EMDR With Children in the Play Therapy Room

An Integrated Approach

ANN BECKLEY-FOREST, LCSW, RPT-S
ANNIE MONACO, LCSW, RPT

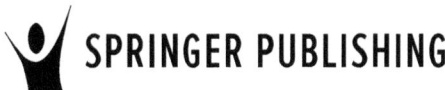

Copyright © 2021 Springer Publishing Company, LLC
All rights reserved.

No part of this publication may be reproduced, stored in a retrieval system, or transmitted in any form or by any means, electronic, mechanical, photocopying, recording, or otherwise, without the prior permission of Springer Publishing Company, LLC, or authorization through payment of the appropriate fees to the Copyright Clearance Center, Inc., 222 Rosewood Drive, Danvers, MA 01923, 978-750-8400, fax 978-646-8600, info@copyright.com or on the Web at www.copyright.com.

Springer Publishing Company, LLC
11 West 42nd Street, New York, NY 10036
www.springerpub.com
connect.springerpub.com/

Acquisitions Editor: Kate Dimock
Compositor: Amnet Systems

ISBN: 978-0-8261-7592-2
ebook ISBN: 978-0-8261-7593-9
DOI: 10.1891/9780826175939

Printed by LSI

The author and the publisher of this Work have made every effort to use sources believed to be reliable to provide information that is accurate and compatible with the standards generally accepted at the time of publication. The author and publisher shall not be liable for any special, consequential, or exemplary damages resulting, in whole or in part, from the readers' use of, or reliance on, the information contained in this book. The publisher has no responsibility for the persistence or accuracy of URLs for external or third-party Internet websites referred to in this publication and does not guarantee that any content on such websites is, or will remain, accurate or appropriate.

Library of Congress Cataloging-in-Publication Data

Names: Beckley-Forest, Ann, editor. | Monaco, Annie, editor.
Title: EMDR with children in the play therapy room : an integrated approach / [edited by] Ann Beckley-Forest, Annie Monaco.
Description: New York, NY : Springer Publishing Company, 2020. | Includes bibliographical references and index.
Identifiers: LCCN 2020010093 (print) | LCCN 2020010094 (ebook) | ISBN 9780826175922 (paperback) | ISBN 9780826175939 (ebook)
Subjects: MESH: Eye Movement Desensitization Reprocessing—methods | Child | Psychological Trauma—therapy | Play Therapy—methods
Classification: LCC RJ505.P6 (print) | LCC RJ505.P6 (ebook) | NLM WS 350.3 | DDC 618.92/891653—dc23
LC record available at https://lccn.loc.gov/2020010093
LC ebook record available at https://lccn.loc.gov/2020010094

Contact us to receive discount rates on bulk purchases.
We can also customize our books to meet your needs.
For more information please contact: sales@springerpub.com

Ann Beckley-Forest: https://orcid.org/0000-0001-5161-5193
Annie Monaco: https://orcid.org/0000-0002-1637-1207

Publisher's Note: New and used products purchased from third-party sellers are not guaranteed for quality, authenticity, or access to any included digital components.

Printed in the United States of America.

Contents

Contributors   xi
Foreword   Ana M. Gomez, MC, LPC   xiii
Preface   xvii
Acknowledgments   xix

SECTION I   MODELS FOR INTEGRATION

1   Using Both EMDR and Prescriptive Play Therapy in Adaptive Information Processing: Rationale and Essential Considerations for Integration   3
Ann Beckley-Forest

    Two Communities of Therapists With One Goal   3
    For EMDR Therapists: Understanding Play Therapy as a Clinical Approach   4
    For Play Therapists: Understanding EMDR as a Clinical Approach With Children   5
    Taking the Next Steps in Integration: The Eight Essentials   6
    Essential 1: Safe Alliance Through Play   8
    Essential 2: Holding Space for Posttraumatic Play   10
    Essential 3: Playing EMDR With Prop-Based Bilateral Stimulation   13
    Essential 4: Expanding Capacity for State Change   15
    Essential 5: Expanding and Assessing Memory Targets in the Posttraumatic Play With EMDR   17
    Essential 6: Build Bridges From Implicit to Explicit Trauma Work   20
    Essential 7: Ongoing Reevaluation of Memory Targets   24
    Essential 8: Involving Parents Throughout Treatment   24
    Potency of Integrated Models of Treatment in Complex Posttraumatic Stress Disorder and Dissociation   28
    Conclusion   28

2 TraumaPlay and EMDR: Integration and Nuance in Holding Hard Stories 33
Paris Goodyear-Brown and Eleah Hyatt

TraumaPlay 33
Integrating EMDR and TraumaPlay 37
Assessment 39
Enhancing Safety and Security 41
Safe Place in TraumaPlay 42
Contamination of Safe Place 43
Soothing the Physiology and Parents as Partners 45
Assessment and Augmentation of Coping 47
Soothing the Physiology 49
Assessment Phase in EMDR 51
Parents as Partners 55
Relational Resourcing 55
Increasing Emotional Literacy 56
Posttraumatic Play and Play-Based Gradual Exposure 58
Experiential Mastery Play 59
Trauma Narrative Work 59
Nurturing Narration 62
Scaling 63
Addressing the Thought Life During Reprocessing 65
Titration and the Dance Toward and Away From Trauma Content 67
Somatic Experiencing With Trauma Targets 67
Making Positive Meaning of the Posttrauma Self 69
Conclusion 72

3 Room for Everyone: EMDR and Family-Based Play Therapy in the Sand Tray 75
Marshall Lyles

Adaptive Information Processing in a Family/Play Therapy Context 75
Sandtray as the Modality 78
Weaving EMDR, Sandtray, and Family Play Therapies 84
Phase 1: History and Treatment Planning 85
Phase 2: Preparation 95
Phase 3: Assessment 99
Phases 4 to 7: Densensitization, Body Scan, Installation, and Closure 101
Phase 8: Reevaluation 103
Conclusion 104

4 Synergetic Play Therapy Combined With EMDR Therapy   109
Jan Schaad and Lisa Dion
    SPT and EMDR: Long-Lost Best Friends   109
    The Foundation   111
    Synergetic Play Therapy and EMDR   114
    The Therapist as an Instrument of the Regulation of the Child's Autonomic Nervous System   117
    Becoming the External Regulator   117
    Dual Awareness   119
    Therapist Activation   120
    The Mirror Neuron System   120
    Therapist Authenticity   121
    The Synergy Between SPT and EMDR in the Playroom   123
    Assessment: Is the Child Ready?   130
    The Parent–Child Dyad in the Playroom   134
    Developing Emotional Resources   137
    Reprocessing Trauma With SPT/EMDR   138
    Conclusion   142

5 Treating Trauma in Young Children: Integrating EMDR, Child-Centered Play Therapy, and Developmental Play Therapy   145
Roxanne Grobbel
    A Case Study for Integrating CCPT, DPT, and EMDR: Introducing Peter   146
    EMDR and Children   154
    Play Therapy and EMDR History/Case Conceptualization   155
    Conclusion   176

6 EMDR and Creative Arts Therapy: How Creative Arts Therapies Can Extend the Reach of EMDR With Complex Clients   183
Elizabeth Davis
    The Development of Art Expression and Experience   184
    Evidence for Using a Creative Arts Approach for Healing   187
    MBT and Mentalization   190
    Expressive Therapy as Mentalization Therapy   194
    EMDR, Art Therapy, and Maximizing Mentalization for Processing   197
    Integrating Creative Arts and EMDR: The Case of Ella   198
    Conclusion   219

7 Playful and Creative Approaches for EMDR Therapy With Latinx Children   223
Viviana Urdaneta and Viviana Triana
    Background and Latinx Term Clarification   223

Culture and Cultural Competence   224

Generational Differences and Acculturation Levels   227

Integrating Playful and Culturally Relevant Interventions Throughout the EMDR Phases   229

Additional Ideas: Group Protocol   246

Conclusion   247

8 Understanding and Responding to Dissociation in Children With Play-Based Approaches   251
Annie Monaco

Using the Lens of Dissociation   251

What Is Dissociation, Why Does It Occur, and What Are the Theories?   256

Treatment   268

The Playroom Parts-of-Self Process   275

Treatment Examples   283

Integration   286

Conclusion   287

SECTION II   PLAY-BASED INTERVENTIONS FOR EMDR PHASES

9 Taking a Play-Based Trauma History   293
Ann Beckley-Forest and Melissa LaVigne

Description of Intervention   294

Step-by-Step Directions   295

Modifications   296

Considerations   297

Case Example   297

10 Building a Calm/Safe Place in the Play Therapy Room With the Fort Tent   301
Alice Stricklin

Description of Intervention   303

Step-by-Step Instructions   303

Modifications   306

Considerations   306

Case Example   306

11 Using Trauma-Sensitive Yoga and Embodied Play Therapy for Stabilization and Resourcing   311
Jennifer Lefebre

Interventions   315

Case Example   320

12 The Pocket Smock as a Preparation Phase Resource   325
Faith Thompson-Lee

Description of Intervention   327
Step-by-Step Instructions   327
Modifications   332
Case Example   335

13 The "Lemon Squeezies" Metaphor for EMDR Processing With Children   339
Kristen Hurvitz

Description of Intervention   340
Step-by-Step Instructions   340
Modifications   344
Considerations   344
Case Example   344

14 EMDR-Infused Theraplay®   349
Faith Thompson-Lee

Description of Intervention   352
Step-by-Step Instructions   353
Modification: Predictability   358
Considerations   359
Case Example   361

15 Resource Wand for Bilateral Stimulation in EMDR Therapy   365
Annie Monaco

Description of Intervention   366
Step-by-Step Instructions   366
Modifications   367
Considerations   368
Case Example   368

16 Using the Superhero Shuffle for Bilateral Stimulation in EMDR With Children   371
Tyne Potgieter

Description of Intervention   372
Step-by-Step Instructions   373
Modifications   374
Considerations   375
Case Example   376

17 "Splatting" Out the Trauma With Movement in EMDR Processing   379
Alice Stricklin

Description of Intervention   381
Step-by-Step Instructions   381
Modifications   383
Considerations   384
Case Examples   384

18 Using the Color Hands Approach to Bilateral Stimulation   393
Tyne Potgieter

Description of Intervention   394
Step-by-Step Instructions   394
Modifications   396
Considerations   396
Case Example   397

19 Play Therapy Targets for EMDR Processing: How to Get a "Bulls-Eye"   401
Victoria McGuinness

Step-by-Step Instructions: Explaining EMDR   403
Step-by-Step Instructions: In the Assessment Phase   403
Considerations   404
Case Example   405
On a Personal Note   410

20 Effectively Managing the Closure and Reevaluation Phase With Parents   413
Annie Monaco

Description of the Intervention   415
Step-by-Step Instructions: Closure Phase   416
Step-by-Step Instructions: Reevaluation   418
Modification: Caregivers Who Are Not Available   418
Considerations   419
Case Examples   419
A Creative Alternative to the Popcorn Night   420
Conclusion   421

Index   427

Contributors

Elizabeth Davis, MFA, MS, LCAT, ART-BC, Director, Trauma Institute and Child Trauma Institute, Satellite Amherst, New York (Based in Northampton, Massachusetts)

Lisa Dion, LPC, RPT-S, Founder and President, Lead Instructor, Synergetic Play Therapy Institute, Boulder, Colorado

Paris Goodyear-Brown, MSSW, LCSW, RPT-S, EMDRIA, Clinical Director of Nurture House, Executive Director of the TraumaPlay Institute, Creator of TraumaPlay, Franklin, Tennessee

Roxanne Grobbel, JD, LCSW, RPT-S, Insight Counseling Center, Boca Raton, Florida

Kristen Hurvitz, LCSW, RPT, Berkeley Play Therapy, Berkeley, California

Eleah Hyatt, MA, LMFT, RPT, Senior Clinician and Intern Director of Nurture House, Franklin, Tennessee

Melissa LaVigne, LCSW, RPT, Private Practice, Buffalo, New York

Jennifer Lefebre, PsyD, RPT-S, TCTSY-F, Healing the Child Within, New Hartford, Connecticut

Marshall Lyles, MA, LMFT-S, LPC-S, RPT-S, EMDRIA-Approved Consultant; Sandtray Faculty, Institute for Play Therapy-Sandtray Therapy Certification, Texas State University, San Marcos, Texas

Victoria McGuinness, LMHC, Bayside Therapy Associates, LLC; North West Independent Behavioral Practitioners, Inc.

Tyne Potgieter, MS, LMHC, NCC, CCMHC, Licensed Mental Health Counselor; Director, The Living Practice, South Africa

Jan Schaad, LCSW, Approved Credit Provider, EMDR International Association, Austin, Texas; Regional Trainer, EMDR Institute, Watsonville, California

Alice Stricklin, LMFT, Private Practice, Lebanon, Tennessee

Faith Thompson-Lee, MEd, LMHC, South Country Central School District, Pupil Personnel Services, East Patchogue, New York

Viviana Triana, MDiv, LCSW Supervisor, Program Director, South Dallas Counseling Center, Family Place, Dallas, Texas

Viviana Urdaneta, MDiv, LCSW, Private Practice, Oakland, California

Foreword

Play is central in the development of the child's identity and the process of self-definition. In the safety of the parent–child relationship, play emerges as a powerful self-shaping force. Through play, infants and children begin to experience others, supporting the brain in its transformation into a social structure (Cozolino, 2010).

Panksepp's brilliant work elucidated the existence of seven emotional systems at birth, one of which is play (Panksepp & Biven, 2012). No longer is play seen as a random activity in which mammals engage, but instead it is a biological need and a drive that moves humans toward transformation and growth. Through playful interactions, the brain and the nervous system of infants and children develop. The energy and containment emerging from play provide the nervous system with the playground, where various levels of arousal can be experienced, experimented with, and ultimately modulated.

When it comes to trauma, play becomes the vessel and vehicle for self-expression that allows children to communicate what otherwise could be overwhelming. Children, especially young ones, cannot verbalize their innermost states. However, they are able to tell their stories through drawings, storytelling, expressive arts, and symbolic play. Play supplies children with the necessary distance to explore, access, and express what sometimes is inexpressible using words or too painful and shameful to understand and verbalize.

To facilitate the healing of children, we must honor their developmental demands, qualities, needs, tendencies, capacities, and neurobiological maturity. Embracing the forces of play—and the child's natural tendencies toward play—is vital throughout the eight phases of eye movement desensitization and reprocessing (EMDR) therapy. The addition of play in EMDR therapy provides containment and safety as memories of trauma and adversity are identified, explored, and processed (Gomez & Shapiro, 2012).

This book marks an important historic moment in the recognition of therapeutic and intentional play as a crucial and essential component that is interwoven within the eight phases of EMDR therapy with children.

The play themes of traumatized children are full of cognitive, emotional, somatic, and behavioral elements that are reminiscent of the traumatic events they experienced as well as the legacy of what these experiences did to their neurobiological systems. For children with sensitized sympathetic or parasympathetic systems, fight, flight, and collapse responses may become activated during their play. Puppet shows, sand tray worlds, and stories may reflect the child's most inner conflicts, shame, and fears as well as their deepest longings and unmet needs. These stories and play themes with an EMDR framework also hold the possibility for completing truncated defenses and accomplishing new and empowering actions that could not be executed during the traumatic event. They also provide the ground for recovering dissociated cognitive, affective, and somatic material, challenging representations of the self and others, meeting unmet needs, utilizing new resources, and reconnecting to the mind, the heart, and the body in novel and creative ways.

In *EMDR With Children in the Play Therapy Room: An Integrated Approach,* the authors offer enormous alternatives and ingenious ways of using the playroom to provide a fertile ground where the child can play out explicit material as well as implicit urges. Quite often these impulses exist below awareness in the nonconscious mind in somatic and emotional states. In the first part of the book, the authors offer models of integration and significant insight into the blending of two approaches while maintaining the heart and essence of each. They beautifully incorporate creativity and imagination combined with attunement and synchronicity. Grounded in the latest literature and research, the authors provide numerous play-based interventions and a how-to approach to assist children as they work through their multiple adaptations to trauma. This volume is infused with metaphors, analogies, and inviting stories that playfully reach the mind of the child. They transform complex constructs into child-friendly and easily digestible material that make the process comprehensible. Clinicians reading this book will find numerous child-friendly means of providing dual attention stimuli (DAS) as well as inspiring and innovative ways of navigating through the eight phases of EMDR therapy while honoring what it means to be a child.

The authors of *EMDR With Children in the Play Therapy Room: An Integrated Approach* furnish us with incredible insight into the richness and possibilities that play therapy in its various forms provides to EMDR practitioners. They invite play therapists to immerse into the wealth, power, and complexities of EMDR therapy. At the same time, they offer a depth of understanding into the challenges of utilizing both. They provide numerous portals and access routes into the traumatogenic memory networks that validate and honor the child's biology and dance with implicit and explicit data.

This book invites therapists to embrace connection, resonance, and synchrony with the child while maintaining a close connection with their own internal states. The therapist takes the role of an external psychobiological regulator of the child's system (Schore, 2012) and is informed in their decision-making process by the data broadcasted by the child at any given moment in the therapeutic process. EMDR therapy becomes a piece of art where the child and therapeutic companions join forces as they embrace deep states of activation while receiving the gift of containment that play often provides.

Multiple chapters thoroughly address the continuum from nondirective and child-steered activities to more directive approaches and therapist-guided interventions—a beautiful dance that joins the child and meets them where they are while gently inviting them to visit the various layers left behind by trauma. Abundant applications are articulated to work with complex trauma and dissociation that assist children growing up in traumatizing and relationally impoverished environments that did not support integration. As a result, these children had no other choice but to move into greater and greater levels of fragmentation in their emerging sense of self.

The work with the family system and the parents is addressed in *EMDR With Children in the Play Therapy Room: An Integrated Approach* from multiple play therapy modalities, some of which work on strengthening the parent–child bond by increasing the parent's capacity to connect, mentalize, synchronize, and attune to the child's needs. The use of family-based play therapy in the sand tray, TraumaPlay, and Theraplay® in conjunction with EMDR therapy offers multiple opportunities to engage the parents and work systemically to support the healing of the child and the parent–child bond. These approaches carry on the important goal of reestablishing the parent's role as the bigger, wiser, older individual capable of engaging in mutual regulation while responding contingently to the child's needs.

Traumatized children experience delays in language development and skills compared to their counterparts (Sylvestre, Bussières, & Bouchard, 2016). These children may be physiologically activated while being verbally inhibited. Areas in the brain actively involved in language shut down as a result of emotional activation resulting from trauma (van der Kolk, 2014). Additionally, children are just developing their linguistic capacities and are too young to convey needs, thoughts, and feelings into words. Art representations and creations provide children with a doorway and a window into their inner reality. Expressive arts possess a prolific number of possibilities from movement to dance, drama, and music. Across the eight phases of EMDR therapy, children can experience regulation, safety, and homeostasis through the practice of art in all its forms. This volume presents how art therapy and expressive arts can become a road and a pathway into the inner world and internal milieu of the traumatized child so the processing, and ultimately the integration of memory within an EMDR framework, can be facilitated.

Ann Beckley-Forest, Annie Monaco, and all the contributors to this book offer abundant and valuable discernments, and this book will be indispensable to beginning and experienced child therapists. Dr. Francine Shapiro's vision was for EMDR therapy to reach every wounded heart and every human being trapped in the agony left by trauma. Her dream and the arduous work throughout her life were directed to alleviating human suffering in all corners of the world. The richness offered in this book will certainty support this vision and will accompany child therapists and the children they serve in their journeys toward finding healing, integration, and wholeness.

Ana M. Gomez, MC, LPC
AGATE Institute Founder and Director
Phoenix, Arizona

REFERENCES

Cozolino, L. (2010). *The neuroscience of psychotherapy: Healing the social brain.* New York, NY: W. W. Norton.

Gomez, A. M., & Shapiro, F. (2012). EMDR therapy with children: Journey into wholeness. *Child & Family Professional Journal, 15*(3), 20–30.

Panksepp, J., & Biven, L. (2012). *The archaeology of mind: Neuroevolutionary origins of human emotions.* New York, NY: W. W. Norton.

Schore, A. N. (2012). *The science of the art of psychotherapy.* New York, NY: W. W. Norton.

Sylvestre, A., Bussières, È. L., & Bouchard, C. (2016). Language problems among abused and neglected children: A meta-analytic review. *Child Maltreatment, 21*(1), 47–58. doi:10.1177/1077559515616703

van der Kolk, B. (2014). *The body keeps the score: Brain, mind, and body in the healing of trauma.* New York, NY: Penguin Books.

Preface

The book you are holding began as a conversation that turned into many years of conversations and collaboration.

We first crossed paths in a training by Ricky Greenwald. Each of us had our different ways of conceptualizing how to help children overcome trauma, and we were fascinated by our questions of how to really make eye movement desensitization and reprocessing (EMDR) work with children while remaining faithful to Dr. Francine Shapiro's protocol. Eventually we organized our own series of workshops on using EMDR with children, which ultimately led to this book.

Our conversations were about how to engage children effectively and how to teach other therapists to use playful and skillful interventions with this population. In our most exciting and intense conversations, we attempted to bridge what we perceived as a gap in treatment between our two home bases as therapists—the world of play therapy and that of EMDR. Along that journey, as we have become respectively cross-trained and fully credentialed as consultants and trainers for other therapists in both play therapy and EMDR, the conversation about how to help children heal from trauma, attachment, and dissociation has continued.

As we have held trainings around the country and the world, we hear many of the same things: Play therapists are encountering children who are hurting and want to use EMDR to help them toward healing as quickly as possible, but without giving up the character of their play therapy relationship; EMDR-trained therapists struggle to work with children who are hard to engage, distrustful of adults, and have very narrow windows of tolerance for therapy; and trauma therapists are curious as to what play therapy might offer as a therapeutic space for trauma work. All these therapists want to be faithful to the theoretical models that underpin their work.

Ann's background was in child-centered play and was more nondirective, Annie's approach was more directive, but we both recognized that providing good EMDR therapy with children encompasses much more than just learning the protocol. We recognized the need to teach therapists about early childhood trauma, attachment wounds, and dissociation because these complexities can easily sabotage progress in therapy regardless of the approach.

The result of all of this talking is this book. As editors we have tried to seek out some of the innovators in play therapy and EMDR to write about their own journeys toward an integrated approach that holds the promise of extending the benefits of EMDR to even the youngest children, and within the emotional safety of the play therapy room.

To truly benefit, the reader must first have access to high-quality EMDRIA-approved basic EMDR training and child-sensitive consultation. An intentional approach to play therapy rooted in theory and applied under supervision (such as the process leading to a play therapy credential) is also the ideal path to becoming qualified to provide the kind of play therapy environment that is the safest haven for trauma work.

In the first chapter, Ann lays out some of the essential considerations for a fully integrated approach that considers how posttraumatic play makes memory networks available for EMDR reprocessing. In Chapters 2 to 6, we invite some leading innovators to describe in depth their approach to integration of their modalities with EMDR, encompassing TraumaPlay, sandtray, art therapy, synergetic play therapy, child-centered, and developmental play therapy approaches. In Chapter 7, we ask the authors to use their journey as therapists within the Latinx community as an example of how to explore playful approaches that enhance cultural sensitivity in EMDR. In the final chapter of Section I, Annie uses the lens of dissociation to make sense of how children exposed to complex early trauma behave in the playroom and how to begin their preparation for EMDR therapy.

Section II offers a series of shorter intervention-based chapters, organized according to the eight phases of EMDR, which describe each author's contribution to the repertoire of play-based EMDR interventions.

All of these authors have been inspired by the work of pioneers in both play therapy and EMDR with children, and whose names appear throughout these pages. In particular, we feel a great debt to the work of Violet Oaklander, Eliana Gil, and Paris Goodyear-Brown on the play therapy side and the creative geniuses of Bob Tinker, Ricky Greenwald, Ana Gomez, Robbie Adler-Tapia, Carolyn Settle, and Frankie Klaff, among others, in the EMDR world. We also owe a debt to Victoria McGuinness, whose early efforts at integrating play therapy and EMDR have inspired many and who graciously agreed to contribute a chapter to this book.

Finally, we acknowledge our true inspiration, the children who let us into their worlds and whose bravery in the face of adversity has pushed us all to become the best healers we can possibly be.

Ann Beckley-Forest and Annie Monaco

Acknowledgments

Ricky Greenwald was one of the first people to make EMDR comprehensible to children and to many child therapists. He came to Buffalo, New York, many times to train therapists and allowed us to be his assistants. Eventually we became trainers under the Trauma Institute and Child Trauma Institute. Were it not for his trust and his example, we would not be the editors of this book. We thank him for his mentorship and his guidance and his friendship.

We also want to thank the EMDRIA Child Special Interest Group for having amazing leaders who, since its inception, have pushed hard for more training and more research of EMDR with children.

Section I
Models for Integration

1

Using Both EMDR and Prescriptive Play Therapy in Adaptive Information Processing: Rationale and Essential Considerations for Integration

ANN BECKLEY-FOREST

INTRODUCTION

Despite the potential benefits, children are often very reluctant to participate in eye movement desensitization and reprocessing (EMDR) therapy. Children may accomplish some digestion of traumatic experiences in play therapy, a naturalistic setting in which children participate eagerly. Prescriptive play therapy for trauma involves a phase-based approach where the activities within the playroom may vary from less directive to more directive with the goal of supporting trauma exposure/trauma narrative work. Trauma-informed prescriptive play therapists guide play in the avenues that will support trauma digestion and emotional regulation. Integrating play therapy within Francine Shapiro's adaptive information processing (AIP) model with a flexible approach to the EMDR protocol holds promise in using play to enter the memory network and promote healing. This chapter establishes eight essential considerations in fully integrating EMDR in a play therapy setting and examines the idea that play may be the preferred avenue to access and reprocess with EMDR the implicit memories involved so often in complex trauma in children.

TWO COMMUNITIES OF THERAPISTS WITH ONE GOAL

A newly trained therapist, well versed in the most current understanding of how trauma and adversity affect the long-term emotional and physical health of children, sets out on a career oriented toward helping children to heal. But where to begin? How can therapists best learn to provide the kinds of experiences within treatment that will help children to feel competent, loved, and optimistic despite the wounds to their neurobiological development from trauma? In my career, I have had the privilege of operating within two different professional communities both focused on improving outcomes for such children—play therapy and EMDR therapy. I have developed a firm belief that cross-discipline conversation will lead to more fully integrated models and deeper healing. These communities must understand the contributions made by each respective field and ultimately develop ways of integrating on both a theoretical and practical level while remaining faithful to each approach.

FOR EMDR THERAPISTS: UNDERSTANDING PLAY THERAPY AS A CLINICAL APPROACH

The term "play therapy" broadly describes a variety of models and theoretical approaches that clinicians use to create opportunities for therapeutic change, learning, and healing among children. What sets play therapy apart from other child therapies is the *intentional*, not accidental or incidental, use of play. Play therapists see play as "the specific change agent" that initiates, facilitates, or strengthens the therapeutic effect. Regardless of the play therapy model, play therapists understand play itself to produce change, beyond being merely a way of making treatment more accessible or palatable (Schaefer & Drewes, 2014). Traditionally, notions of play therapy were associated with child-centered play therapy or CCPT, which developed from the early work of Virginia Axline (1964) and was further developed by Gary Landreth (2012) and others. CCPT relies on the therapist providing an environment for expressive play in which the child's activities are noticed and supported in a calm, neutral way by a therapist who respects the child's own power in using the experimentation of play to resolve emotional difficulties. In CCPT's companion filial approach, child–parent relationship therapy (CPRT), parents are coached to provide the acceptance and reflecting statements that a play therapist would use (Landreth & Bratton, 2019). Over time, play therapy as a clinical approach has developed to include evidence-based approaches along a continuum from child-led to therapist-led, also described as the continuum from nondirective to directive play therapy, including Adlerian play therapy (Kottman, 2013) and cognitive behavioral play therapy (Knell, 2009) among others.

The term *prescriptive play therapy* (Schaefer, 2011) describes a theoretical approach to play therapy that draws from a variety of modalities and approaches within play therapy in an integrated manner to develop a comprehensive assessment and treatment plan. This plan applies the healing power of play through a variety of child-led and adult-influenced activities. Prescriptive play therapy is being widely applied in the treatment of trauma, as it balances both the establishment of a CCPT relationship where posttraumatic play can emerge (Gil, 2006; Terr, 1990), with the urgent need for the therapist to direct children along the path of trauma digestion and exposure work. Phobic avoidance of trauma triggers might make a purely child-centered approach ineffective, as many clinicians who use CCPT have observed that when the child is so defended from the traumatic memories, their play in the therapy room feels superficially cheerful. Prescriptive play therapists rely heavily on a foundation of CCPT, especially in the earliest phases of treatment, to establish the relationship, increase attunement, and develop a case conceptualization of the child's unique needs and responses. In tandem with this free play, the prescriptive therapist would use additional directive strategies to accomplish therapeutic purposes, such as teaching self-soothing and nervous system regulation, or addressing specific therapeutic needs, such as the digestion of an overwhelming or upsetting event, using a trauma protocol such as EMDR.

Play therapy as a discipline within psychotherapy places a large emphasis on a therapeutic environment that promotes the therapeutic benefits of play in the presence of a play therapist trained to respond deliberately to the child in accordance with the specific play therapy approach. While play therapy environments do vary, a typical play therapy room offers many options for dramatic and role play, such as props, simple costumes for role playing, household items, a doctor's kit, dolls, expressive art materials, simple musical instruments, puppets, items for active play such as balls, and items that are interesting to touch and hold such as items from nature (Landreth, 2012). In addition, many play therapists also have a sand tray and an assortment of miniature figures to use in projecting "worlds" expressively in the sand, including human and animal figures, miniature versions of everyday items as well as fantasy and iconic symbols, and landscape props such as trees and bridges and other items (Homeyer & Sweeney, 2016). Younger children tend to use the sand tray as a miniature world in which to play actively, whereas older children respond to prompts to use the sand tray and miniatures as an expressive space for projection of feelings and experiences.

However, not all play therapy approaches emphasize the provision of toys and props for projective play. Some are more game-based or focused on an interactive approach and may use few or no props, such as Theraplay™ (Jernberg & Booth, 2001) or developmental play therapy (Brody, 1997).

Play therapists are informed by a variety of theoretical models and vary in terms of the emphasis placed on verbal expression of feelings and developing insights versus experimentation and experiences kept in the metaphor of the play with little or no explicit self-reflection. Over the past decade, increasing emphasis on establishing the research support for various play therapy approaches has led to many published studies and meta-analyses affirming the clinical efficacy of using play therapy to treat a variety of childhood mental health conditions, despite the difficulties in studying what is often a nonprotocolized and highly individualized approach to intervention (Bratton, Ray, Rhine, & Jones, 2005; Lin & Bratton, 2015; Ray, Armstrong, Balkin, & Jayne, 2015).

FOR PLAY THERAPISTS: UNDERSTANDING EMDR AS A CLINICAL APPROACH WITH CHILDREN

Francine Shapiro's AIP model proposes that the integration of both positive and negative experiences into our nervous system is the healthy process by which we grow. When an acutely negative or traumatic event occurs, this information processing is sabotaged by our own neurobiological effort to cope with the trauma by isolating the related associations, images, feelings, and so forth (Shapiro, 2017). Our own phobic avoidance of reminders of the pain, fear, and shame of the traumatic experience contributes to further isolation of this network of related associations. The more severe and complex the trauma, the more elaborate this isolation becomes, even resulting in dissociation and the exiling of the part of self that had the traumatic experiences from present awareness (Gomez, 2012). EMDR's potency in entering this isolated memory network and enabling the client to begin the adaptive process of integration is well established in the literature (Chen et al., 2014) and has been listed as an evidence-based treatment for posttraumatic stress by Substance Abuse and Mental Health Services Administration (SAMHSA) since 2010 (SAMHSA, 2012).

In order for EMDR to be effective in helping the client to "digest" the trauma—or in AIP language, remove blocks to allow adaptive information to reach the memory network or node—we have to be able to reach and activate the memory and its related associations. The therapy has to allow the resurfacing of disturbing images, sensory data, emotions, body sensations, and the co-occurring cognitions without overwhelming clients and causing their systems to shut down. The eight phases of the EMDR protocol guide the clinician in first identifying these memory nodes or touchstone memories, then preparing the client to manage the intensity of the stored emotions and sensory data, followed by facing and digesting the upsetting elements of the trauma while using eye movements or another form of bilateral stimulation (BLS), and finally attaching more adaptive self-referential beliefs to the experience to promote full integration of this memory into the client's own narrative. EMDR emphasizes attention to the somatic experience of the trauma throughout this processing (Shapiro, 2017).

Since the earliest days of EMDR, practitioners have attempted to extend the benefits of EMDR to children (Greenwald, 1999; Tinker & Wilson, 1999), and there is a growing body of evidence in support of the outcomes of this treatment with trauma-exposed children (Adler-Tapia & Settle, 2008; de Roos et al., 2010; Fleming, 2012; Kemp, Drummond, & McDermott, 2010; Moreno-Alcazar et al., 2017). In considering what AIP looks like in children versus adults, we recognize that children do the majority of their learning through action and imaginative experimentation—also known as "play"—not through the verbal reflection or even the visual imagery that is the primary portal of processing for most adults using EMDR. There is wide acceptance that the therapist must include movement, props, and other aspects of play into child-friendly EMDR. Some examples would include having the child draw images from the target memory (Adler-Tapia & Settle, 2016; Tinker & Wilson, 1999), using sensory experiences to evoke the safe/calm state in the preparation phase (Gomez, 2012), using the sand tray to create a narrative of the trauma experience during reprocessing (Gomez, 2012), or using BLS to install positive experiences of attachment during baby role play (McGuiness, 2003). These authors have established the need for EMDR with children to be adapted to make EMDR more appealing as well as more comprehensible.

TAKING THE NEXT STEPS IN INTEGRATION: THE EIGHT ESSENTIALS

This chapter represents an effort to advocate for an even more intentional and systematic integration of EMDR therapy with established play therapy principles and approaches on the basis of understanding several ideas: (a) The therapeutic alliance available to children in a play therapy context, especially in CCPT, expands the emotionally safe space that is needed for trauma work. (b) The AIP described by Shapiro will be most fully realized in children who are actively engaged in dramatic and expressive play, as the neural networks the therapist is trying to reach are mostly available during play. Children are often already engaging in posttraumatic play if only the therapist is able to enter the metaphor, understand this communication, and invite processing. (c) A thoughtful integration of play therapy strategies with EMDR will reduce the risk of flooding children with traumatic material too soon, by building the bridge between the metaphor of the play and their own first-hand experiences gradually, staying within their ability to tolerate, even while engaging in reprocessing with EMDR.

In clinical work with children and as a trainer and consultant within both the EMDR and play therapy communities, I have struggled alongside my colleagues to articulate a comprehensive approach to integrating the best of both approaches in meeting the needs of the individual child survivors of trauma. In this context, I have developed a series of eight essential considerations for fuller integration of play therapy with EMDR therapy based on a paper previously published on this topic (Beckley-Forest, 2019; see Figure 1.1).

This working model of the eight essential components is not rigidly hierarchical but builds gradually over time, beginning with a more nondirective stance on the part of the therapist and layering in essential skills before more actively engaging the child in explicit first-person trauma work using EMDR. It is most compatible with a prescriptive play therapy approach, where the therapist flexibly uses a mixture of child-centered playtime along with child-responsive interventions from the therapist, using the lightest touch possible with these insertions and suggestions, such as wondering aloud—"I wonder what would happen if. . . ." Using these kinds of observations in place of more didactic teaching or even gentle questioning can help shifts in thinking to be more congruent, much as the gentle language EMDR therapists would use along with interweaves in EMDR processing. In addition, prescriptive play therapists use information gained through observing and attuning to the child's play to develop a menu of play-based skill-building activities for the child and family to complement the play in which the child is already engaging. A prescriptive approach to play therapy is quite compatible with integration with the eight phases of EMDR. Paris Goodyear-Brown (2010a) proposes a model for flexibly sequential play therapy, a phase model that she now calls TraumaPlay™ (Goodyear-Brown, 2019), as an integration of directive and nondirective play therapy activities. Her model is an example of a play therapy approach, which is quite compatible with these eight essential considerations for integration of play therapy with EMDR.

To the child's own preferred play themes, the therapist must add a gradual introduction to EMDR-specific tools, props, and activities. We will also need an approach to enhancing the child's ability to self-soothe and change their state from agitated/upset to calm by using play that involves the parts of their neurobiology affiliated with social engagement and present time orientation.

A word about the eighth essential is needed, as it represents the overarching consideration of how to develop and maintain a parallel process with parents and the care-giving family system at all points during the course of treatment. Family involvement is associated with the best outcomes in child treatment in

I. MODELS FOR INTEGRATION

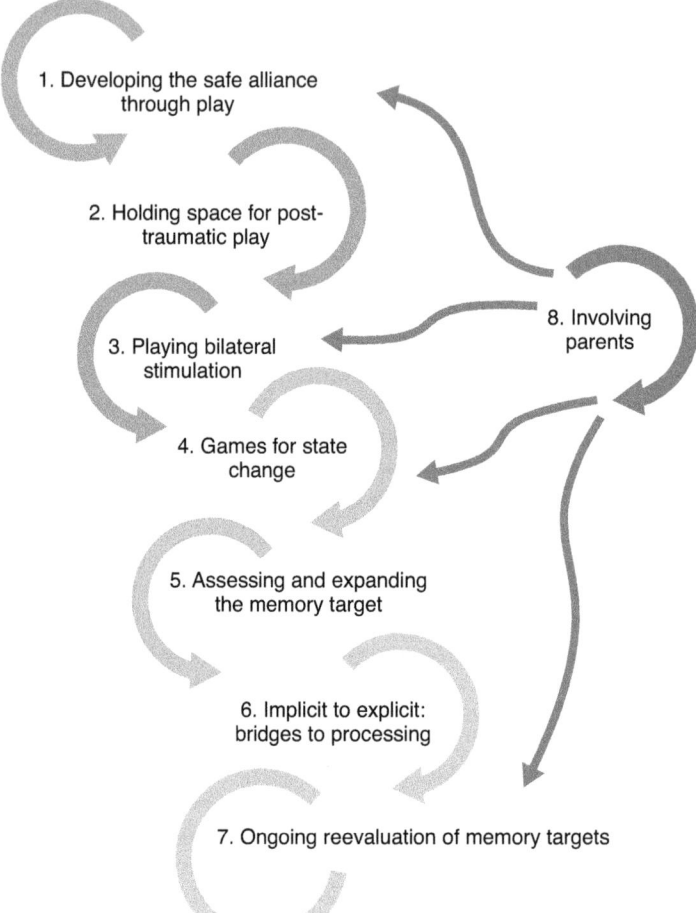

Figure 1.1 *The Eight Essentials for Integrating Eye Movement Desensitization and Reprocessing and Prescriptive Play Therapy*

both the play therapy literature (Lin & Ray, 2015) and EMDR literature (Gomez, 2012; Lovett, 1999; Wesselman, Schweitzer, & Armstrong, 2014).

ESSENTIAL 1: SAFE ALLIANCE THROUGH PLAY

CCPT is the foundation of the relationship between the therapist and the child in play therapy, and its unique features set it apart from other ways of being with children in treatment. In a CCPT relationship, the child is offered the opportunity to access troubling emotions and upsetting memory networks at their own pace and from a safe emotional distance. The therapist's participation in the form of tracking and reflecting statements delivered with calm, dispassionate interest is also regulating for the child (Landreth, 2012). Researchers describing and understanding the mechanism of how this child-centered environment helps the child to unfold and access material safely have noticed the importance of the neutrality of this arrangement in reducing the power differential in the relationship. Badenoch (2008) noted that adult directives can be experienced by the child's nervous system as a threat and activate rage in a sensitive child's limbic system (p. 302). Establishing the kind of authentic emotional safety, which enables clients to respond to therapist requests and questions honestly and without transference, has long been seen as an important process in adult therapy. In child therapy, the power differential is inherent to the relationship, as children obviously have less power than adults. Children are more likely than adults to respond to therapist directives or questions with either adult-pleasing or adult-defying behaviors, which are already part of their primary attachment repertoire. In a relationship where the therapist will ultimately be leading the child toward exposure to traumatic material, these power differences have the potential to cause great harm.

> *Brenda, aged 7, is brought to treatment by her parents 6 months after a coercive sexual assault by an adolescent neighbor. She originally had coped well with parent support but over time the parents accepted her request to "stop talking about it all the time." She has become more isolated, anxious, avoidant of new situations, and has great trouble sleeping, so the parents sought treatment. She is a cooperative and highly verbal child without a significant history of disruption or adversity.*

While the therapist may conclude quite readily that there is still material related to the trauma that is troubling to this child, moving too quickly to trauma work will likely backfire, even though this obedient child would possibly comply. The adult-pleasing dynamics will make it difficult for her to be honest about the intensity of her distress. If she is dissociating or flooding, the therapist may miss it, as Brenda is reading her therapist's reactions and trying to give the "right" answer. Or the opposite situation:

> *Sam is an 8-year-old who struggles with rules and self-regulation despite having been in a stable foster home for 3 years where he is about to be adopted. The case worker and soon-to-be adoptive parents are well informed of the impact of the trauma of removal from his biological parents 3 years earlier, and subsequent termination of contact due their inconsistency and substance abuse. They are anxious for him to receive trauma treatment to "get over" his earlier experiences and be able to flourish in his current family. He is suspicious of new people and new experiences and reacts aggressively in these instances.*

While the therapist might rightly conclude that this child needs to be able to digest his own memories of neglect and removal in order to move forward, efforts to engage him directly around this kind of work will almost certainly fail, not only because he may have developed some layers of protection through dissociation, but any attempt at therapist direction will be likely met by him with suspicion leading to adult-defying behaviors in an effort to control the course of the session.

Scenarios such as these might be very challenging in a directive or protocol-driven model of treatment, but play therapists frequently rely on CCPT to establish an egalitarian therapeutic relationship. In CCPT, the therapist invites the child to "use these things in any way that you want" and accepts the child's process without challenging it. Over a period of sessions conducted in this way, the child may at first test this dynamic and then visibly relax and become increasingly engaged in the play therapy space, constructed to elicit the full breadth of emotion and human experience. Without the need to earn the adult's approval—or establish independence by defying the norms the child sees the adult as enforcing—the play therapy space becomes a more purely projective-holding environment for the child's own ideas about the world and a safer place to experiment with the mastery of feelings and experiences, including traumatic experiences. The narrative themes that emerge in the play may contain metaphors, which reflect the child's emotional landscape, communicate about how the child views the world and their place in it, and contain sensory pieces of traumatic memories or even literal reenactments of the trauma. The autonomy of the child in the playroom is a felt experience of empowerment, which is essential to therapeutic change.

In order to help children who have been affected by adverse experience to move forward in therapy as quickly as possible, quite paradoxically the therapist should initially "slow down" and use CCPT to establish therapeutic safety. In addition to helping establish the egalitarian relationship, this child-led dynamic may allow for the emergence of play already activating the trauma memory network and providing information to the therapist about the child's experiences of the trauma, especially where verbal disclosure may be difficult, if not impossible. This material is allowed to emerge congruently, without activating the child's defenses.

ESSENTIAL 2: HOLDING SPACE FOR POSTTRAUMATIC PLAY

The term "posttraumatic play" is credited to the groundbreaking work of Lenore Terr in the 1990s. Her extensive work studying and interviewing children who had survived significant trauma led her to conclude that not only are trauma-exposed children often affected by a lingering sense of terror without words, but that the "fear of further fear" will lead them to avoid accessing support from caregivers. Instead, elements of the trauma are approached in reenactive play, which she noted was often done in secret, "grim and monotonous, obsessively repeated, and may not relieve anxiety" (Terr, 1990, p 238).

Eliana Gil (2006) describes posttraumatic play as a repetitive and often rigid type of play initiated by children who are trying to "expose themselves to the literal aspects of the trauma which cause them despair" (p. 184). The AIP model would describe these elements in the play as connected to the memory node, which holds the trauma, and thus offering a possible pathway into the associated neural network. If the child is able to gradually move in and out of this processing in a dynamic way, the brain's own drive toward integration will promote healing. Gil's work within play therapy has been significant in helping with the complexities of recognizing and supporting *dynamic* play, which may be posttraumatic in nature, providing options for intervening to prevent the play from becoming static and potentially retraumatizing as well as using play to ground children who begin to

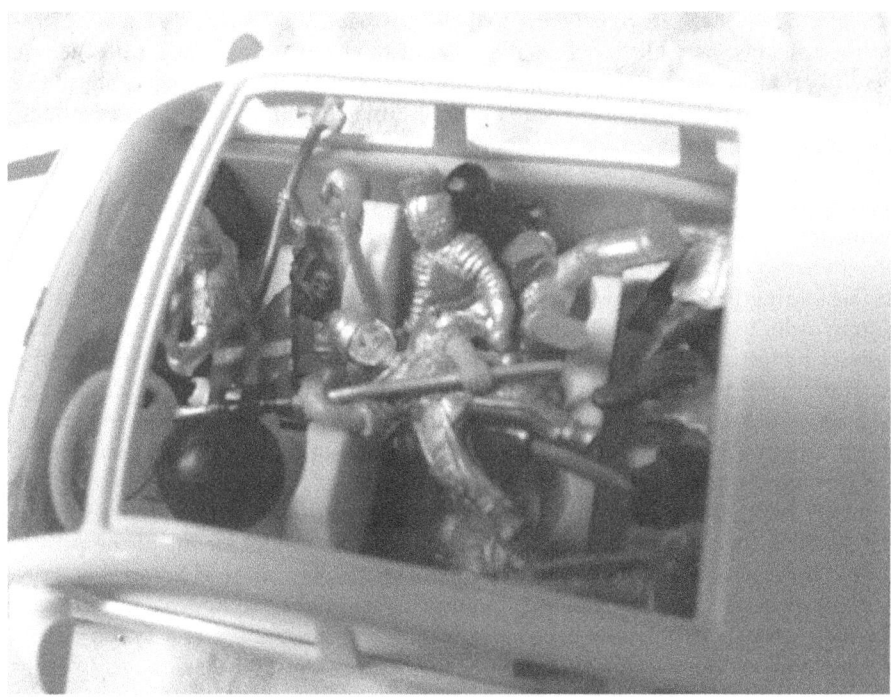

Figure 1.2 *The Trauma Memory Network: "They Can't See, They Can't Get Out, They Can't Get Away"*

dissociate (Gil, 2016). We can use this framework to recognize when themes in a child's play may be literal or metaphoric reenactments of traumatic experiences.

Missy was an 8-year-old child who had been adopted as a toddler. She came to therapy after a minor car accident appeared to have had a major impact on her day-to-day behavior and well-being. Offered the opportunity for CCPT in the playroom, she returned again and again to a story she created about a litter of puppies. Missy's story was enacted with the same materials each week, in the sand tray and in the dollhouse.

> Missy: *These are the puppies. They are being kidnapped. No one can hear how they are barking and crying.* (Pitiful barking and whimpering.)
>
> Therapist: *The puppies cry and no one hears them.*
>
> Missy: *Yes, and they all get stuffed in the car like this* (see Figure 1.2). *They can't breathe, and they can't get out.* (The child herself breathed more rapidly and shallowly here, and her voice rose with anxiety.)
>
> Therapist (intervening to keep Missy regulated, but within the metaphor): *Hey puppies, I see you under there. You need a deep breath.* (Therapist breathes audibly.) *Can we both take a breath for the puppies?*
>
> Missy (after breathing): *They are stuck in here, they can't see out* (piling more figures on top).

When children return urgently to the same materials and themes over a number of sessions, as well as when the content of the play feels upsetting versus playful and fun, we are alert to the possibility that aspects of the metaphor in the play may have begun to hold some of the trauma content (Gil, 2016). Sometimes, the therapist has to employ a fair degree of creativity and speculation in order to understand the clues that are available in the play, which can help with the gradual exposure work. In Missy's case, I began to suspect that there may have been elements of the trauma of her removal from her biological family that were available to her in the "kidnap" metaphor in the play. Once the posttrauma metaphors are unfolding in the play, we can add this information to our case conceptualization in order to begin considering how to enter this memory network to allow the flow of adaptive information. We return to this idea later when we discuss the essential consideration of expanding the target. As the therapist, I could engage in a series of speculations about the information available within the metaphor. In Missy's case, pairing the story about being kidnapped by car with elements of the trauma memory network, both the traumatic experience of being removed from her biological parents and the recent trigger experience of being trapped in her seatbelt after the car accident became a working model for me of the activation of this memory network. The distancing of the play allowed her to stay more present even as traumatic intensity emerged. The ability to approach traumatic intensity from a distance is especially important when there is a lot of fear of the memory or the memory is beyond the child's current awareness, as in early attachment trauma. When the intensity of the play is overwhelming or at risk of becoming toxic or retraumatizing to the child, a light touch with reflections and child-responsive invitations can help the play to move along dynamically, such as in the earlier example when Missy was invited to breathe during the play.

Gil's distinction between dynamic and toxic posttraumatic play is important in guiding the therapist along the continuum of in-session activities from child-centered to more directive. The autonomy of the child in the rich sensory environment of the playroom helps to mitigate the risk of children becoming overwhelmed and dissociated during posttraumatic play. If the child has internalized the belief that they have the power to decide in the playroom what to do next, they are more likely to move away from the intensity on their own to avoid being flooded by traumatic content. This possibility is one of the key reasons why the play therapy room makes an ideal setting for approaching and digesting trauma content. Another check on therapist interference considers that attempts to introduce adaptive information too soon can shut down the child's own processing, interfering with the child's opportunities for expressive release through exposure (Gil, 2016, p. 19). Trauma-exposed children already have messages in their environment from parents and others, which increase phobic avoidance of exposure to traumatic elements such as "just don't think about it" or "it wasn't so bad." When the posttraumatic play is dynamic and shows evidence of movement toward digestion, nondirective CCPT can hold the space for the play to begin the exposure and also show the therapist where directive support may be needed once the child is ready for a more explicit digesting of the experience, such as with EMDR processing added to the play.

Some children exhibit repetitively reenactive play related to the trauma, which is static and unchanging, resembling Terr's "grim and monotonous" description

(1990). Many years ago, I worked in a Head Start setting with a young boy who, unbeknownst to anyone at the program, had witnessed a particularly frightening episode of domestic violence between his parents. Three weeks in a row, he reenacted the experience in the dollhouse, mimicking the words and actions used and grimly repeating them over and over. The play never varied in location or materials, and the emotional content was flat. This was play that did not feel at all like play or experimentation, or mastery of any kind. In addition to spurring me to action outside of the play sessions with regard to ensuring the safety of the family members, I was not able to continue as a bystander to merely track and reflect the content of this narrative session after session and needed to respond along a continuum of interventions, such as described by Gil (2016, pp. 47–48). The continuum encompasses everything from the lightest touch of verbalizing some additional descriptions and asking children to give their characters a voice, along the continuum to more directives such as asking children to change the order of events by starting the story in the middle or showing the ending first. We also can ask the child to breathe or move, or involve another medium such as drawing the story or photographing the sequence of play. I did not know EMDR in those days, but now in a similar scenario, I would add to that list the possibility of using reflections to invite *moments of noticing* how the characters felt or where those feelings are in their bodies as another possible way of helping move the play along in a more dynamic direction. These moments of noticing help prepare the child for EMDR processing.

ESSENTIAL 3: PLAYING EMDR WITH PROP-BASED BILATERAL STIMULATION

BLS, also called dual attention stimulation, is a unique feature of EMDR, setting it apart from other trauma-digestion approaches. In adult EMDR therapy, we emphasize eye movements following the therapist's fingers or using a light bar or other device as the primary way of delivering the BLS. With children, a wider variety of options have developed. Using magic wands, toys, or comfort items is a common strategy for the eye movements, but EMDR therapists sometimes use purely tactile BLS (Shapiro, 2017). Some options include "tappers" developed for the EMDR community. These are handheld tactile vibration devices, some with headphones, which offer alternating auditory tones. At other times, the therapist may gently tap the child with puppets, use hand claps, bang drums, or coach the child to use the "butterfly hug" (Jarero, 2002). These all represent innovations now in wide use in EMDR with children, as the need for tactile BLS arises primarily from the difficulty younger children have sustaining attention to eye movements (Tinker & Wilson, 1999). The novelty of having a variety of methods can help engage a reluctant child. For example, having recently added some light-up drum sticks to the playroom options (inspired by Swinden, 2018), I noticed that several child clients were more engaged and interested in returning to the trauma-focused narrative play that they sometimes try to avoid. Taking a kinesthetic or full-body approach inspires the use of large muscles for the BLS, here demonstrated by a young friend of mine (not a client) with a foam sword (Figure 1.3) or a ribbon wand (Figure 1.4).

Short episodes of therapist-led activities are needed to introduce this novel way of playing to the child early in treatment. These introductions to BLS or "back

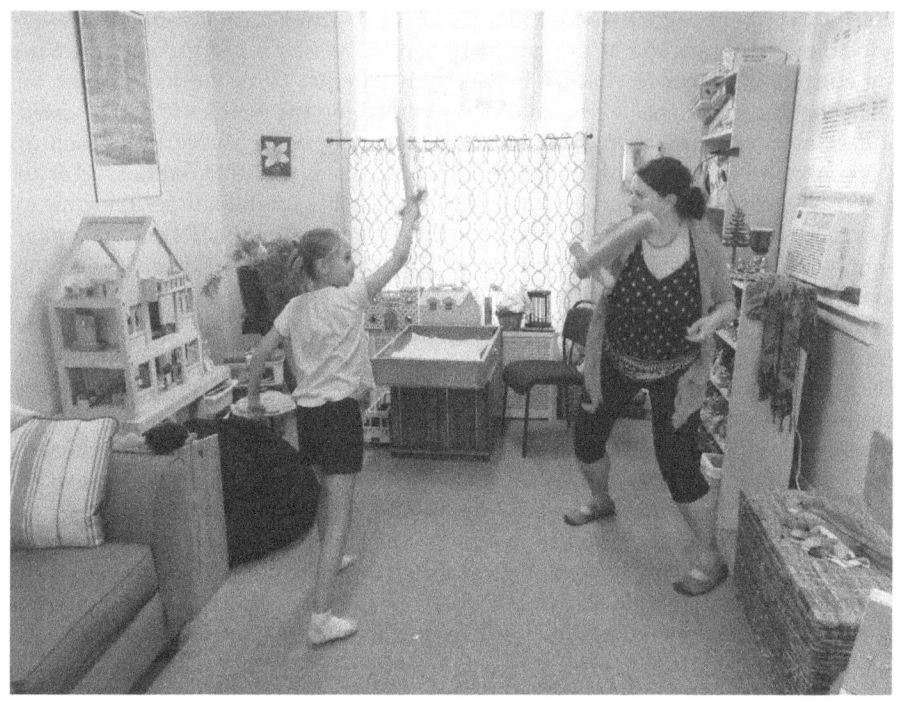

Figure 1.3 *Foam Swords for Full-Body Bilateral Stimulation*

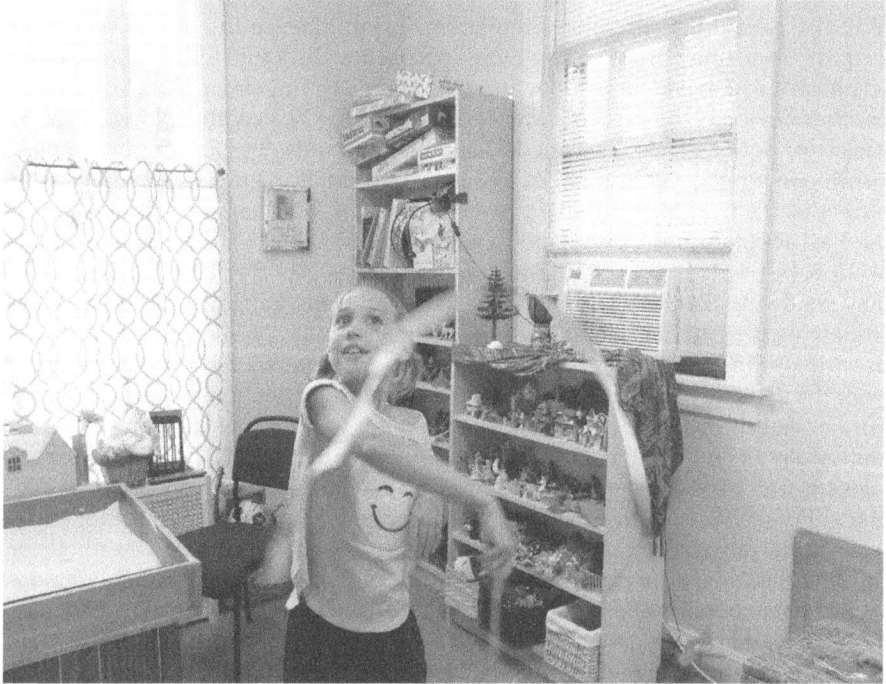

Figure 1.4 *Ribbon Wand for Bilateral Stimulation*

and forth games" are an important part of the preparation phase for children. Using BLS (brief sets of 5–10 slow saccades, or back and forth passes) to install positive feelings and notice body sensations for a moment before, during, or after other play activities in the playroom sets the stage for their later use in processing. The novelty of introducing a *wide variety* of ways of using BLS to children eventually helps expand their capacity to sustain and reenter processing. In the earliest stages of therapy, such as during engagement with the child and family system, we can use brief directives to teach self-soothing and install positive feeling states using the BLS props and games in the context of the play therapy session. Some examples include:

- Inviting children to use sand trays and expressive materials to create positive images, including constructions of safe spaces, and then using the "back and forth" movement of BLS to "find how it feels in your body/tummy/heart to see what you made."
- Role playing versions of installing positive self-statements as resources. For example, with a young client with very low frustration tolerance, we developed a sword fight game using pool noodles as the swords (the full-body BLS initiated by the therapist) and the positive cognition "I can handle it" to practice and reinforce this self-talk as a resource in challenging situations. In the playfully aroused state of the sword fight, her repetition of "I can handle it" again and again helped this adaptive belief to more fully enter her nervous system where it could be more available to her during other times of hyperarousal (intervention inspired by a story in *The Worry Wars*, Goodyear-Brown, 2010b).
- In play that is taking place within the parent–child dyad, such as in a Theraplay™ or other dyadic play therapy moments as in role-playing baby care, we can use brief sets of BLS to help the child and parent notice or tune in to the attachment experiences as an internal resource.

In fidelity to the EMDR protocol, I am not in favor of the practice of some child therapists using BLS by "letting the buzzers just run" continuously during play. The therapist should be using BLS with intention, to promote the linking of adaptive information with the memory networks, whether that information is noticing a body sensation, having an experience of orienting in the present, or an experiential moment of mastery in the play. I think about inserting BLS as a way of inviting the child to *notice* what is happening in the moment. Later, in treatment, when I am trying to facilitate reprocessing, I use expressions such as "let's tap on that big feeling/big thought" to create pauses in the narrative for longer and faster sets of BLS during moments of trauma digestion in the play narrative. BLS should make sense to the child as a way of calming and "looking inside" or noticing what is going on within, to whatever degree that is developmentally possible.

ESSENTIAL 4: EXPANDING CAPACITY FOR STATE CHANGE

Our emerging understanding of the neurobiological impact of trauma on the developing brains of children has a significant effect on the prioritizing of somatosensory experiences in the play therapy approach. Some children will seek this kind of self-regulating play on their own in the playroom, whereas others may need structure and invitation. Using a neurosequential approach (Gaskill & Perry, 2014) helps the therapist to justify to caregivers and others why the child is "not ready to just talk about it" and why a verbal, narrative approach to trauma work is premature for many children. We seek consistent opportunities within the play to model experiences that are soothing and regulating and use repetition and cycles of excitation and modulation to "teach" the child's nervous system about calm in order to move up the neurobiological hierarchy to the more relational and reflective potential of the higher brain functions.

Within each session, either before or after (or sometimes in the midst of) the child-centered playtime, I introduce more directive miniactivities, which promote state change from distress to calm as well as generally developing resources as preparation for approaching the trauma. Games that teach and reinforce deep breathing, progressive muscle relaxation, and "bottom-up" neurobiological self-regulation are part of the play prescription for these children (see Table 1.1). Daniel Siegel (1999) first used the term "window of tolerance (WOT)" to describe the capacity of a person to remain engaged in the face of internal and external stimuli and perceived threat. Modeling and encouraging playful activities that help keep the child in the WOT is highly needed by these children. Many of these

Table 1.1 *Playful Activities for State Change*

Breathing	**Balancing and Movement**
Deep breaths with: Blowing bubbles Blowing feathers Blowing pinwheels Blowing on imaginary butterflies Blow-pens Inhaling favorite scents	Balance boards Balancing peacock feathers Yoga poses Stretching Rocking Swinging Playing catch
Deep Pressure	**Tactile**
Being wrapped in a blanket Being swung gently in a blanket or swing Weighted items, such as stuffed animals, blankets Being held gently by parent	Slime Clay Wet or dry sand Finger paints Holding stones
Oral	**Auditory**
Gum, mints, water, snacks	Musical instruments and singing

This list is original to this author, but inspired by numerous sources (especially Gaskill, R., & Perry, B. [2014]. The neurobiological power of play: Using the neurosequential model of therapeutics to guide play in the healing process. In C. Machoidi & D. Crenshaw (Eds.), *Creative arts and play therapy for attachment trauma*. New York, NY: Guilford Press; Goodyear-Brown, P. (2010a). *Play therapy with traumatized children: A prescriptive approach*. Hoboken, NJ: Wiley; Najavits, L. M. (2002). *Seeking safety: A treatment manual for PTSD and substance abuse*. New York, NY: Guilford Press; Van der Kolk, B. A. (2015). *The body keeps the score: Brain, mind and body in the healing of trauma*. New York, NY: Penguin).

ideas are based on sensory experiences. The play therapy literature offers many directive options compatible with these goals, including many activities within Theraplay™, and other approaches (Hong & Mason, 2016).

Once BLS has been introduced to the child, these moments of state change offer opportunities to notice the body during short, slow sets of BLS. The key to using these very short and often only momentary interventions to gradually impact the arousal level of the child is to keep the activities novel and to use a child-responsive approach to teaching them, avoiding power struggles with the child. As Gaskill and Perry (2014) point out, the therapist should advocate with caregivers and teachers for carryover of these activities outside of the weekly therapy session for the intended results of beginning to establish new patterns within the child's arousal system.

ESSENTIAL 5: EXPANDING AND ASSESSING MEMORY TARGETS IN THE POSTTRAUMATIC PLAY WITH EMDR

Initial EMDR processing of trauma content can occur in the context of the play metaphor using the characters in the story for the initial assessment of the target and beginning reprocessing. In particular, the metaphors in the posttraumatic play may give the clinician clues about the feelings, negative cognitions, and body sensations in the memory network. Because it is difficult for children to identify negative cognitions in the ways that adolescents or adults are capable of as part of the EMDR Phase 3 assessment of the target, it is often up to the therapist to guess or suggest what negative beliefs may be stored in that network. A thoughtful consideration of the themes in the posttraumatic play can provide information about the child's sense of ongoing danger, helplessness, and self-blame.

A young client with insecure attachment stemming from her addicted mother's inconsistent care in infancy used the CCPT time to again and again reenact a similar story. She played the role of a baby figure who is alternately cared for and threatened by the imaginary characters in the room played by the therapist and various stuffed animals and toys at her direction. Over time, as she was allowed to remain in charge of the play as the director, she added more and more elements of the ambivalent attachment into the play. For example, she had the therapist act as the mother, sometimes taking care of her and feeding her, and so forth, while at other times she instructed the therapist to play the role of the mother to accuse the child of lying, to deny her the things she wanted, or to be sleeping or distracted while threats came to bother the child in the context of the developing play narrative.

> Child: *I'm the baby, you pretend to be the mother.*
>
> Therapist: *You want me to be the mother.*
>
> Child: *Yes. First you have to cover me with the blanket and feed me some of the crackers.*
>
> Therapist: *Okay, baby, I am taking care of you; here is a snack for you* (playfully feeds the baby the crackers one by one).
>
> Child: *Now, you have to go away and the bad guy comes.*

Therapist: *Baby, I am going to go over here and . . .* (stage whispers: what shall I be doing?)

Child (shrugs): *On your phone.*

Therapist: *Okay, I'm talking on my phone. . . .*

Child (gives therapist a puppet): *Now be the bad guy.*

Therapist (now has a puppet the child chose as the bad guy, and it is a scary alligator puppet): *I'm coming over to the Baby now.*

Child (screams): *Help Mommy help!*

Therapist (stage whisper): *Does the mom come?*

Child: *No. She never hears.*

This drama has many of the qualities of dynamic posttraumatic play, including urgency to the child, a sense of felt reality and emotional intensity, as well as thematic parallels to the child's own experience. In this setting, the child was able to convey the negative beliefs and emotions and body sensations experienced by the "Baby."

Therapist: *That baby is feeling afraid and also alone.*

Child: (Now whimpering quite realistically.)

Therapist (stepping in now with some EMDR processing): *She might feel it in her heart, her stomach, her throat. . .*

Child: *Yes, her throat!*

Therapist: *Let's do a few patty cakes and see where that feeling is in her throat.*

The child and therapist previously developed a "game" of using patty cakes for BLS, with a "patty cake" type of hand claps bilaterally across the line of sight (Tinker & Wilson, 1999). During patty cake BLS, she was able to notice the distress in her own body. Jumping ahead for a moment to Essential 6, described more fully later, the self can be brought explicitly into this processing using the bridge of the moment in play, initially just momentarily until the therapist can see how much the child is ready to tolerate.

Therapist: *You were a once a baby who knows what that lonely feeling is like.*

Child: *She thinks the Baby is already grown up.*

This shift in awareness represents some important adaptive information entering the memory network. This child has uncovered in the play a moment that quite accurately represents the misattunement of her biological mother who did not consistently grasp and respond to her baby needs.

Therapist: *Let's patty cake on that idea . . .* (BLS hand claps). See Figure 1.5 for a (nonclient) *recreation of that moment in the play session.*

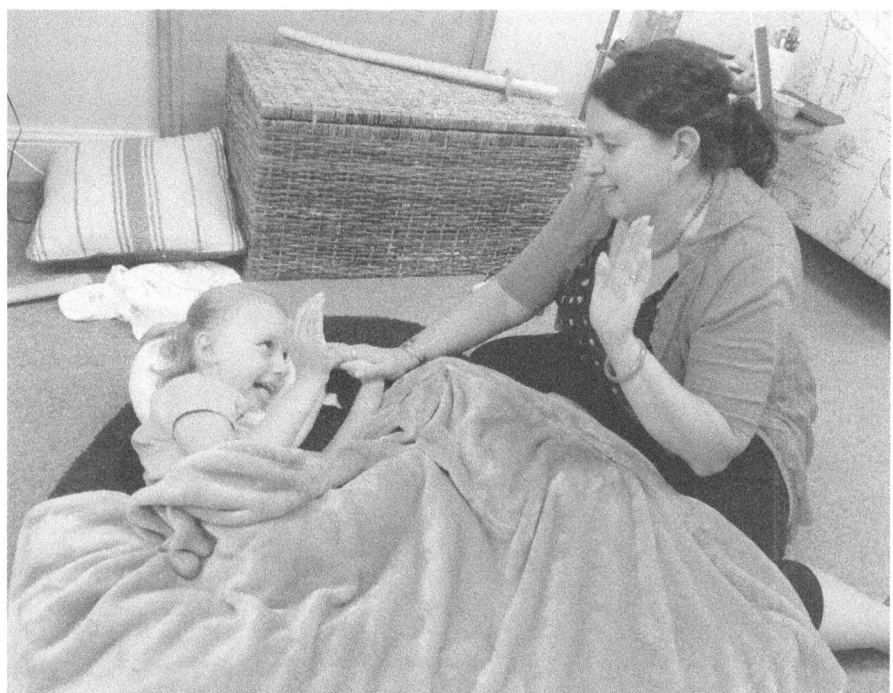

Figure 1.5 *Processing Baby Memories With "Patty Cake" Bilateral Stimulation*

Child: *Now the mom is coming and she is mad at the bad guy—they are fighting!* (Child thrusts a foam sword into the therapist's hand.)

Therapist (hitting the alligator puppet with the sword): *Like this?*

Child (calming, smiling): *Yes, yes!*

Therapist: *Take that, bad guy! Leave my baby alone!* (See Figure 1.6 of therapist hitting alligator with sword.)

Child: *Let's play the whole thing again.*

Therapist: *Patty cake with me and see how your body feels, so we can play it again* (BLS).

This child could not have tolerated a standard protocol approach, and as much of the trauma was pre-verbal, she would not have had the words to convey the magnitude of her experience. Yet, through the play, she was able to not only activate that memory network but also use the opportunity to begin noticing her anger and fear in an embodied way. By using the BLS to focus her moments of noticing, the posttraumatic play remains more dynamic and within her ability to tolerate. By drawing the parallel to her own experience, the target network is more fully activated. This flexible approach to desensitization and reprocessing must be grounded in all the elements of the standard EMDR protocol, with attention

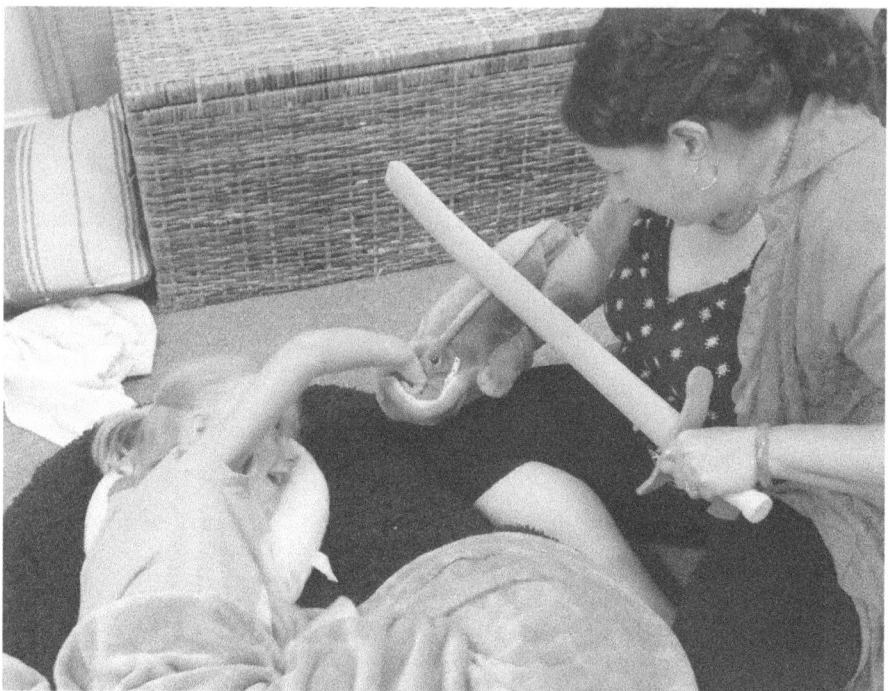

Figure 1.6 *Fighting the Alligator*

paid to the images, emotions, negative beliefs, and body sensations present in the network. The process is spontaneous and driven by the narrative of the play and over time may weave in and out of the child's awareness of the story as a first-person narrative. Swimm (2018) recently published a case study in the *Journal of EMDR Practice and Research* in support of this kind of developmental play context for processing attachment targets.

ESSENTIAL 6: BUILD BRIDGES FROM IMPLICIT TO EXPLICIT TRAUMA WORK

When adequate relationship and preparation are in place, we do look for opportunities to build bridges of self-awareness from the play to the child's own experiences, using short episodes of EMDR processing. In these episodes, the child is invited to use BLS for "noticing" the upsetting body responses, beliefs, and so forth in a child-responsive but not highly directive way.

For example, a child who witnessed domestic violence developed a drama in the dollhouse using superheroes and villain figures. On the surface, it might seem like a fairly simplistic replay of action scenes from superhero movies. However, his persistence in frequently returning to this play when offered CCPT allowed the narrative to unfold and begin to carry meaning and content from his trauma experiences. He eventually expanded the story to include a helpless younger sister figure whom his hero character needed to rescue from bullying by the villain over and over again.

Applying Essential 5, using the posttraumatic play to inform my assessment of the target memory, I could begin to recognize how this urgent narrative carried the trauma content of standing helpless while his mother was beaten and wishing to be strong enough to protect and defend her. I began developing an assessment of this trauma target over the sessions in which he returned to this narrative while still within the metaphor of the play. In this assessment, I understood that "I am helpless" was a significant negative cognition within this memory node, and the physical feeling of pent up/frozen rage was a relevant body sensation for him.

This sixth essential consideration of looking for and acting upon opportunities to bridge from the play into explicit trauma work is a challenging and perhaps novel extension of the idea of full integration of EMDR processing into the posttraumatic play. In these moments, I began by asking him to notice his own intolerance of bullying, his physical desire to defend the helpless, and accompanied these moments of noticing with BLS on drums, a favorite activity. Making the child's own self present in an explicit way offered a momentary window or bridge in which to invite him to remember his own experience of helplessness in the face of the violence and bullying directed toward his mother.

> Therapist: *I am noticing how much your guy hates this bully, how much anger he has. . .*
>
> Child (smashing his figure into the bully character): *I. Hate. Him. I hate him.*
>
> Therapist: *You have seen bullies too. I know you saw your Mom get bullied and hurt. Come bang on the drum with me for a minute so we can get that big feeling out, too* (BLS). *You wanted to save her* (BLS).
>
> Child: *If I was bigger I could have. I wanted to.*
>
> Therapist: *That's a big thought, let's drum on that one* (BLS). *Your muscles were all tight because you wanted to, but you had to keep still.* (More BLS, his intensity increases.) *Whew, we need a deep breath!*
>
> Child (titrates the intensity by going back into the play narrative): *Leave her alone. You need to move out of this neighborhood. We do not want you!!!* (Throws bully figure across the room.)
>
> Therapist: *Now he is far away from them.*
>
> Child: *Yes.* (To girl doll) *You don't have to be afraid, he's gone.*
>
> Therapist: *He is gone and it is safer now. Let's breathe. What does that feel like? Let's hug our bodies and really feel what they are feeling when he is gone* (BLS with butterfly hug).
>
> Child: *I will never let any bullies hurt anyone ever again.*
>
> Therapist (reflects as a positive cognition): *You want everyone to be safe now.* (Butterfly hug.)
>
> Child: *He might come back next time.* (Child gets up and paces across the room.)
>
> Therapist: *You and Mom are safe now, though. Let's drum on that.* (Offers light up drum sticks for BLS.)
>
> Child (drums for a few seconds, exhales): *I want to play something else.*

The positive cognition is still incongruent, so he shifts uncomfortably out of processing, and I follow his lead and "allow" this distancing by responding with a CCPT reflection, instead of pushing to remain in the trauma network.

> Therapist: *You know just what you want to do next.*

EMDR Phase 4 (desensitization and reprocessing) as described in this case example is very short, may be only 5 to 10 minutes out of an entire session. But this bite-size approach to processing is important for several reasons. In the context of this therapist–child relationship, the child has a felt sense of control over the narrative. We recognize that approaching a terrifying memory such as this one goes against the child's own instincts for self-protection, what Struik (2018) calls "waking the sleeping dogs." The children most in need of trauma processing, those with a history of chronic exposure to adversity, have a neurobiology that is very resourceful in avoiding trauma triggers. Digesting a small bite of trauma work builds distress tolerance, and over a period of time, if the therapist respects the child's movement in and out of intensity, they often are able to process bigger "bites" and sustain longer episodes of Phase 4 desensitization and reprocessing. Gradually, the child becomes occupied more fully in the role of first-person narrator of his own experience. Situating these bites of processing in the context of longer play therapy sessions also helps the child to contain the processing.

Reflecting on these brief episodes of EMDR Phase 4 (desensitization and reprocessing) situated in larger sessions of primarily CCPT can help the therapist to be ready to invite the child back into the processing toward the yet-unprocessed channels. Continuing with the boy described earlier, I recognized that the block was related to his current internal awareness of feeling safe. For him, some interweave relating to the idea and/or felt experience of the danger being truly over was needed.

When he returned in the next session to the superhero drama, I was able to use a light touch to suggest some ways in which the play could carry this needed experience of safety.

> Therapist: *You are able to throw that bully guy all the way across the room.*
>
> Child (repeating the action of throwing the figure again and again): *You are a goner!!*
>
> Therapist: *That feels really big—let's smack the drum on that* (BLS). *I'm wondering how to keep him from coming back? I'm wondering if any of these jails could hold him?*
>
> Child (testing the bully figure and the jails): *He fits in here and I can get these dragons to guard him* (see Figure 1.7). (Child visibly relaxes.)

With signs that the child is having a felt experience of safety from this interweave within the play metaphor, I bridged again to the first-person trauma memory.

> Therapist: *The guy who bullied you and mom is in a jail like this I bet. Let's hit the drum while we notice how that feels* (BLS).

1. USING BOTH EMDR AND PRESCRIPTIVE PLAY THERAPY   23

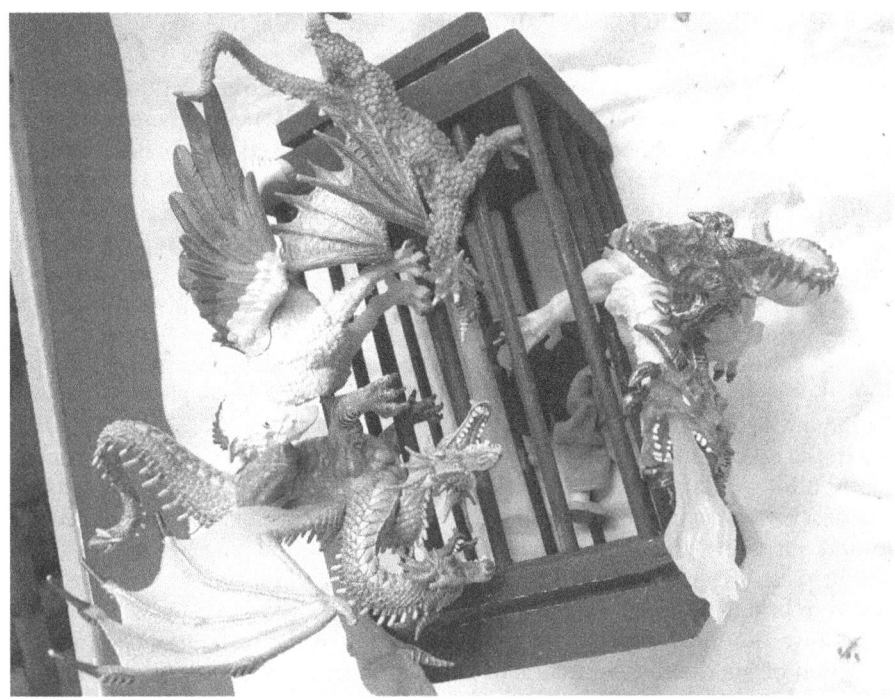

Figure 1.7 *Mastery of Threat: "The Bully Is in Jail"*

Child (laughing): *No dragons though. Policemen.* (Puts a toy policeman on the pile.)

Therapist: *They are safe now.*

Child (accepts positive cognition for the first time): *Safe . . . yeah . . . for now.*

Therapist: *Let's do that butterfly hug and see what that safe feeling is like in our bodies.*

For clinicians with experience in using the standard EMDR protocol with children, there is an all-too familiar sense that we are not always really in the memory network when we ask kids to bring up the disturbing images. Processing ends up feeling superficial. As we move through the Phase 3 assessment questions from the standard protocol, the child might shrug or answer "I don't know." When children are engaged in posttraumatic play such as this example illustrates, which explicitly or metaphorically reenacts elements of the trauma experience, we are more fully in the trauma network of associations and more likely to help them take the "right bites" that will help the memory shift. When the therapist uses the light touch of a play therapy reflection to try out a possible positive or negative cognition or interweave that might or might not fit, the child can go back into the play as needed without getting overwhelmed.

ESSENTIAL 7: ONGOING REEVALUATION OF MEMORY TARGETS

How much reprocessing is enough? As challenging as it is to answer this question in trauma work with adults, it is even harder to ascertain whether there is remaining distress in the memory network based on a child's self-report. Because it is quite challenging for young children to use the Subjective Units of Disturbance Scale accurately, and they tend to report everything as either a 10 or 0, we must rely more heavily on the external evidence such as through the use of caregiver interviews for Phase 8 reevaluation of targets (Beckley-Forest, 2015; Beckley-Forest & Monaco, 2016). We can ask the caregivers to keep track of the child's moods, eating and sleeping patterns, any nightmares, or improvement of functioning. The therapist should continue to return to processing in small chunks as needed as well as attending to the shifts in the child's play themes as a clue about the remaining distress.

In the case of the boy described earlier, the superhero play narrative continued to orbit similar themes of helplessness and the desire to rescue over many sessions. I was able to help him and his mother develop some increased resources around felt safety, then-and-now time orientation, and helping her to reflect on how helplessness had remained a trigger for episodes of rage for him. As we continued to bridge between the play metaphor and his own story, we were able to move toward a more explicitly first-person narrative about the trauma, and the reduction of his distress became more apparent. In the play metaphor, the boy began on his own to incorporate more adaptive solutions to the dilemmas of the characters, for example, creating an elaborate courtroom scene, before losing interest in the story altogether. With this shift in the play, accompanied by remission of some symptoms, we can feel more certainty that the target memory is no longer as distressing to him. In this case, as the play themes became less important to him, his night fears decreased and he began sleeping in his own bed.

In the case of very early trauma, such as pre-verbal attachment experiences, some younger children may never really engage in extensive explicit trauma work around events that "happened to me" as they have great trouble connecting to these events. Instead, we would look for the shifts in intensity, interest, and content of the play themes. Also, due to their emerging development of abstract thought, some children who have done significant trauma digestion through play therapy in earlier childhood may need return episodes of processing as they mature and begin to ask questions that were not available to them in the earlier episode of treatment. An example of this would be a young child who does some processing of an experience of sexual abuse but may need a return to treatment in puberty as an emerging awareness of age-appropriate sexual expression begins to develop.

ESSENTIAL 8: INVOLVING PARENTS THROUGHOUT TREATMENT

The final of these eight essential considerations is the most complicated to apply. Every child therapist has to explore their own theoretical orientation and countertransference around how and when to integrate parents into children's treatment. The context for these decisions is further complicated by children who have not had consistent caregivers, such as foster children who have had multiple placements or children with parents whose capacity for attachment and support is compromised by their own trauma or attachment history. Therapists may struggle to find ways to include parent figures in the safe therapeutic alliance and may have ambivalence about them based on the nature of the child's trauma, the parents' own role in failing to adequately protect the child, and the impairments in the parental attachment pattern, which are negatively impacting the child. Despite the complexity, the literature is clear that parents (by which we also mean other caregivers including foster and adoptive parents, and grandparents; even possibly extending to residential direct care workers in some cases) *must* be involved in therapy as a resource and for fullest benefit of trauma processing with EMDR (Gomez, 2012; Lovett, 1999; Wesselman et al., 2014). Likewise, a significant factor in the research that established the evidence base for play therapy was the finding that the benefits of play therapy were markedly enhanced when parents were fully involved in treatment (Lin & Ray, 2015).

CPRT is an example of a filial approach within play therapy, which attempts to extend the attuned relationship that the play therapist has with the child to the parent–child system (Landreth & Bratton, 2006). In the play therapy environment, the parent and child have the opportunity to experiment more flexibly with attunement in their social engagement with one another. The child has the opportunity to be enjoyed and fully seen by the parent, increasing what Fonagy, Gergely, Jurist, and Target (2018) called mentalization, or the parent's ability to "hold another's mind in mind." Whenever possible, we try to model and coach parents to enter the play therapy space with their child and assist them in expanding their capacity to witness and notice their child and their play. When parents have the capacity to be child-centered even for short periods of time, they are encouraged in this role, as it will promote an expanded capacity for mentalization over time.

We know through the work of Stephen Porges on the polyvagal theory that trauma and its aftermath tend to disengage the social engagement system in response to threat. Chronic trauma represents an ongoing suppression of the brain's own ability to form and sustain attachments and regulate the neurobiology in the face of moment-to-moment challenges. The problematic symptoms in children described by their parents as the impetus for treatment can often be explained as failures of their social engagement system (Porges, 2011).

The attachment trauma of the parent may be echoed in the attachment disruptions the child is experiencing, and the child's posttrauma symptoms may trigger traumatic material for the parent (Gomez, 2013). Parallel comprehensive treatment for the parent–child dyad must of necessity be a component of healing, and there are models for this in both the EMDR therapy and play therapy literature. The Integrative Attachment Trauma Protocol (Wesselman et al., 2014) incorporates family therapy and EMDR processing in a multimodal, multitherapist approach. Naturally, the child therapist is often in the position of wishing the parent was engaging in their own trauma therapy. Even when involved with the family system as a single practitioner, there are treatment plan benefits from conducting a thorough assessment of the parent's own attachment pattern (consider tools such as the Adult Attachment Interview [George, Kaplan, & Main, 1996], or the Family Experience in Childhood Scale [Gonzalez, Mosquera, & Leeds, 2011]) to help the therapist make decisions on how to involve the parent in the child's play therapy and how much structure the parent will need to be successful and recommendations to parents about how their own attachment needs may be impacting the child.

For example, some years ago, I worked with an adoptive mother and the son she adopted through the foster care system using a filial approach to play therapy. This mother was coached on the basic rules of reflecting and responding to the child's imaginative play, primarily on how to stay connected through observations instead of asking or answering questions, teaching, or influencing the play. Over several sessions she watched as I modeled these responses, gradually taking over this role while I receded to more of an observer or facilitator role. One of the greatest difficulties for parents in play therapy is to avoid coaxing the child to be more prosocial (such as by saying—"Oh, we shouldn't hit the baby doll like that, we should play nice"), which has the effect of shutting down the often-intense posttraumatic themes in the play. This mother found the intensity of the child's play dramas with themes of abandonment and rage to be upsetting at times, but she made good use of support from me and from her own therapist and partner and so was able to remain present to the child and play out the narratives as the child directed them. This is the type of parent who might be able to be present throughout the various phases of treatment and enhance the therapeutic safety of the play.

It is not always advisable to have parents present in each play therapy session. In particular, when the content of the child's play has the potential to carry the posttraumatic content, as described earlier (Essentials 5 and 6) and when the therapist is trying to hold the space for this play and expand it through a child-centered approach, parents may not be ready to collaborate, as they may be too triggered themselves. Often children's play is quite different when parents are in the room and the child may be trying, whether consciously or unconsciously, to protect the parent from their distress. There may be implied cognitive distortions around shame and blame that the therapist or the parent has not yet addressed.

Another case example serves to illustrate when it might be a good idea to limit the presence of the parent. In this case, the trauma history for the child was parallel to that of the mother, as there had been several incidents of domestic violence between the parents. This very committed and attuned mother had taken all the steps to get her and her young child to safety, but the loss of regular contact with the father had a very different meaning for her than for the child, and her presence in the play therapy room during play therapy and trauma digestion that included themes of missing his father might have created loyalty binds for him. In this case, I chose not to have her in the room for the CCPT or explicit trauma work, but she was still very actively engaged in the therapy in learning coping skills as described later.

When using games and play strategies to promote state change (see Essential 4), we want parents to be playing and learning alongside their children. Theraplay is an example of a directive play therapy approach to recreating or enhancing basic relationship engagement between the parent and child in a context that helps children to oscillate between excitement and calm, while promoting engagement with the parents and the child's acceptance of nurturing, structure, and challenge. The Theraplay approach is planful and directive and relies on repetition and systematic modeling and feedback to the parent delivered on a moment-to-moment basis. It is associated with positive outcomes in the interaction patterns in the parent–child dyad (Jernberg & Booth, 2001). Theraplay and EMDR are highly compatible approaches, and the full integration of these approaches is well established among therapists who are trained in both (Gomez & Jernberg, 2012).

An educational approach that helps parents understand their child's (sometimes quite narrow) WOT and how to use playful coregulation to expand this window and reestablish calm is invaluable to parents and other caregivers. I limit problem talk in front of the child and try to help parents shift from a solely cause-and-effect behavioral approach to one based on an understanding of the hyper- and hypoaroused states and their child's threat response system. I use playful engagement of the parent in coregulating their child with lots of repetition and practice. Activities that were described in Essential 3 earlier should include the parent or other caregivers such as prop-based ways of breathing (e.g., feathers, pin wheels, bubbles), using soothing sensory input (e.g., lotions, essential oils, relaxing music), tastes (e.g., cold drinks, mints, ice, small snacks), and physical activity (e.g., large muscle activity, deep pressure, nature). These game-based "experiments" are offered as an adjunct to the main body of the play therapy sessions while treatment is getting established, often as rituals in the opening or closing of the session, and help the parent and child increase their repertoire of state-change activities. Empowering parents to become coregulators of their children has important benefits in carrying over in-session experiences and can help with the stabilization that supports progress in therapy, especially if we want children to risk venturing into trauma content. Goodyear-Brown (2010a) describes numerous additional activities to encourage this kind of coregulation. Engaging families in this kind of play offers moments to install shared delight as adaptive information using slow, short sets of BLS. For example, I have had parents and children tap using the butterfly hug while laughing at something together, rock back and forth while mirroring each other's facial expressions, and adding a brief set of eye movements or tapping to a moment when the child is enjoying being held/rocked like a baby by the mother.

Each child's progress through therapy demands an ongoing individualized assessment of how best to involve parents as a resource. As a general rule, when the traumatic elements of the memories are still in the metaphor of the play, I am more cautious about having parents witness this play unless they have shown they are able to attune and contain their own reactions to a sufficient degree as not to compromise the emotional safety the child needs to expand these themes and enter the traumatic memory network. As digestion of the trauma moves toward the more explicit first-person narratives, I am more likely to invite the child to include the parent as a way of not only integrating the experience, but also potentially using the parent as a source of adaptive information and interweaves. Including the parent necessitates preparation sessions with the parent to help them to digest their own emotional reactions sufficiently to be present to the child without overreacting or oversoothing. Lovett (1999) describes a step-by-step approach to preparing parents in using a storytelling approach to EMDR processing of targets with children, and this can be enhanced through the addition of playful props for acting out the story. The investment of time in the relationship with the parent is worth it when we see the shifts in the day-to-day interactions between the parent and child that are indicative of increased emotional safety as we move through the phases of EMDR treatment. Also, caregiver input is needed in order to evaluate the success of both the EMDR protocol and play therapy interventions as discussed in Essential 7.

POTENCY OF INTEGRATED MODELS OF TREATMENT IN COMPLEX POSTTRAUMATIC STRESS DISORDER AND DISSOCIATION

Therapists who work with children, especially children with complex, early trauma, are well aware that even the best, most developmentally accessible interventions will not offer a quick fix to the traumatized child and their wounded nervous system. My efforts to articulate the urgency of a sophisticated use of play therapy as the best context for EMDR have been significantly influenced by Knipe's concept of the Constant Installation of Present Orientation and Safety, or CIPOS (2018). Knipe's emphasis on helping clients with dissociative symptoms establish and maintain continual here-and-now orientation led me to think more deeply about how play therapy serves as the best way of delivering CIPOS to younger children. The attunement and acceptance delivered via reflective feedback of a trained play therapist in the presence of posttraumatic play is a form of child-friendly CIPOS and over time will help child clients build capacity for desensitization to trauma content using EMDR by an accumulated sense of felt safety in the here-and-now experience of the therapy room.

For the most vulnerable and damaged children, innovation and integration are essential to cope with the intensity of their symptoms, in particular the managing and healing of dissociative states. A full clinical literature to address structural dissociation in children is still emerging. Frances Waters's landmark book, *Healing the Fractured Child* (2016), resonated deeply with every clinician who has spent considerable time with traumatized children. The incredible potential of applying classic structural dissociation theory in a practical and integrative way in child therapy settings is still being unpacked and realized. Using the lens of structural dissociation theory to comprehend the intense experiences of posttraumatic play in the therapy room generates even more questions than answers. Obvious opportunities to use creative and dramatic play to recognize and work with the child's dissociative self-states represent an amazing frontier for further integration of play therapy as the setting for this particular kind of trauma work, such as Monaco's use of a playroom metaphor as a "conference room" for a child's self-states to meet and initiate cooperation (Beckley-Forest, Goodyear-Brown, & Monaco, 2018).

CONCLUSION

In any blending or integrating of models, fidelity to the original and purest version of the contributing models must be an important consideration. CCPT, other models of play therapy, and the EMDR standard protocol each have processes and procedures developed over time, and the evidence that supports their efficacy is based on a faithful adherence to their application under controlled circumstances.

Adler-Tapia and Settle (2008), while articulating the difficulties of manualizing EMDR with young children, found that "children were much less likely to produce all the phases of the protocol verbally but instead were successful with expressive techniques, including play therapy and art therapy. Offering alternative methods for expression did not preclude the therapist from demonstration of fidelity to the eight phases" (p. 105).

When research-supported models of care are modified or adapted in any way, we must do so with intention and purpose and engage in a continual evaluation of the benefits to the client, ideally with the help of good clinical consultation. We must also construct sequences of treatment experiences with an eye on the neurobiology of posttrauma and make continually attuned adjustments based on the child's felt experience of safety. Eliana Gil (2016) speaks to a client-centered approach to treatment integration when she states that "posttraumatic play advances therapy goals and prepares children for specific techniques such as Trauma-Focused Cognitive Behavioral Therapy (TF-CBT) and EMDR" (p. 19).

High-quality research, which can offer more information on how best to harness the clinical benefits of integrating specific models of play therapy and EMDR, would improve the efficiency of such an endeavor, but until such time as that specific research emerges, we must use the best clinical instincts of highly trained child therapists as the guide for how to best integrate these evidence-based approaches. With that in mind, the next steps in fuller integration must include increasing the numbers of therapists trained and credentialed in *both* play therapy and EMDR, and those qualified to provide specialized consultation in both fields, in order to respond with skill and flexibility to the complex needs of the children.

REFERENCES

Adler-Tapia, R., & Settle, C. (2008). *EMDR and the art of psychotherapy with children: Treatment manual*. New York, NY: Springer Publishing Company.

Adler-Tapia, R., & Settle, C. (2016). *EMDR and the art of psychotherapy with children* (2nd ed.). New York, NY: Springer Publishing Company.

Axline, V. (1964). *Dibs in search of self*. New York, NY: Random House.

Badenoch, B. (2008). *Being a brain-wise therapist: A practical guide to interpersonal neurobiology*. New York, NY: W. W. Norton.

Beckley-Forest, A. (2015). Play therapy and EMDR: A conversation. *Play Therapy, 10*(3), 10–14.

Beckley-Forest, A. (2019). Exploring the intersection of EMDR and play therapy. *Go With That, 24*(1), 7–11.

Beckley-Forest, A., Goodyear-Brown, P., & Monaco, A. (2018, October). *EMDR and play therapy: A powerful combination*. Presentation at the 23rd EMDR International Association Conference, Atlanta, GA.

Beckley-Forest, A., & Monaco, A. (2016, August). *Teaching kids to play EMDR therapy*. Presentation at the 21st EMDR International Association Conference, Minneapolis, MN.

Bratton, S., Ray, D., Rhine, T., & Jones, L. (2005). The efficacy of play therapy with children: A meta-analytic review of treatment outcomes. *Professional Psychology: Research and Practice, 36*, 376–390. doi:10.1037/0735-7028.36.4.376

Brody, V. A. (1997). *The dialogue of touch: Developmental play therapy* (2nd ed.). Northvale, NJ: Jason Aronson.

Chen, Y. R., Hung, K. W., Tsai, J. C., Chu, H., Chung, M. H., Chen, S. R., . . . Chou, K. R. (2014). Efficacy of eye-movement desensitization and reprocessing for patients with posttraumatic-stress disorder: A meta-analysis of randomized controlled trials. *PLoS One, 9*(8), e103676. doi:10.1371/journal.pone.0103676

De Roos, C., Greenwald, R., den Hollander-Gijsm, M., Noorthoorn, E., van Buuren, S., & de Jongh, A. (2011). A randomized comparison of cognitive behavioral therapy (CBT) and eye movement desensitization and reprocessing in disaster-exposed children. *European Journal of Psychotraumatology, 2*, 5694–5704. doi:10.3402/ejpt.v2i0.5694

Fleming, J. (2012). The effectiveness of eye movement desensitization and reprocessing in the treatment of traumatized children and youth. *Journal of EMDR Practice and Research, 6*(1). 10.1891/1933-3196.6.1.16

Fonagy, P., Gergely, G., Jurist, E., & Target, M. (2018). Attachment and reflective function: Their role in self-organization. In P. Fonagy, G. Gergely, & E. Jurist (Eds.), *Affect regulation, mentalization and the development of the self* (pp. 21–63). New York, NY: Routledge.

Gaskill, R., & Perry, B. (2014). The neurobiological power of play: Using the neurosequential model of therapeutics to guide play in the healing process. In C. Machoidi & D. Crenshaw (Eds.), *Creative arts and play therapy for attachment trauma*. New York, NY: Guilford Press.

George, C., Kaplan, N., & Main, M. (1996). *Adult attachment protocol* (3rd ed.). Unpublished manuscript, Department of Psychology, University of California at Berkeley.

Gil, E. (2006). *Helping abused and traumatized children: Integrating directive and non-directive approaches*. New York, NY: Guilford Press.

Gil, E. (2016). *Posttraumatic play in children: What clinicians need to know*. New York, NY: Guilford Press.

Gomez, A. M. (2012). *EMDR therapy and adjunct approaches with children: Complex trauma, attachment and dissociation*. New York, NY: Springer Publishing Company.

Gomez, A. M., & Jernberg, E. (2012). Using EMDR therapy and theraplay. In A. M. Gomez (Ed.), *EMDR therapy and adjunct approaches with children: Complex trauma, attachment and dissociation*. New York, NY: Springer Publishing Company.

Gonzalez, A., Mosquera, D., & Leeds, A. (2011). *Family experiences in childhood scale*. Retrieved from https://docplayer.net/147066497-Family-experiences-in-childhood-scale-fecs.html

Goodyear-Brown, P. (2010a). *Play therapy with traumatized children: A prescriptive approach*. Hoboken, NJ: Wiley.

Goodyear-Brown, P. (2010b). *The worry wars*. Nashville, TN: Author.

Goodyear-Brown, P. (2019). *Trauma and play therapy*. New York, NY: Routledge.

Greenwald, R. (1999). *EMDR in child and adolescent psychotherapy*. Northvale, NJ: Jason Aronson.

Homeyer, L., & Sweeney, D. (2016). *Sandtray therapy: A practical manual* (3rd ed.). New York, NY: Routledge.

Hong, R., & Mason, C. M. (2016). Becoming a neurobiologically informed play therapist. *International Journal of Play Therapy, 25*(1), 35–44. doi:10.1037/pla0000020

Jarero, I. (2002). The butterfly hug: An update. *EMDRIA Newsletter, 7*(3), 6.

Jernberg, A., & Booth, P. (2001). *Theraplay*. San Francisco, CA: Jossey-Bass.

Kemp, M., Drummond, P., & McDermott, B. (2010). A wait-list controlled pilot study of eye movement desensitization and reprocessing (EMDR) for children with post-traumatic stress disorder (PTSD) symptoms from motor vehicle accidents. *Journal of Clinical Child Psychology and Psychiatry, 15*(1), 5–25. doi:10.1177/1359104509339086

Knell, S. M. (2009). Cognitive behavioral play therapy: Theory and applications. In A. A. Drewes (Ed.), *Blending play therapy with cognitive behavioral therapy: Evidence-based and other effective treatments and techniques* (pp. 117–133). Hoboken, NJ: Wiley.

Knipe, J. (2018). *EMDR toolbox: Theory and treatment of complex PTSD and dissociation* (2nd ed.). New York, NY: Springer Publishing Company.

Kottman, T. (2013). *Partners in play: An adlerian approach to play therapy* (3rd ed.). Alexandria, VA: American Counseling Association.

Landreth, G. (2012). *Play therapy: The art of the relationship* (3rd ed.). New York, NY: Routledge.

Landreth, G., & Bratton, S. (2019). *Child parent relationship therapy (CPRT): A 10 session filial model* (2nd ed.). New York, NY: Routledge.

Lin, Y., & Bratton, S. C. (2015). A meta-analytic review of child-centered play therapy approaches. *Journal of Counseling and Development*, 93(1), 45–58. doi:10.1002/j.1556-6676.2015.00180.x

Lovett, J. (1999). *Small wonders: Healing childhood trauma with EMDR*. New York, NY: Free Press.

McGuiness, V. (2003). *Integrating play therapy and EMDR with children*. Bloomington, IN: AuthorHouse.

Moreno-Alcazar, A., Treen, D., Valiente-Gomez, A., Sio-Erlos, A., Perez, V., Amann, B. L., & Radua, J. (2017). Efficacy of eye movement desensitization and reprocessing in children and adolescents with post-traumatic stress disorder: A meta-analysis of randomized controlled trials. *Frontiers in Psychology*, 8(1750), 1–10. doi:10.3389/fpsyg.2017.01750

Najavits, L. M. (2002). *Seeking safety: A treatment manual for PTSD and substance abuse*. New York, NY: Guilford Press.

Porges, S. (2011). *The polyvagal theory: Neurophysical foundations of emotions, attachment, communication and self-regulation*. New York, NY: W. W. Norton.

Ray, D., Armstrong, S., Balkin, R., & Jayne, K. (2015). Child centered play therapy in the schools: Review and meta-analysis. *Psychology in the Schools*, 52, 107–123. doi:10.1002/pits.21798

Schaefer, C. (2011). Prescriptive play therapy. In C. Schaefer (Ed.), *Handbook of play therapy* (pp. 365–377). Hoboken, NJ: Wiley.

Schaefer, C., & Drews, A. (2014). *Therapeutic powers of play: 20 core agents of change*. Hoboken, NJ: Wiley.

Shapiro, F. (2017). *Eye movement desensitization and reprocessing (EMDR) therapy, third edition: Basic principles, protocols and procedures*. New York, NY: Guilford Press.

Siegel, D. (1999). *The developing mind: How relationship and the brain interact to shape who we are*. New York, NY: Guilford Press.

Struik, A. (2018). The sleeping dogs method to overcome children's resistance to EMDR therapy: A case series. *Journal of EMDR Practice and Research*, 12(4), 224–241. doi:10.1891/1933-3196.12.4.224

Substance Abuse and Mental Health Services Administration. (2012). *Comparative effectiveness research series: Eye movement desensitization and reprocessing therapy: An information resource*. SAMHSA's National Registry of Evidence-based Programs and Practices. Retrieved from https://cdn.ymaws.com/www.emdria.org/resource/resmgr/research/treatment_guidelines/samhsa.2012.nrepp-comparativ.pdf

Swimm, L. (2018). EMDR Intervention for a 17-month-old child to treat attachment trauma: Clinical case presentation. *Journal of EMDR Practice and Research*, 12(4), 269–279.

Swinden, C. (2018). The Child-centered EMDR approach: A case study investigating a young girl's treatment for sexual abuse. *Journal of EMDR Practice and Research*, 12(4), 282–295.

Terr, L. (1990). *Too scared to cry*. New York, NY: Basic Books.

Tinker, R. H., & Wilson, S. A. (1999). *Through the eyes of a child: EMDR with children.* New York, NY: W. W. Norton.

Van der Kolk, B. A. (2015). *The body keeps the score: Brain, mind and body in the healing of trauma.* New York, NY: Penguin.

Waters, F. (2016) *Healing the fractured child: Diagnosis and treatment of youth with dissociation.* New York, NY: Springer Publishing Company.

Wesselman, D., Schweizer, C., & Armstrong, S. (2014). *Integrative team treatment for attachment trauma in children.* New York, NY: W. W. Norton.

2

TraumaPlay and EMDR: Integration and Nuance in Holding Hard Stories

PARIS GOODYEAR-BROWN AND ELEAH HYATT

INTRODUCTION

An integration of TraumaPlay and eye movement desensitization and reprocessing (EMDR) functions as a one–two power punch combination as the power of play is recognized as the child's most natural form of adaptive information processing (AIP) and encourages the full-body somatic experiencing of new neurophysiological states while desensitizing and reprocessing hard things. The overarching goals of TraumaPlay include leaching the emotional toxicity out of clients' traumatic experiences, creating a more coherent narrative of these life events, and deepening relational resources. Getting through the child client's layers of protection requires developmental sensitivity, titration, and creativity. Unlocking a traumatized child's healing may take more than one key, so pairing TraumaPlay and EMDR together can maximize the effectiveness of each.

TRAUMAPLAY

TraumaPlay™ is a flexible, sequential, play therapy model designed for treating traumatized and attachment-disturbed children and teens. TraumaPlay has evolved over the course of 20 years of direct clinical work with hundreds of children who present with complex trauma histories and significant attachment disruptions. The wisdom and experience of other clinicians whom we have come alongside in supervision have further informed the model resulting in real-world application of these concepts with thousands of children and teens. The overarching goals of TraumaPlay include leaching the emotional toxicity out of clients' traumatic experiences, creating a more coherent narrative of these life events, and deepening relational resources. TraumaPlay identifies seven key components of treatment, informed by the evidence base for best practices in the treatment of

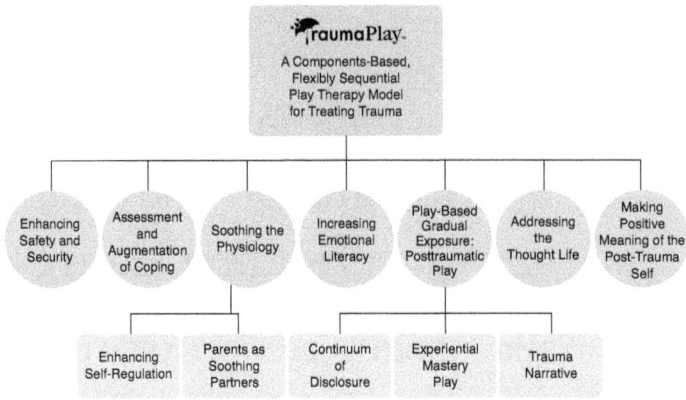

Figure 2.1 *The TraumaPlay Flowchart*
Source: Goodyear-Brown, P. (2019b). *Trauma and play therapy: Helping children heal* (p. 2). New York, NY: Routledge. Copyright 2019. Reproduced by permission of Taylor & Francis Group, LLC, a division of Informa PLC.

childhood trauma. TraumaPlay is informed by our current understandings of the neurobiology of play and the neurobiology of trauma and is built on the power of one to heal the other. Grounded in attachment theory, the child or family is met moment-to-moment as therapeutic needs are assessed. The framework of seven therapeutic treatment goals serves as the umbrella under which clinicians have freedom to employ a variety of interventions. A subset of goals related to enhancing the role of parents as partners expands clinicians' finesse in integrating parents into trauma treatment. TraumaPlay allows room for both nondirective and directive approaches to be employed and incorporates clinically sound elements of other evidence-based treatments such as child-centered play therapy (CCPT), Theraplay™, and cognitive-behavioral play therapy, while offering original interventions that were developed in real-world clinical settings to maximize therapeutic absorption through every play-based learning portal. See Figure 2.1 for a better understanding of the treatment continuum.

The key components of TraumaPlay include enhancing safety and security, assessing and augmenting coping, soothing the physiology, increasing emotional literacy, using play-based gradual exposure, addressing the thought life, and making positive meaning of the posttrauma self. Two of these components offer multiple pathways to achieving the therapeutic goal. The goal of soothing the physiology can be pursued by teaching play therapy interventions that help with clients regulating, moving back into their window of tolerance from states of either hyper- or hypoarousal, or by enlisting parents as soothing partners. When a child presents with complex trauma or has had multiple caregiver disruptions, the Parents as Partners piece of TraumaPlay becomes central to the child's recovery. In these cases, a child's chronological age is often vastly different from their developmental age. Additionally, these children have had limited ability to experience the benefits of a regulating, connected adult. The younger the child is developmentally, the more important it becomes to help parents see themselves as coregulators of the child's arousal states. In TraumaPlay, the coregulating adults are given the label Safe Boss, and support is provided to parents and teachers in learning how to become uniquely Safe Bosses for the children in their care. At the same time, support is given to clients as they learn to trust their caregivers more deeply. TraumaPlay offers a best practice framework for trauma work with families while encouraging ongoing assessment and offering flexibility to the clinician to tailor treatment to the needs of individual families.

Two-dimensional graphics, such as the TraumaPlay Flowchart in Figure 2.1, can be misleading, in that they project a linear flow, making it appear that you must do the first thing first, the second thing second, and so forth. However, far from being protocolized, the TraumaPlay model is meant to put best practice components for treating traumatized children into an umbrella framework that gives clinicians a developmentally sensitive road map for treatment while allowing the clinician to remain in the driver's seat. TraumaPlay clinicians make treatment choices based on their understanding of the child's moment-to-moment needs during the therapeutic process and may switch gears within a single treatment session if the need of the child calls for it (Goodyear-Brown, 2019b).

ONGOING ASSESSMENT AND THE TraumaPlay MAPPING TOOL

The TraumaPlay Mapping Tool, seen in Figure 2.2, was created to help track the dynamic therapeutic movement that occurs during treatment. A seasoned therapist may have spent ample time developing safety and security, soothing the physiology, and so forth prior to beginning a narrative process and still have a child become dissociative as soon as the scariest stuff, the most toxic content, is touched. In this case, a wise therapist may bounce back up to one of the earlier treatment goals to help the child regulate. This does not mean that the therapist did anything wrong, or did not work long enough in a certain area, but is a reminder that a child's window of tolerance for distress may not be clearly delineated until the invitation into hard things is extended. Another situation that often arises is that the TraumaPlay therapist is prepared for a certain aspect of therapeutic work to be the focus of the next session, but the family arrives to the next session with the crisis of the week that may derail progress along the treatment continuum. In using this mapping tool, TraumaPlay clinicians notate the number of sessions spent in pursuit of each goal along a treatment continuum. Tracking in this way can help therapists and their supervisors begin to notice patterns in derailment that may actually be avoidance symptoms of posttraumatic stress disorder (PTSD). This tool can also help TraumaPlay clinicians quickly notice any components that may require a deeper dive therapeutically.

Both the amount of time spent in pursuit of each treatment goal, and the order in which they are pursued may vary from client to client. When a child has been sexually abused for several years by various caregivers and is developing felt safety with a new therapist, this process might take months, while some children may respond to a therapeutic environment with felt safety in just a few sessions, or even in the first session. A child who has experienced a discrete traumatic incident, such as a car accident or a painful but accidental burn, might have a soothing, supportive family system and high emotional literacy and therefore will not need to spend much time on shifting parenting paradigms and very little time on increasing emotional literacy prior to beginning play-based trauma narrative work. In contrast, the child

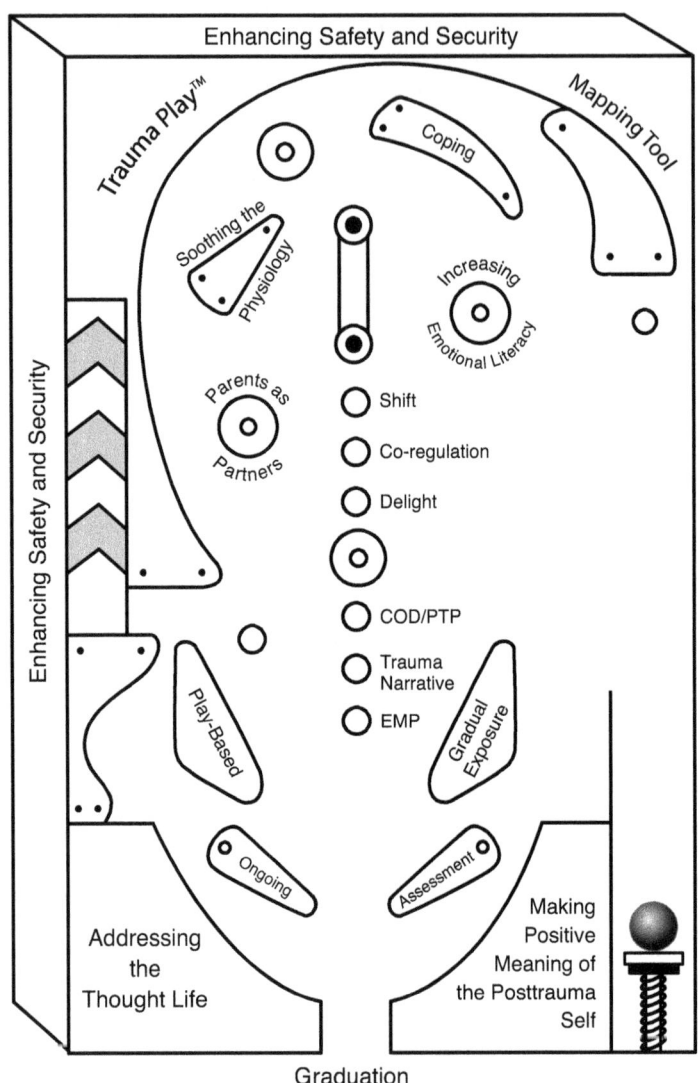

Figure 2.2 The TraumaPlay™ Mapping Tool
COD, continuum of disclosure; EMP, experiential mastery play; PTP, post-TraumaPlay.
Source: Goodyear-Brown, P. (2019). *The TraumaPlay treatment manual* (p. 117).
Self-Published. Reproduced with permission.

who has had multiple caregiver disruptions and may also struggle with features of autism spectrum disorder may have a great deal of difficulty identifying internal feeling states, using feelings vocabulary, expressing emotions appropriately, or pairing situations with the emotions they tend to engender. The child who presents with this set of challenges may need significant time spent with increasing emotional literacy prior to trauma narrative work so that the naming of emotions experienced at different points in the experience can be nuanced and integrated more fully.

INTEGRATING EMDR AND TRAUMAPLAY

The eight phases of the EMDR protocol align well with the goals of TraumaPlay, making an integration of TraumaPlay and EMDR fairly seamless. In order for EMDR to effectively reprocess traumatic memories, these targets must be identified and activated (Shapiro, 2017). Both the process of identification of trauma targets and the process of activation are invited most effectively through the developmental language of the child: play. The first four components of TraumaPlay (enhancing safety and security, assessing and augmenting coping, soothing the physiology, and increasing emotional literacy) fully support the goals of the preparation phase of EMDR. In TraumaPlay, play is seen both as the natural language of children and also as the primary mitigator toward and away from the trauma content. TraumaPlay therapists recognize the neurochemical boxing match that is taking place continually with traumatized children, and work intentionally to pair the approach to hard content (that will result in an elevation of cortisol, the stress hormone) with play, which results in the release of oxytocin and dopamine in the brain. The AIP model that is central to EMDR identifies past experiences that are currently contributing to a client's difficulties, maladaptive response patterns that are being triggered in the here-and-now, and aim at fostering adaptive neural networks so that future response patterns are ones that embrace health (Shapiro & Laliotis, 2011). Play in itself is adaptive for children, helping them build attachments, try on various roles, experience a variety of neurophysiological states with full-body expression, and practice new skill sets. So, when we pair EMDR with experiential mastery play (competency enhancement experiences) and relational resourcing, we get maximized effects, and when we pair EMDR with posttraumatic play and play-based trauma narrative, we get maximized reprocessing and desensitization effects.

We begin introducing the idea of chewing up the trauma early on in the therapy process so that preparation is happening as soon as treatment starts. The well-used toy pictured in Figure 2.3 was purchased at an after-Halloween-clearance sale 15 years ago.

This battery-operated brain opens and closes in the middle, exposing teeth that chew up trauma memories, cognitive distortions, and anything else that needs to be digested. We then introduce clients to a variety of playful ways to do the bilateral stimulation (BLS) of EMDR. In addition to more traditional methods, such as tracking a laser pointer between two points, tapping on their hands or knees, using the "buzzies" or vibrating electronic therapeutic tappers in socks or pockets, or having a client track a finger puppet, sword, or wand with their eyes while crossing the midline of the face, we introduce a variety of drumming techniques, play Patty Cake, and use Devil Stixx™ (a pair of long sticks between which a third, shorter stick is bounced back and forth) and poi balls (balls that have been covered in fabric and long ribbons that are worn by the child through finger grips, which allow the child to complete full rotations of their arms with rapid, full-body bilateral motion to help clients engage more of their bodies). We may also have them walk a slackline and of course go on therapeutic walks. One of our clients was fearful about EMDR but was comforted by having the buzzies put inside two birds in our bird's nest puppet (see Figure 2.4). She held onto these and was able to do her work in this way. Once we have entered into processing, if processing appears to be stuck, we already have a list of mediums that may restart processing through a different portal for integration.

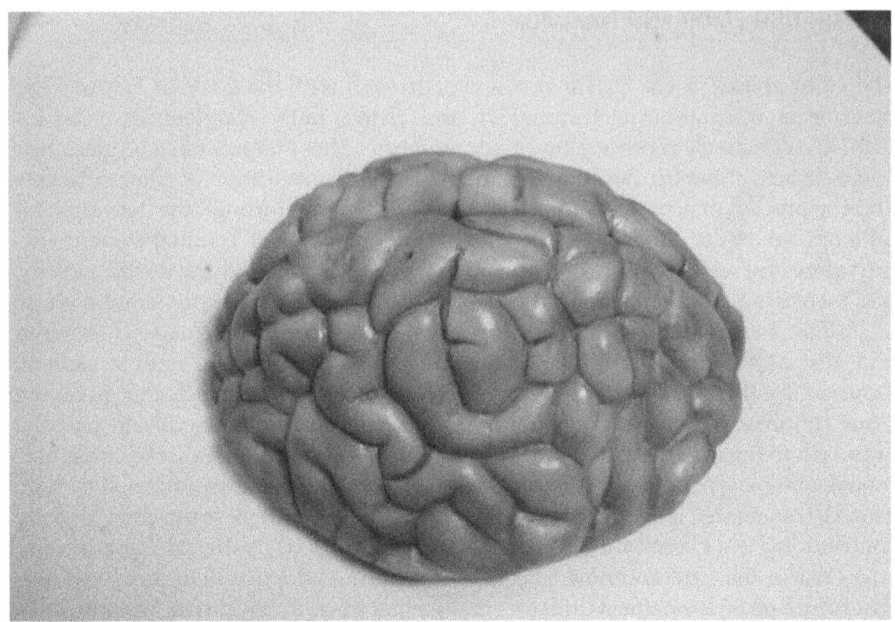

Figure 2.3 *The Toy Brain*

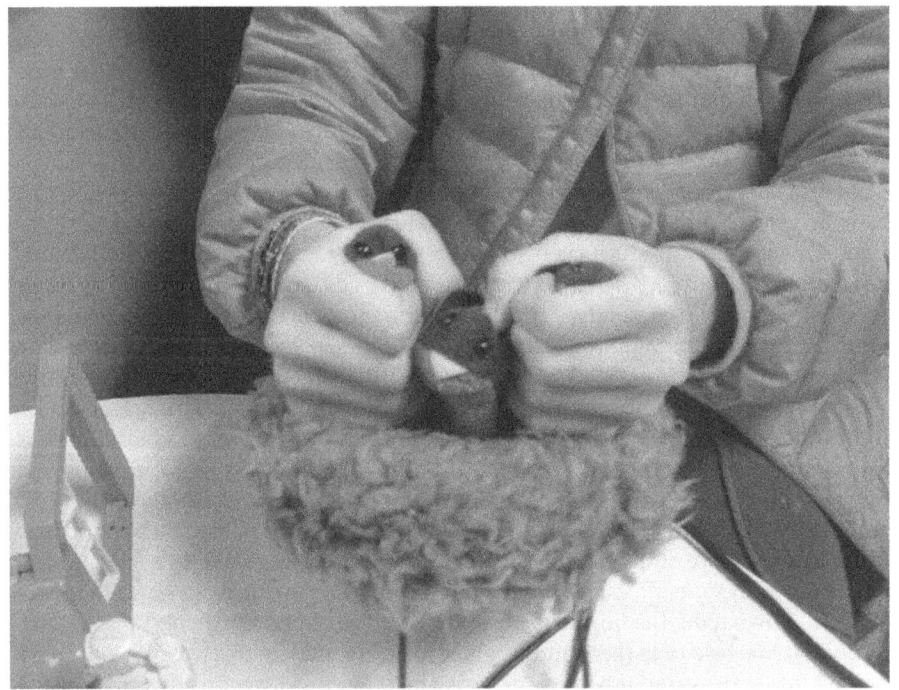

Figure 2.4 *Tappers in Bird Puppet for Bilateral Stimulation*

ASSESSMENT

TraumaPlay therapists view the overall assessment of the child as ongoing and value the richness of knowledge that becomes the scaffolding for case conceptualization when both caregivers and children are involved in the assessment phase of treatment. Therefore, TraumaPlay embraces a developmentally sensitive assessment process that encourages clinicians to enter into the family's experience from several directions (not to be confused with Phase 3 of EMDR, which involves target assessment and activation). The initial biopsychosocial intake interview is completed with adult caregivers only. Therapists who work in third-party payment situations are often forced to see parent and child together at intake. These therapists face the additional challenge of attempting to join with the parent, helping the parent feel seen and heard, without endorsing the child's "badness" or seeming to collude with the parent. When parents are seen first, they are able to express concerns without censoring themselves, and the therapist is able to begin building relationships with parents while laying the groundwork for any paradigm shifts that may need to occur later in treatment.

The intake session is followed by two sessions in which the Nurture House Dyadic Assessment (NHDA) is completed with the child and each parent. NHDA observations begin with the clinician observing the dyad in the lobby . . . are they sitting close together or far apart? Are they engaged in a shared activity or each doing their own thing? Does the dyad transition easily to the playroom? If the transition is difficult, is the parent able to provide support and comfort or does the parent seem to watch helplessly? Once inside the playroom, there are proscribed time frames in which the child gets to be in charge and the parent gets to be in charge, reminiscent of the Dyadic Parent-Child Interaction Coding System (DPICS), which is designed to assess parent–child social interactions, providing a guide for treatment decisions and measure of behavioral change in Parent-Child Interaction Therapy (UC Davis PCIT Training Center, 2013). Then they move to a series of tasks on cards that include tasks from the Marschak Interaction Method (Jernberg & Booth, 1999) and other tasks that help us assess how each member of the dyad handles an approach to slightly more difficult material. The NHDA helps clinicians better understand how caregivers may need to be trained/shifted in order to become more effective anchors and coregulators for their child during trauma narrative work/trauma reprocessing. Integrating this work with EMDR helps us understand what parents and children may need during the preparation phase.

In addition to these dyadic assessments, TraumaPlay clients often have three individual sessions with the following goals: (a) to build rapport while entering the child's world through play and (b) to invite developmentally appropriate play-based exploration of the child's current emotional literacy, current coping, their perceptions of their family dynamics, and, depending on the age of the child, initial assessment of potential cognitive distortions. The specific TraumaPlay assessment tools used during this phase of treatment include the Family Play Genostory, a Color-Your-Heart, a Three Wishes Prompt, and possibly a Coping Tree. When TraumaPlay and EMDR are being combined, TraumaPlay therapists may also be doing preparation-phase work, including identifying various forms of BLS and which tools are most comfortable for the child and identifying targets. These activities are typically completed over the course of three sessions that are divided into half. For half of each session, the TraumaPlay therapist is employing CCPT, following the child's lead, and inviting the following therapeutic powers of play into the space: self-expression, access to the unconscious, therapeutic relationship, attachment, and self-regulation. An understanding of the therapeutic powers of play is foundational to TraumaPlay, and Exhibit 2.1 can serve as an introduction for those less familiar with these core change agents.

Exhibit 2.1 *Therapeutic Powers of Play*

A list of the therapeutic powers of play was first presented, in 1993, by Dr. Charles E. Schaefer, Association for Play Therapy (APT) cofounder. It has since been expanded based on clinical experience and research to include 20 core agents of change. The principle underlying the therapeutic powers of play is that the play itself is the source of change, not the medium or the moderator by which change occurs.

This important distinction and its transtheoretical approach are at the heart of how play therapy is defined by APT. The following is a list of the therapeutic powers of play as identified by Dr. Charles E. Schaefer and Dr. Athena A. Drewes:

I. **Facilitates Communication**
   A. Self-Expression
   B. Access to the Unconscious
   C. Direct Teaching
   D. Indirect Teaching

II. **Fosters Emotional Wellness**
   A. Catharsis
   B. Abreaction
   C. Positive Emotions
   D. Counterconditioning Fears
   E. Stress Inoculation
   F. Stress Management

III. **Enhances Social Relationships**
   A. Therapeutic Relationship
   B. Attachment
   C. Social Competence
   D. Empathy

IV. **Increases Personal Strengths**
   A. Creative Problem-Solving
   B. Resiliency
   C. Moral Development
   D. Accelerated Psychological Development
   E. Self-Regulation
   F. Self-Esteem

Source: Reproduced with permission from Schaefer, C. E., & Drewes, A. A. (Eds.). (2014). *The therapeutic powers of play: 20 core agents of change* (2nd ed.). Hoboken, NJ: Wiley.

Sometimes, the core targets for EMDR work are approached during CCPT as the child begins engaging in posttraumatic play. The other half of each session is given over to one of the specific assessments mentioned earlier. The child is given the choice of which happens first, through the therapist's prompt, "Today, you get to be in charge of the play for part of the time and I get to be in charge of the play for part of the time. Do you want to be in charge first or would you like me to lead first?" Once we have completed the dyadic assessments, the structured play-based assessments, and joined with the child through CCPT, we have a parent feedback session in which we give synthesized information and lay out a treatment plan moving forward.

ENHANCING SAFETY AND SECURITY

Establishing a child's sense of safety in the person of the play therapist and in the environment of the playroom is at the forefront of the TraumaPlay therapist's mind, beginning with their very first encounter. TraumaPlay therapists increase a child's sense of safety in these experiences by "following his lead, reflecting his talk, describing his play, and generally 'being with' him, being attuned to his communications in the space" (Goodyear-Brown, 2010a, p. 51). These experiences establish the play therapist as a secure base for the child, a safe presence from which they can explore and return to for comfort, welcome, or soothing as they move through the harder parts of their work.

The importance of the presence of the therapist has been regarded as a crucial factor in building a therapeutic relationship and shown to be an essential ingredient of therapeutic change (Crenshaw, Kenney-Noziska, & Demanchick, 2014). CCPT further reiterates the importance of play in the context of a secure environment and within the presence of an accepting therapist as the primary mechanism for change (Schultz, 2016). Geller and Greenberg (2002) define therapeutic presence as bringing one's whole self into the encounter with clients by being completely in the moment on multiple levels: physically, emotionally, cognitively, and spiritually. TraumaPlay therapists intentionally work to communicate safety to the child by following their "need" (Goodyear-Brown, 2010a) and "fidelity to the model is defined as fidelity to the child—to the need being expressed and the most appropriate way for [the clinician] to meet it at each moment within the session" (Goodyear-Brown, 2019a, p. 8). This empathetic approach to connection with a child is supported by psychotherapy outcome research (Duncan & Moynihan, 1994), which reveals that it is the client's experience of the therapist that is strongly associated with session outcome and the quality of the therapeutic relationship. TraumaPlay emphasizes the importance of the play therapists' use of self to create a feeling of safety in the play therapy room (Goodyear-Brown, 2019b) and encourages therapists to continually engage in a self-reflection process as a way to alleviate the effect of any intrapersonal influences that may hinder the therapeutic safety of the playroom.

Some of the traumatized children we see do not even have a template for safety when they begin treatment. Some children have predominantly experienced pain at the hands of their caregivers, and they, understandably, perceive true safety as devoid of human interaction. Jimmy, a 15-year-old foster child, showed me this dynamic during an expressive arts activity called *Postcards in Motion* (Goodyear-Brown, 2002). I gave Jimmy a postcard that was blank on both sides. I asked him to imagine or identify a place that he would like to visit, a vacation spot that would feel safe and peaceful (sometimes clients are not able to imagine or identify one on their own and we will look up pictures of vacation spots in magazines or on the computer). Jimmy thought about it for a few minutes and then began drawing a small structure on an island. I thought that this was going in a good direction until he began filling in visual details. He explained that he was creating a desert island "with no people anywhere to be seen." This part I understood, as Jimmy had often found his greatest sense of felt safety in isolation. As he continued to draw, what emerged was rather alarming. When I asked him to describe the structure, he said "it's a rat-infested hut with holes in the roof." This was the extent of Jimmy's current template for safety. It would be slow going with him to create felt safety together.

SAFE PLACE IN TRAUMAPLAY

TraumaPlay therapists enhance safety and security through both nondirective play therapy methods (CCPT) and directive play therapy interventions. One of the most typical prompts in this phase of treatment involves asking a child to create a Safe Place in the sand tray. A core concept in TraumaPlay is that a child may have no concrete or experiential template for felt safety when beginning treatment. Based on this understanding, we never ask a child to remember a place where they felt safe, but to imagine or create a Safe Place in the sand. We maximize the potential of kinesthetic involvement in creating a Safe Place in three dimensions in the sand. Once the Safe Place has been built, the child has an external, fully concrete representation of safety that can be further installed (internalized and expanded) using BLS in slow short sets. The TraumaPlay Safe Place Sandtray Exercise has a number of exploratory prompts, aimed at harnessing sensory experiences in relation to what they have made. Children imagine being in the Safe Place and are asked, "What can you smell in your Safe Place? What can you hear in your Safe Place?" I (Paris) once had a very withdrawn, defensive 9-year-old client, who had refused any other form of mindful engagement, but after he had created a beach scene, I had him imagine being in the scene while I did several slow short sets of BLS. Then I asked him what he could smell in his Safe Place, and he identified the smell of the ocean. I had him focus on this smell and did several more slow, short sets. Then I asked him what he could hear at his beach. He said he heard the sound of the waves . . . and then the seagulls calling. We enhanced these sounds with slow, short sets. Lastly, I asked him what he could feel in his Safe Place, and he surprised me by closing his eyes. His eyes popped open as he exclaimed, "My feet being scratched by the sand." We installed and further enhanced this pleasant sensation with more slow, short sets of BLS. This young man left the session with Safe Place imagery that could more easily be accessed and that was tied to full-body soothing based on our expansion of the sensory experiences with BLS. This standard TraumaPlay tool also functions as a resourcing intervention during resource development and installation in EMDR. When children are unable or unwilling to create a Safe Place, we will work with other interventions specific to soothing the physiology in TraumaPlay. When integrated with EMDR, we refer to these as Safe State work.

CONTAMINATION OF SAFE PLACE

A common issue that arises during supervision is how to handle Safe Place work when elements of danger are present. Sally was a 7-year-old child who had been traumatized by her father's repeated promises to come and see her, the hope and excitement she would experience each time as she waited for him and the crushing disappointment and rejection she felt when he did not show up. Given subsequently is the excerpt from the session in which she created a Safe Place in the sand:

> Paris: *You talked about all these other parts of the sand tray . . . the birds, the animals . . . and then you mentioned the Shadowman. When you look at the Shadowman and think about him, does he make you feel good and safe and happy on the inside, or does he give you that kind of worried feeling?*
>
> Sally: *Not very worried. He's kind of cute and handsome.*
>
> Paris: *He's kind of cute and handsome.*
>
> Sally: *Yeah, so I put him on there . . . he looks kind of like my dad.*
>
> Paris: *He does look kind of like your dad?* (Sally nods). *Hmmm . . . and is daddy someone you can make be in your Safe Place? Can we make him? If we say, "Come here and be in Sally's Safe Place!"*
>
> Sally (her face falling): *No.*
>
> Paris: *So what do you think? For our Safe Place in here, do you think we should have him in there or we should have him out?*
>
> Sally: *Maybe out.*
>
> Paris: *Maybe out. We can find another place to put him and we can work with him later.*
>
> Sally: *How about . . . in the end* (circling her hand in a repetitive motion)*?*
>
> Paris: *In the end, we'll work with him.*
>
> Sally: *Because he's so far away I can't even see him.*
>
> Paris: *You can't even see him. Why don't you put him* (holding the Shadowman figure [Figure 2.5]) *somewhere in the room where you want him to go.* (Sally moving over to the sand tray shelves.)
>
> *You found a place for him on that shelf.*
>
> Sally: *Protected by this man.*
>
> Paris: *He's protected by a police officer.*
>
> Sally: *So he won't get hurt.*

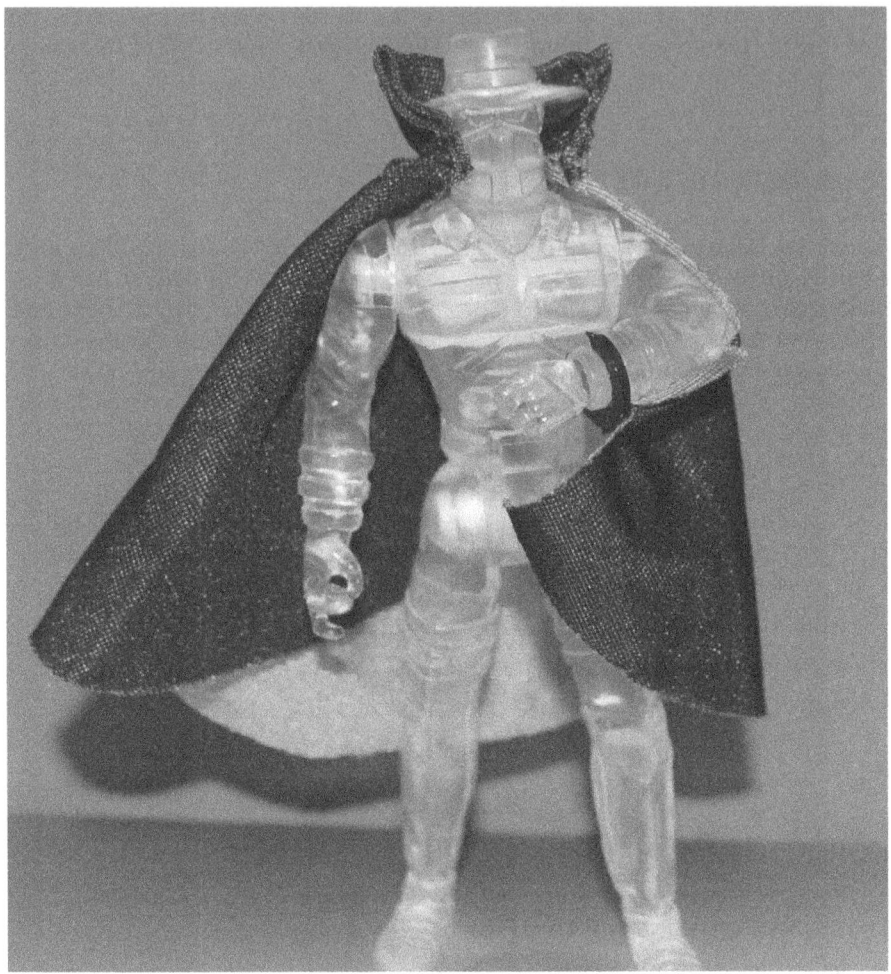

Figure 2.5 *The Shadowman*

Paris: *You want to make sure that he doesn't get hurt . . . while he's up there waiting.*

Sally: *Well, he can get invisible.*

Paris (giving the buzzies to Sally for BLS): *Now that your Safe Place feels safer, try noticing any new smells, tastes, sounds in your Safe Place.*

Sally (after focusing her eyes on the tray and letting the buzzies work): *I hear birds chirping.*

We continued in this manner until we had enhanced installation of as many sensory aspects of safety related to her tray as we could.

SOOTHING THE PHYSIOLOGY AND PARENTS AS PARTNERS

Children who have experienced chronic neglect or maltreatment are often so neurocompromised that experiences of safety and security must be targeted first at the reptilian brainstem (Corrigan & Hull, 2015; Sahar, Shalev, & Porges, 2001).

Recapitulating Natural Rhythms of Regulation becomes the first intersection of TraumaPlay and EMDR and is best accomplished in tandem with an available comforting caregiver. In a good enough caregiving system, the infant is wholly soothed by the mother thousands and thousands of times in the first year of life. The baby is hungry and the mother feeds the baby. The baby is cold and the mother warms the baby. The state of distress or dysregulation is a fully-body state for infants, and it is the baby's ability to cue their parent that they are in a state of crisis and to receive help over and over again that begins to provide the scaffolding for later self-regulation. It is counterintuitive to some, but we must first be wholly reliant on another to eventually become autonomous beings. Moments as simple as having the parent read a story to the child while holding a bag of a preferred food that the child can eat can be installed and enhanced with BLS. We really like *The Invisible String* (Karst, 2000) as one of our first reads when we are enhancing attachments. Resulting cognitions from these kinds of experiences, such as "I can get what I need," "I am cared for," and "I am lovable," can also be installed and further expanded using BLS. Nurturing dyadic games are foundational in TraumaPlay and are offered with the facilitation of the therapist, who delights in both the parent and child as they delight in each other. Powerful work is happening when laughter is occurring. Any time that a TraumaPlay therapist recognizes genuine laughter and delight between a parent and child is a good time to incorporate BLS, aiding in the expansion of the child's positive neural net related to caregiving. Powerful cognitions here, such as "I am delightful" and "I am safe," can also be further enhanced with BLS.

We also work on regulation and soothing the physiology through swinging and jumping, activating our proprioceptive and vestibular systems, and playfully managing our sympathetic and parasympathetic responses while playing in these ways. We have several swings at Nurture House, as well as slack lines, rope tunnels, and so forth and often have the TheraTappers™ in the child's pockets while they are using this play equipment, in order to reinforce healthy rhythms and moments of interaction that require trust (walking the slack line) and result in a neurochemical reward of intense pleasure as the child accomplishes the task.

Sometimes, we ask the parent to tell a story of a time the child "did a hard thing anyway this week" or a "time when they took a risk" or "a time when they did something delightful." We will turn on the buzzies and let them do their work while the child is being pushed on the swing and listening to stories about their goodness. Other times, we wait until a child risks something new on their own, often on the swing. A child might move from laying down on their stomach to sitting up in the middle of the swing, moving it back and forth with their core. Our favorite moments are when a child risks standing up and rocks their body backward and forward. At these times, we encourage a child to pay attention to their interoception . . . what their bodies are telling them from the inside out. Sometimes, we will ask them to give the somatic experience words . . . "I can do it!" is the most frequent response. In TraumaPlay, we call this the *competency*

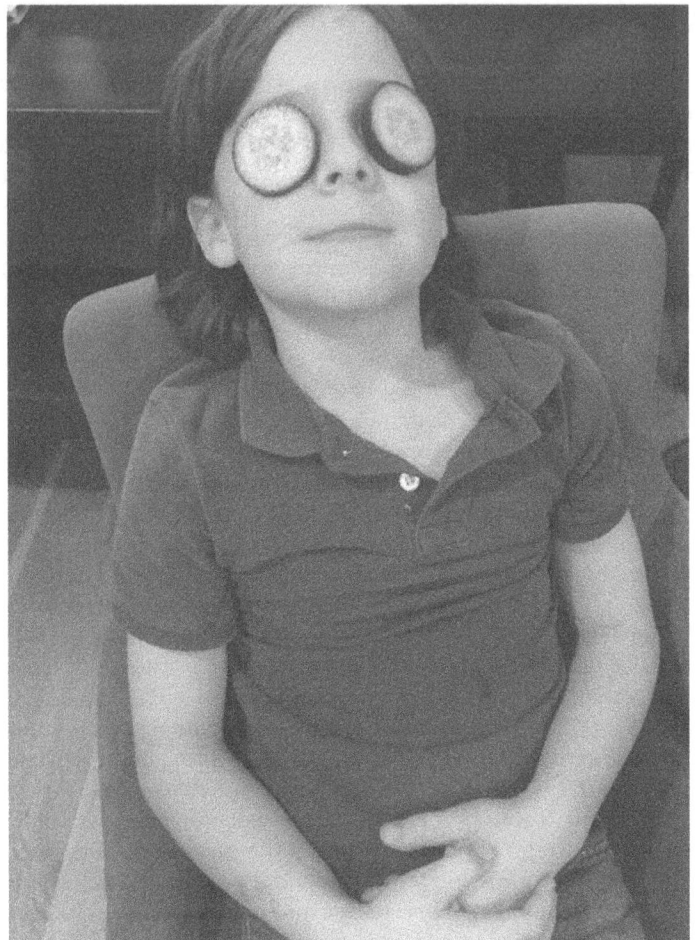

Figure 2.6 *Cool as a Cucumber Intervention*

surge and equate these experiences with the strengthening of positive neural networks, the release of oxytocin and dopamine in the brain, and the building of shared delighting-in memories between a parent and child.

While some children need to have the physiology upregulated, others need experiences of downregulation. We offer dozens of interventions in TraumaPlay that pair the relaxation response with playful props. Figure 2.6 is an example of Cool as a Cucumber (Goodyear-Brown, 2002), a play-based intervention in which children get an in vivo experience of intentionally calming the body, often with the aid of a caregiver.

Some neglected and maltreated children come to us in such a state of dysregulation that they cannot even sit through a story read to them by an adoptive parent. Expanding the child's window of tolerance for physical proximity is often aided by creating small doses of joint attention to a restful task. For example, the seemingly simple task of sitting close to a parent while listening to a story being

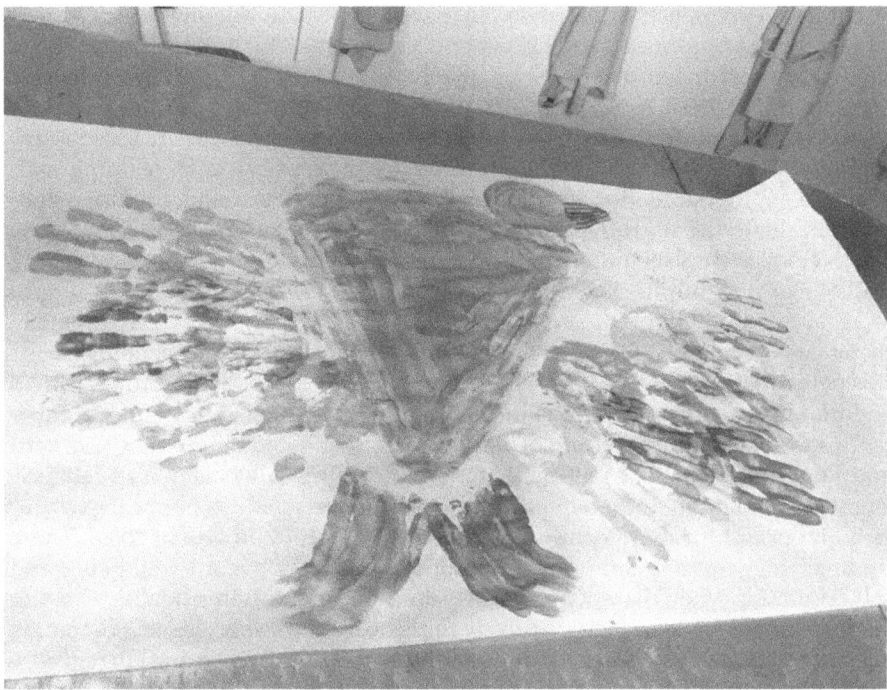

Figure 2.7 *Bird Created by Mother–Son Dyad With Nurturing Touch*

read can become another portal for enhancing safety and security while amplifying the role of parents as soothing partners.

The child holds the buzzies or has them in their socks/pockets. As both parties move into their window of tolerance, we enhance the feelings of connection and shared rest with BLS. We often choose anchoring books that allow for delight and shared narrative between parent and child. We then build a kinesthetic, nurturing play therapy intervention around this bibliotherapy prompt. I (Paris) invited mom to read the book *Beautiful Hands* (Baumgarten & Otoshi, 2015) to her son. When he was able to relax into a snuggle, molding to her body, I further enhanced this experience with BLS. The book itself has stunning art created from colorful fingerprints and handprints. I invite the dyad to choose an image from the book that they wish to recreate (and sometimes pairs come up with uniquely new expressions). The dyad chooses the paint colors, they spend time painting each other's hands and pressing them to the paper, inviting lots of nurturing touch, and encouraging delight to be exchanged between parent and child. Figure 2.7 is a bird created by an adoptive mother and son.

ASSESSMENT AND AUGMENTATION OF COPING

Stress is a normal part of the human experience, and how one learns to cope with that stress can have a profound impact on one's overall quality of life. Children who are raised in environments saturated with severe stress oftentimes experience impairment in psychological development and result in biological consequences. The experience of child maltreatment has been shown to exert harmful effects on the brain as well as on neuroendocrine regulation (Cicchetti & Rogosch, 2001). These stressful or threatening experiences can have profound negative effects on a child's ability to create adaptive coping skills. In addition, young children are susceptible to developing maladaptive coping skills due to their lack of life experience and cognitive ability to evaluate the usefulness of their own coping responses (Baggerly, 2006). TraumaPlay therapists understand the importance of assessing a child's coping skills before beginning the work of processing trauma content, being careful to avoid any potential iatrogenic effects (Goodyear-Brown, 2010a). TraumaPlay therapists' use of play-based interventions provides a developmentally sensitive pathway for assessing a child's coping repertoire (Goodyear-Brown, 2010a) and building adaptive coping skills, thereby, enhancing a child's inner competence and resilience. In a study of resilience in maltreated children by Cicchetti and Rogosch, aspects of self-organization, including self-esteem, self-reliance, emotion regulation, and adaptable yet reserved personalities, appear particularly important for more competent coping (Cicchetti & Rogosch, 2009). These findings suggest that children show improvements in overall well-being and self-regulation when therapeutic work is done around building adaptive coping skills. TraumaPlay therapists positively mitigate a child's approach to the trauma content by supporting the child through the process of augmenting current coping skills, extinguishing maladaptive responses, and developing new, healthy coping strategies (Goodyear-Brown, 2010a). TraumaPlay therapists value kinesthetic involvement in the exploration and identification of current coping. To this end, we offer exercises like the Coping Tree, CopeCakes (Goodyear-Brown, 2010b), and Coping Umbrellas (Goodyear-Brown, 2010a) to get children involved in full-body engagement in their coping work. Sometimes, children bring their own metaphors for coping and healing. For example, a young man who has experienced early medical trauma and abandonment by his biological parents brought in one of the first loveys he received in his forever family. For the first few sessions, this young man had clung to his mother, demanding she meet his needs in ways that an ambivalently attached infant would do. As we worked on enhancing competencies and accessing the big boy self, mom told the story of when he first received this lovey. Joey blurted out, "he's broken . . . his stuffing is falling out." I asked if they could bring the lovey and some needle and thread to the next session. Joey seemed astonished that I would trust him with needle and thread, but I kept supporting mom's position as his Safe Boss. She showed him how to stitch the lovey, and he did several stitches on his own, with her helping hands readily available if he needed her. After about 10 minutes of this, a very interesting thing happened. Joey noticed that one of my pillows was ripped and that the stuffing was falling out. He asked if he could stitch it up . . . and as he used this newfound competency to restore his own lovey and an important item in the playroom, his sense of helpfulness and value was reinforced internally as mom and I both delighted in him in a fully authentic way.

SOOTHING THE PHYSIOLOGY

One of the most devastating effects of trauma is the many ways in which it alters brain development, specifically in areas such as the amygdala, hippocampus, and prefrontal cortex, resulting in dysregulation that manifests in a child's physiology (Goodyear-Brown, 2010a). Children exposed to trauma are frequently scanning their environment, looking for signs of danger (Garaven, Pendergrass, Ross, Stein, & Risinger, 2001). "Chronic stress and trauma can result in a brain trained to exist in a state of hyperarousal. In such a state, children cannot concentrate and become easily frustrated, more impulsive, and moody. Their sleeping and eating patterns may become irregular" (Stewart, Field, & Echterling, 2016, p. 9).

TraumaPlay therapists recognize that children who have experienced trauma have a heightened physiological reactivity, which makes it challenging for them to calm down (Goodyear-Brown, 2010a). Therefore, it becomes pivotal to soothe a child's physiology before approaching any other treatment goals. Research by Bartz et al. reports that neurochemical underpinnings such as oxytocin can increase interpersonal trust and reduce anxiety (Bartz, Zaki, Bolger, & Ochsner, 2011). Stewart et al. (2016) describe play in the therapeutic relationship with the therapist as "an emotionally engaging and creative experience that increases levels of oxytocin" (p. 5). Oxytocin enhances feelings of emotional well-being and trust, helping to create an environment of felt safety and soothing. Once a child's overactive nervous system has been soothed, integration of sensory content and factual accounts of the trauma can be used to explore the child's maladaptive thoughts, provide gradual exposure to the trauma content, or build coherent narrative work (Goodyear-Brown, 2019b).

TraumaPlay offers dozens of regulation activities, some of which provide full-body somatic grounding, some of which invite the use of caregivers as coregulators, and some of which embrace elements of the natural environment to help children regulate. One seminal TraumaPlay concept is that children do not need to be calmed so much as they need to understand the signals their bodies are giving them that they are outside of their optimal arousal window. They can then use this valuable information to upregulate or downregulate according to their need. TraumaPlay therapists employ a very simple intervention called the "Balancing Act" (our name for an intervention Paris first learned from Richard Kagan, the author of *Real Life Heroes*, in a live local training), in which a child simply balances a peacock feather. What skill sets are involved in successfully balancing a peacock feather? One has to remain grounded and fluid in their body, planting their feet lightly and bending their knees, following the movement of the peacock feather. One cannot be successful when the body is in a state of rigidity. Clients also find a focal point, often the eye of the peacock feather, and begin to hyperfocus on that spot. This sort of hyperfocus on an element of the here-and-now environment creates a state of child-friendly mindfulness. This often gets paired, over time, with a client's natural drive for competency. Arthur, a 10-year-old boy who had lost his father to amyotrophic lateral sclerosis over the course of several months of slow decline, was brought to therapy by his mom. Arthur had watched his father die a slow, painful death in a special bed in the living room, and when Arthur and his mother came for their first session, they carried their sadness and grief in a palpable way. After several sessions of work, Arthur still manifested blunted affect. I introduced the Balancing Act and Arthur's brows came together in determined focus as he worked his way up to a balancing time length of 26 seconds. I informed him that he was tied for the record with one other client. The following session, Arthur turned to me as soon as he entered session and said, "Can I try to break the record?" and instructed me to keep time on my phone. The first 26 seconds were quiet and fairly routine for us, but when he reached 26 seconds and was still going, I announced "26 seconds!" He and I were both intensely focused and my announcement was met with a momentary falter in his gate and focus . . . he spun around in a circle and was able to rebalance . . . and for the first time in the whole of his treatment, his dimples creased, and we saw the first hint of positive affect. Baby steps. Immersion in the present moment provided a competency surge for him that allowed him one of his first doses of truly positive experience since his father had died. Having the client further install the somatic experience of competency enhancement, mindful noticing, or delight maximizes therapeutic movement.

Makayla offers another example. She was internationally adopted before the age of 2 and had been in the care of three primary caregivers during her early years of life. Makayla was abandoned as a 3-week-old infant, left on the outskirts of a rural village. Upon being brought to the orphanage, she was soon adopted by a local family only to be returned to the orphanage within the first year of her life. Makayla was a delightful child, but her incessant sensory-seeking behaviors were beginning to cause distress at home and in her preschool environments. Makayla displayed a strong need for sensory input—being very attracted to loud noises, rough play, jumping, hopping, and crashing into things or people around her. She reflected an unusual tolerance for pain and difficulty understanding the concept of personal space. It became very clear that sensory input was very soothing for Makayla, helping her feel more organized in her body. This would become the portal through which she would learn how to become more attuned to her body and discern her body's needs for upregulating or downregulating stimulation. Sessions intentionally began with sensory activities that provided powerful and lasting *proprioceptive input*, providing her with a valuable source of self-regulation and inner sense of competency. On some days, Makayla would choose to begin sessions on the Skycurve® Platform Swing, beginning on her tummy and moving toward a standing position as she experienced an inner competency surge. Upon standing, she would chant the words, "Makayla's body is strong. I can trust my body" as the swing moved back and forth and as she maintained a firm and regulated standing position. Other times, Makayla chose to bury herself in the plastic ball pit in the Nurture House sensory room, where she would lay and practice deep breathing skills until her body was calm and she felt ready to emerge. It was beautiful to witness her inner self emerge as her internal became more regulated. From this regulated state, her mind became more open to learning and she could begin the deeper work of healing from her past traumas.

ASSESSMENT PHASE IN EMDR

In EMDR, the assessment phase is meant to more fully flesh out a target memory. In a standard EMDR protocol, this would include assessing for the specific image, the negative cognition (NC), the positive cognition (PC), the emotions associated with the event, where the client feels it in their body, a Subjective Units of Distress (SUD) level for how they feel in the now when they think about that memory, and a Validity of Cognition number representing how much they believe this new cognition to be true. Even identifying targets can be difficult for our youngest clients and for latency-aged children, who are highly resistant to focusing on any content that may produce a feeling of being overwhelmed. A core tenet of the TraumaPlay model is this: Children can approach trauma content much more quickly when it is paired with play. The play itself becomes both a mitigator for the approach to scary things and a powerful combatant in the neurochemical boxing match between cortisol (the stress hormone that gets released in a child's body as they refocus on the scary thing) that is combated by the release of oxytocin and dopamine that happens when children play. Full-body, kinesthetic involvement that allows for a competency surge to be experienced in the child's body is one way to mitigate the approach to trauma content. Joint attention to external, playful props while approaching hard material is a second form of titration. Pairing the naming of treatment targets and the targeting sequence with play and kinesthetic involvement is the goal of the TraumaPlay activity *Tell Me the Targets*. A dart board is one of the tools in a TraumaPlay-equipped playroom. When identifying targets for play-based gradual exposure and/or EMDR work, the therapist draws at least three rings of a dart board on a piece of paper while the child begins throwing darts at the dart board. With teens, we may allow for the sharply pointed "real deal" darts, but with smaller children, we use either rubber-tipped dart boards where the dart becomes embedded in a field of raised points or magnetic dart boards (see Figure 2.8).

The therapist and client take turns throwing darts as the therapist explains that each ring of the dart board is worth different numbers of points, with the bulls-eye in the middle yielding the most points. The therapist then invites the child to identify the top three hardest things for each of the three darts. We start with the least scary of the child's top three traumatic events (going with the resistance) and then move to the most scary. By the time children hit the bulls-eye, they are often feeling confident and having fun and find it not nearly as hard as they thought it was to verbalize for describing their scariest target. What follows is a transcript of this intervention with a very shut down client who needed to experience strength in his body in order to approach the trauma content. Johnny was an 8-year-old boy who had witnessed years of domestic violence between his parents. The violence ended one night in the death of both parents by murder/suicide. Johnny had been tight lipped about his experience not only because of ongoing police investigation but also because he had been trained, through years of watching his parents lie to the rest of the world about the violence happening in their home, and the direct threats he received that if he talked about what happened in their home he would be taken away or they would go to jail. He was

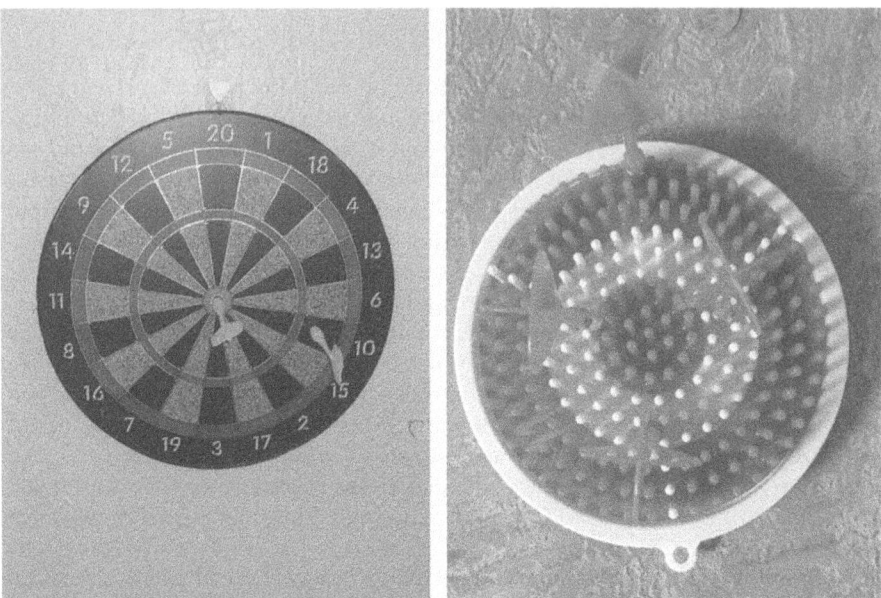

Figure 2.8 *Dart Boards for Tell Me the Targets Activity*

like a sealed vault, although the hurt was sealed inside as well. When I first introduced the dart board, Johnny's eyes lit up.

Johnny: *Can I try?*

Paris: *Yep, you get three and I get three.* (Johnny had shown me in previous sessions that he enjoyed challenge and competition, so this was more alluring to him if we could compete against each other. Fortunately, I am not very good at darts and Johnny ended up laughing at me pretty quickly.)

Johnny: *That's so fun!* (This was the first spontaneous acknowledgment of enjoyment that he had made so far in therapy.)

Paris: *Alright, you're clearly pretty skilled at this, so I'm gonna have you stand at least this far away,* (drawing an imaginary line on the floor. As we are both focused on the dart board, I say....) *What's one thing, one memory that you have that feels kind of bad but not the very worst?*

Johnny (looking down at the floor and then squinting at the dart board): *Uhhh . . . just kind of yelling.* He threw the dart really hard and hit an outer ring.

Paris: *Okay. Mom yelling, dad yelling . . .*

Johnny: *They were kind of yelling at each other. They would get in a fight and I would go upstairs.*

Paris: *Okay, so they would yell, fight, and you would go upstairs. Where should that go on your paper target.*

Johnny pointed to the outside ring.

Paris (while handing him another dart): *Okay. Now we are after something that was a little more scary than that.*

Johnny: *We saw like . . . we would come downstairs and see like a stain on the wall. Like, they had gotten in a fight and there would be, like, broken glass or something.*

Johnny threw the next dart and missed. He and I took a breath together, I gave him another dart, and he hit the second ring.

Paris (crouching down to add the words to his paper target): *Okay, like things on the wall . . . like stains.*

Johnny: *Well, just kind of like broken glass, like they'd gotten in a fight.*

Paris: *They'd gotten in a fight . . . and . . .*

Johnny (picking up a rubber mallet and hitting it on his arm . . . playing out physically the hurt, fear, and dysregulation this is bringing up): *Things would break, you know, accidentally.*

Paris (making direct eye contact for the first time since starting the intervention): *Accidentally.*

Johnny: *Well, you know, they would knock things over.*

Paris (shifting my gaze away, as eye contact itself could be overwhelming and kick him out of his window of tolerance, which for him would trigger hyperarousal and collapse, a complete "turtling" up. This pattern had been established in a previous session): *So just breaking things while they were angry.*

Johnny: *Yes.*

Paris: *And could you hear things breaking upstairs?*

Johnny (still holding the rubber mallet): *Yeah, it would be like crshhhhh . . .* (he made a crashing sound while moving the mallet aggressively). *Then in a whisper voice: I was like, what is happening?*

Paris: *Yeah, kind of double scary because you don't know but you hear something scary.*

Johnny: *Mmm-hmm.*

During this last exchange, Johnny had turned away from the dart board and began hitting the baby dolls with the mallet, first in the feet and then, one by one, he hit the baby dolls in their heads. I shifted focus with him, seeing this as both a self-titrated break from the verbal narrative. What is magical about play therapy is that the communication is continuing to happen in his posttraumatic play engagement. If we perceive the baby dolls as the self-object, he is acting out a situation in which the vulnerable little one is having his head aggressively assaulted. Children who are trying to figure out what to do, how to stay safe, and how to make sense of what they are hearing around them often indicate that their heads hurt from the intense toll that hypervigilance takes during those terrifying moments. Not only is this switch to posttraumatic play another form of expression, but it is also allowing for some cathartic release and self-regulation to occur as he interacts with the tools of TraumaPlay. I follow his need out of his verbalized memories and into his play.

> Paris: *You're smacking all those baby dolls with the wack-a-moler.*
>
> Johnny: *This one's the funniest to smack.*
>
> Paris: *Wonder what makes it the most fun.*
>
> Johnny (Taps it repeatedly with the mallet and the baby's head ricochets back and forth several times. Then he taps the next one, which doesn't move): *It's concrete.*
>
> Paris: *Those babies don't have a lot of protection from the smacking. They've got just kinda sit there and take it.*
>
> Johnny: *They don't. Well, they do by their parents but not by their immune system.*
>
> Paris: *Right. If their parents are protective.*
>
> Johnny (looks up, smiles, and puts the mallet down): *That was fun!* (He glances down at the target.)
>
> Paris: *Okay, we've got one more to do. So this is like, if you had to say what's the worst, the very worst memory that you have—if you took a picture.*
>
> Johnny: *When I woke up that night.* (Johnny gives more detail here then throws a dart and misses. Then he throws another dart and misses.) *Dang it, what is wrong? This is terrible.*
>
> Paris (while moving to pick up the darts): *Well, even talking about it can be a little upsetting—just to think about it long enough for us to talk about it. It might throw your body off a little bit, so take a deep breath—and you have lots of room to use them.*
>
> Johnny (taking a breath with me): *Yah!!*
>
> Paris: *There you go.*

When we had finished the paper dart board, I explained the following:

> Paris: *You get to choose. We can work on the scariest one first, or the least scariest one first. We can go in whatever order you want.*
>
> Johnny: *I choose to go from less intensity to the more intensity.*

Approaching the content at all was very hard for this young man. Pairing the hard work with the mitigating factor of full-body play helped him remain within his window of tolerance for distress. Aided by the play, Johnny won the neurochemical boxing match . . . well, at least this round.

Several other forms of directive targeting are used in TraumaPlay including personalized board game journeys that concretize moments of greatest distress and greatest joy (for later processing). We also keep two Poop Emojis—one that is brown and the other that is golden—and Poop Emoji notepads. Tweeners seem to be especially drawn to this way of identifying the most "crappy" things that have happened to them and the ones that have felt golden. Other forms of identifying targets, such as Beckley-Forest's *Bowl of Light* can also be employed (Beckley-Forest, Goodyear-Brown, & Monaco, 2018).

PARENTS AS PARTNERS

Enlisting parents as coregulators and storykeepers in their child's trauma work is one of the great joys of TraumaPlay therapists. In treatment, we begin educating parents almost immediately about the importance of their role as an external modem for their children. Helping parents shift their paradigms will lead to understanding a harshly stated "no" as a child's descends into a six-foot deep, clay-packed hole out of which there can be no exit until the adult, the Safe Boss involved, offers a way out. The adult makes the first shift, either coregulating, offering delight, or helping the child develop adaptive boundaries.

RELATIONAL RESOURCING

One integration of TraumaPlay and EMDR at Nurture House involves relational resourcing, which we define as enhancing the child's sense of being safely connected to others in the world. Many traumatized children have maladaptive patterns of relating, built on a control foundation versus a trust foundation. Enhancing attachments requires parents to be present in sessions. Sometimes, a traumatized child's caregivers are already a powerful resource for safety, and at other times, parents need some training in attunement, coregulation, or repair prior to being used in this role, but when caregivers are ready, they can quickly help establish new levels of safety or grounding for a child. I will give you a couple of examples. Timmy was a 4-year-old child brought by his parents for treatment after he disclosed that he had been molested by one of his Sunday School teachers. During the preparation phase of EMDR/enhancing safety and security phase of TraumaPlay, Timmy chose two safety symbols from the sand tray shelves and held one in each hand as he crawled up on his mother's lap. I asked mom if they had a special song they would like to sing together, and he immediately started belting out the lyrics, "God Is Bigger than the Boogeyman." This child had experienced his own boogeyman and found this tune comforting. We installed the experience of sitting on mom's lap, singing this song, and holding his safety symbols while I engaged in slow, short sets of BLS. When we began trauma reprocessing, he abruptly stopped at two different points during our work and began singing this song. The simple smell of a mother's hair, or the feel of her fuzzy sweater during a snuggle, or even the sound of her heart beating as he nestles his ear into her chest are all elements of felt safety that can be further installed through BLS. Using Theraplay games (Booth & Jernberg, 2009; Gomez, 2012; Jernberg & Booth, 2009) is one way to create in vivo delighting-in experiences that can be further enhanced with BLS and used to help develop adaptive cognitions as well, such as "I am delightful" and "I am loved." We also recognize parents as offering "parent-assisted cognitive interweaves" as needed during treatment. TraumaPlay therapists also recognize the importance of a child being able to access parental support in times of distress and need. TraumaPlay celebrates parents as the first and most influential modulators of their children's stress reactions (Goodyear-Brown, in press). Perry et al. confirm that "the presence of a healthy caretaker can diminish dramatically the alarm response or the dissociative response in the young child thus supporting the necessity of an available, healthy and responsive caretaker to provide nurture and support for a child after a distressing event" (Perry, Pollard, Blakley, Baker, & Vigilante, 1995, p. 285). Polyvagal theory also supports the powerful role played by parents in regulating children (Porges, 2011). Parent involvement is a crucial aspect of the TraumaPlay process and is augmented early in treatment to provide the scaffolding upon which further repair and healing can be made in the child's treatment process.

INCREASING EMOTIONAL LITERACY

Difficulty with emotion regulation is considered both an outcome of trauma and a predictor of psychopathology (Thornback & Muller, 2015). Traumatized children often have no words for their feelings or have summary words such as "fine" or "bad" or "upset." Helping clients turn inward, acknowledging somatically encoded feeling states, and eventually giving them voice are an important part of treatment. During the assessment phase of EMDR, clients are often asked to name the emotions they experience when they focus on a trauma target. During trauma narrative work in TraumaPlay, emotions are almost always woven into the story of the scary thing that happened. In both models, and certainly in an integration of the two, deepening the emotional granularity and expanding the feelings vocabulary of the client may be a necessary prerequisite to trauma reprocessing. One example of a TraumaPlay tool that expands emotional granularity is shown by the anger volcano. The child and therapist use the volcano metaphor for the way that unprocessed feelings get shoved down and pressurized until they blow; and when they do, the anger is often what is communicated. However, there are many other feelings, sometimes more difficult for our clients to embrace, that are gradations of anger. Figure 2.9 is an example of a fully processed anger explosion using the anger volcano.

Emotional states that are difficult to define are often initially communicated through art or other expressive mediums in the playroom. Oftentimes, children communicate core feeling states more powerfully through their art than through their words (Malchiodi, 2014; Malchiodi & Crenshaw, 2015). TraumaPlay therapists understand that children who have been traumatized need support identifying, articulating, and regulating their emotions (Goodyear-Brown, 2010a), foundational steps that enhance emotional literacy and communication skills. Increasing a child's emotional literacy skills can build a sense of control, competence, and empowerment in their own lives and in the world. Research done by Cicchetti and Rogosch found that "for all children striving to cope with adversity, a greater capacity to modulate the expression of negative emotions fostered resilience" (Cicchetti & Rogosch, 2009, p. 55), supporting the importance of building

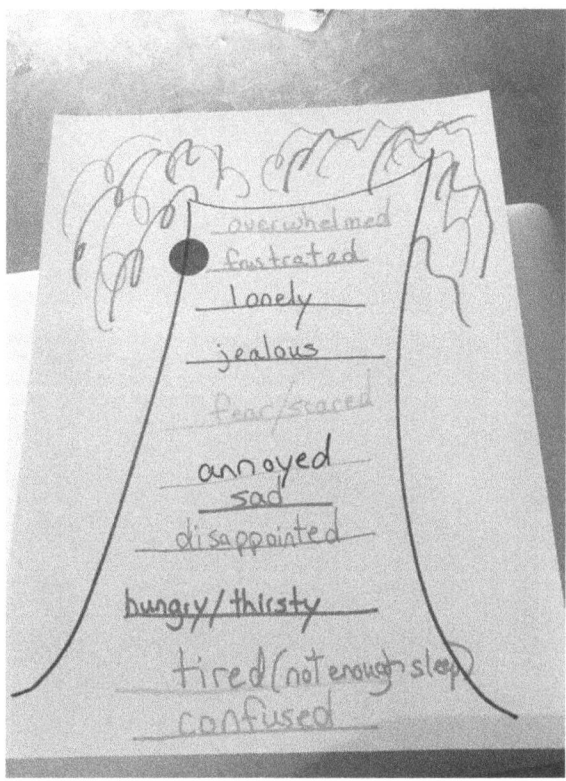

Figure 2.9 *The Anger Volcano Activity*

emotional literacy skills as a way of coping with life stressors. Further, internalizing problems has been found to be a correlate of maladaptive forms of emotional regulation, such as inhibition of anger and dysregulation of both anger and sadness, as well as adaptive forms of emotional regulation, such as constructive coping with anger (Zeman, Shipman, & Suveg, 2002). TraumaPlay therapists work toward building affect-regulation strategies and a healthy understanding of emotions to create a subset of coping skills that provide protection for clients as they are gradually exposed to the trauma content in future treatment (Goodyear-Brown, 2010a). We use interventions, such as Color Your Heart, Mood Music, All Tangled Up (Goodyear-Brown, 2002), and Sands of Time (Goodyear-Brown, 2010a), to help clients reflect on and quantify, nonverbally, the intensity of various emotions. We also have a three-dimensional dry-erase face that is often used when a child is unable to articulate an emotion but can draw it on this projective surface (see Figure 2.10).

These nonlinguistic explorations set the ground work for "naming it to tame it" (Siegel & Bryson, 2012) and beginning to identify the situations that may trigger these emotions and the resulting behavioral responses, both adaptive and maladaptive.

58   I. MODELS FOR INTEGRATION

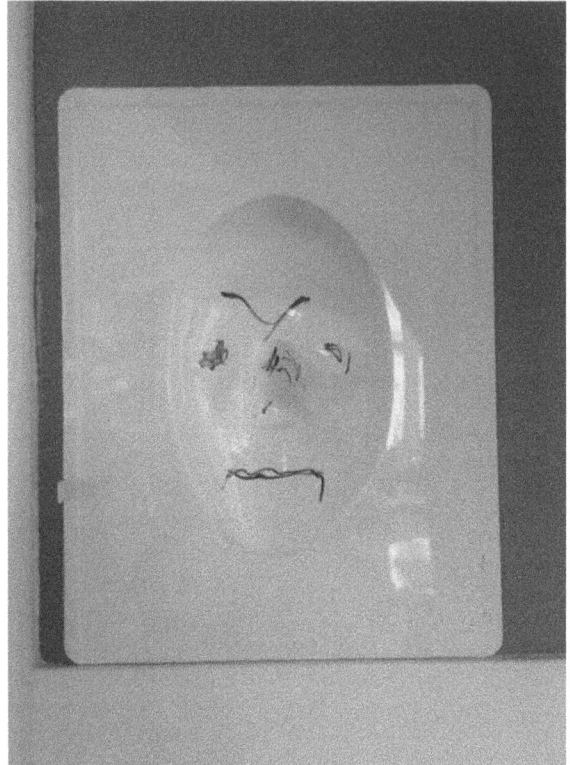

Figure 2.10 *The Dry Erase Face*

POSTTRAUMATIC PLAY AND PLAY-BASED GRADUAL EXPOSURE

Posttraumatic play is a play-based gradual exposure process that many children enter into naturally when given the correct tool. It can be moving, metaphoric, healing play or can be toxic, stuck play (Gil, 2017) for which children sometimes need invitations (Goodyear-Brown, 2010a, 2019b). Trauma-focused cognitive behavioral therapy (TF-CBT) offers children and their nonoffending caregivers a brief form of trauma treatment focused on addressing distorted or upsetting beliefs and attributions and providing them with learning skills to help them cope with ordinary life stressors. Gradual exposure is a core principle of the TF-CBT model (Cohen & Mannarino, 2008), a treatment modality that has been highly effective in treating children suffering from PTSD, anxiety, depression, externalizing and/or sexualized behaviors, and feelings of mistrust and shame as a result of traumatic life events (Weiner, Schneider, & Lyons, 2009). Each TF-CBT component includes graded exposure to the child's traumatic experience; the intensity of the exposure incrementally increases as the child and parent systematically move through the hierarchy.

TraumaPlay therapists use the gradual exposure process, supported by the natural curiosity children have for play, to create shifts in a child's immobilizing fears, distressing sensory impressions, and troublesome thoughts (Goodyear-Brown, 2010a) through their most natural language. The gradual leaching of toxicity from the content through play-based gradual exposure prepares the child for sequencing events and building a coherent trauma narrative. In many cases, children who are offered the magical environment of the playroom, the vocabulary of play tools, and the witness and felt safety of the therapist will move toward their own healing (Axline, 1969). For example, a 4-year-old boy named Billy, who has recently witnessed a moment of interpersonal violence, began playing out his desire to be free from this trauma memory by taking the toy brain and the plastic tweezers from the doctor's kit and repeatedly pretending to pluck out the "hurting thing" from the brain. In TraumaPlay, we refer to this as self-titration of the child's approach to the trauma content.

EXPERIENTIAL MASTERY PLAY

Experiential mastery play is considered a form of gradual exposure, a therapeutic process that captures a variety of ways in which children use the tools of childhood to work through their immobilizing fears while mitigating their approach to scary content with competency surge experiences (Goodyear-Brown, 2019b). Children will sometimes choose perpetrator symbols and act upon them in ways that increase their felt power. Common containments or manipulations of these symbols involve putting them in jails, burying them in the sand tray, dirtying them in some way, aggressing against the symbol in some way, putting it in handcuffs or otherwise confining it, and removing them altogether from the room (Goodyear-Brown, 2010a, 2019b).

In TraumaPlay, experiential mastery play also refers to the process by which children experience more strength, competency, or goodness in themselves and the process by which these competency surges mitigate the approach to trauma content. One of our favorite ways to do this at Nurture House is by introducing children to the magic carpet swing, a long, curved swing that glides. Children often begin by lying down on the swing and being pushed by the therapist or caregiver. As they gain courage, they may sit in the middle of it and use their core to help the swing move. Eventually, the natural competency drive (that has often been shut down due to trauma) is activated, and they attempt standing on the swing. At this point, we often get giant smiles and can almost feel the neurophysiological surge in their sense of competence and joy. They are thrilled that the caregiver (therapist or parent) has witnessed their achievement and sometimes even want to create a lasting representation of this moment.

TRAUMA NARRATIVE WORK

As seen in the picture (Figure 2.11), trauma content can be locked away, sealed tightly behind layers of self-protection. This play creation was the work of a child who had written down a trauma (that was a secret) and had immediately put it into the wooden closet and wrapped it in rubber bands vertically and horizontally.

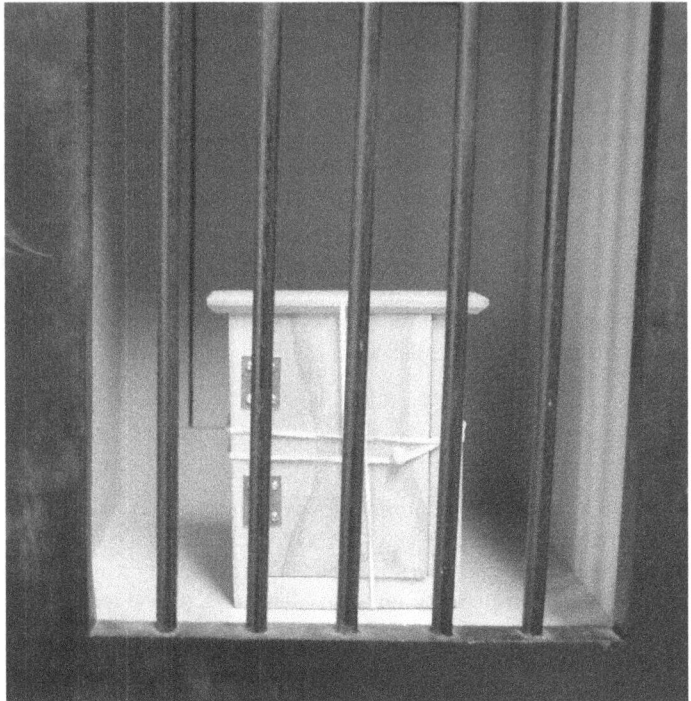

Figure 2.11 *Locking the Trauma Away*

She then looked for another layer of protection and ended up putting the tightly guarded closet inside this jail and locking it as well.

Getting through the protection and unlocking the healing may take more than one key, so pairing TraumaPlay and EMDR can maximize effectiveness. Part of the finesse of integrating TraumaPlay and EMDR involves bridging the space between posttraumatic play, which desensitizes and integrates dimensions of the trauma and EMDR reprocessing of specific thoughts, feelings, and bodily sensations related to the trauma. Play is often the language by which a child creates their trauma narrative in TraumaPlay, and then thoughts, feelings, and sensory impressions related to the trauma can be further reprocessed using EMDR. Abby, a 7-year-old girl was referred after her parents realized she had been sexually reactive with a neighbor boy who was a couple of years her junior. It became clear in the course of work that Abby had been sexually abused by an older neighbor boy a couple of years before. As we began to help Abby connect her reactive behavior with her earlier abuse, I (Paris) invited her to show me what had happened in the sand tray. She used animals instead of people to enact where the abuse happened and gave details related to a parent coming in and finding them. She moved to the dollhouse and spontaneously reenacted the moments in which she hid in the closet to try to hide from him. TraumaPlay pairs posttraumatic work with the healthy, fun medium of play. The desensitization work begins while the client is engaged in posttraumatic play. During the play, she identified the self-object as believing that she is bad. After she had worked through the story in play, during which BLS was added (as buzzies were in her shoes), I invited her to come and sit in the comfy chair, focus on different aspects of the abuse, and let the tapping do its work. She put a pillow on her lap with her hands on top of the pillow, and I began tapping the tops of her hands alternately.

> Paris: *Keep the picture of him putting his fingers inside you in your head, and that thought I am bad; when you think about those things, do you feel it in your body anywhere?*
>
> Addy: *My vagina hurts because he did that to me...*
>
> Paris: *Okay, your vagina hurt.*
>
> Addy: *And my, like, my head started to hurt 'cause I was trying to think, because he was... 'cause I was trying to... we were trying to get away from him but he wouldn't let us.*

Another case example (Eleah's) serves to further explore how this pairing works through a storytelling approach. Andrew was a 4-year-old boy who had witnessed a long season of emotional abuse from his father toward his mother in their home. Andrew was quick to describe his Dad as "happy or mad" all the time with various examples of when his Dad could go from being "hot or cold" without much notice. Clearly, the unpredictability of his Dad and his moods was causing Andrew distress and impacted his sense of emotional felt safety in his Dad's presence. Andrew was asked to write a story about his dad and decided to call his narrative "The Dad With Two Hearts." He began illustrating pictures immediately, and the story unfolded with words and pictures together (see Figure 2.12). The story read as follows:

> *Once upon a time there was a little Daddy who had two hearts, a mad heart and a happy heart. It started to rain and he got mad and had to go home. Then it became sunny and he was happy and played basketball. It started to rain again but he didn't go home. He jumped in the puddles instead.*

Through the lens of his simple story, a deeper understanding of the incongruency and instability that Andrew felt in his Dad's presence was gained. The EMDR and TraumaPlay protocol were used to begin the process of exploring his thoughts, feelings, and sensory impressions related to his experience of his Dad in the home with the hopes of bringing some resolution to the distress he was carrying inside. Eventually, his body relaxed and his affect lightened, evidencing a release of an intense amount of emotional turmoil that his little body had been holding. The competency surge of drawing pictures and writing a whole story "like a big boy" positively filled the internal places where the negative emotion had been discharged.

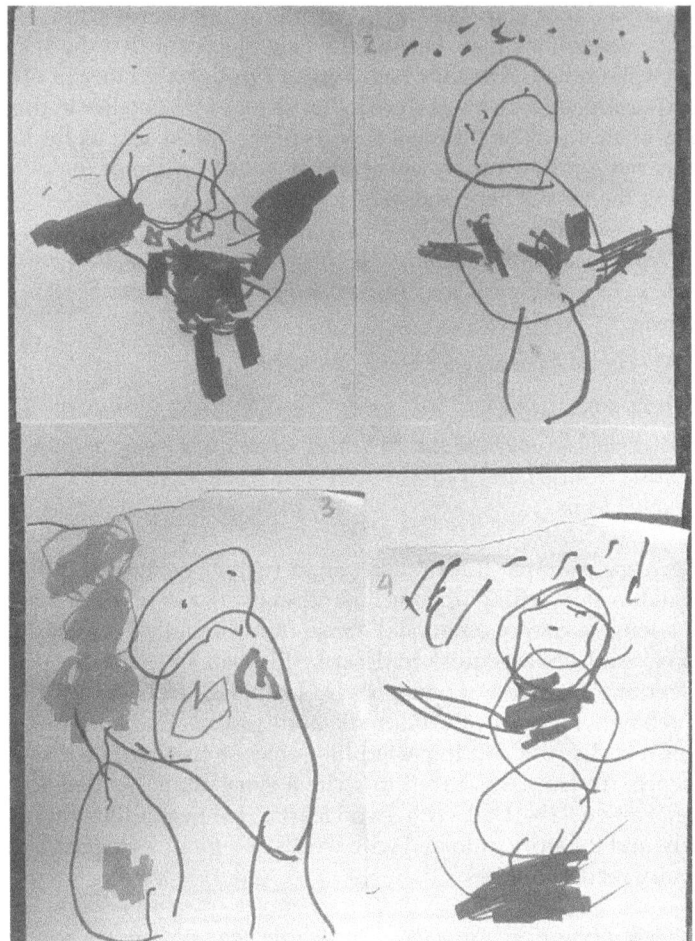

Figure 2.12 *The Story of "The Dad With Two Hearts"*

NURTURING NARRATION

While some children approach their trauma narrative work in a self-titrated way once they have built an attachment to the TraumaPlay therapist (which involves experiencing the therapist as witness, nurturer, and Safe Boss), other times children are so mired in the avoidance symptoms of PTSD that they would have great difficulty building coherence in their narrative without the help of another. One of the forms of play-based gradual exposure in TraumaPlay is directive trauma narrative work. We call this Nurturing Narration (Goodyear-Brown, 2019b) and find this to be easily integrated into EMDR work. Parents or the therapist has often pieced together previous glimpses and snapshots of the trauma, brought their own understanding of details that may not be known to the child, but that may help create a coherent narrative. In these cases, parents and the therapist work closely together to create a timeline and a developmentally sensitive "story of what happened" that may also be augmented with sensory details, articulated emotions, the cognitive distortions that resulted from the trauma, and more recent adaptive cognitions.

SCALING

The use of the SUD scales in EMDR is critical, and yet children may not resonate with simply naming or identifying a number. At Nurture House, we use many different scaling instruments in TraumaPlay, ranging from laminated 0 to 10 charts with feeling faces scaled, to Hoberman spheres in multiple sizes, to slinkies and staircases on which children can position an action figure. It is helpful to have several options available to children so that they can exercise choice and to ensure that a novel way of scaling is available if the child becomes bored with a previous method. In the section on Relational Resourcing, I shared an example of a mom and a child singing "God Is Bigger than the Boogeyman." Even though we had carefully installed and expanded the little boy's sense of safety, as soon as he began to focus on the trauma narrative that mom had written out and was telling, he began to become very dysregulated in his body. I acknowledged what his body was telling me, gave him the slinky, which we had been using as a scaling tool, and said, "Can you show me how big the fear is right now?" He hopped down off of mom's lap, looked relieved, asked mom to hold the one end of the slinky, and walked backward all the way across the room to the other wall—stretching the slinky as taut and long as it could be stretched. I thanked him for showing me, and we decided that we would chunk the scary things from this point forward. A variety of playful containers (Goodyear-Brown, 2010a) can be used when a child is needing to exert more physical control over the trauma content. Additionally, the play therapist and the design of the therapeutic space itself can offer bigness or smallness as we match a child's need for containment (Goodyear-Brown, 2019b).

Sometimes, the child offers us a metaphor that gives us a portal through which to create a developmentally sensitive scaling tool. Emily was a 6-year-old girl who had experienced a traumatic dog bite to her face when she was 3 years old. It required several surgeries and left her with a paralyzing fear of anything or anyone coming in contact with her face. Emily struggled with simple things like bath time and face washing, visits to the dentist, and so forth. This otherwise quiet and polite little girl, who always came dressed up in princess clothes, became full of anger and aggressive meltdowns upon approach to the dentist's office. When I (Eleah) first met Emily, she was very quiet and reflected some resistance to engaging with her story and the memory of the dog attack. She reported being very uncomfortable thinking about the scary thing. Knowing that EMDR would be an important tool in her healing process and being aware of her natural delight of art and the concept "princess," I invited her to draw a picture of a princess whom she believed to be very brave. Emily's face immediately lit up as she moved toward the art supplies and began drawing a picture of Rapunzel. We began exploring her understanding of Rapunzel and her story and what lead her to become so brave. Emily was able to identify some hard and scary things that

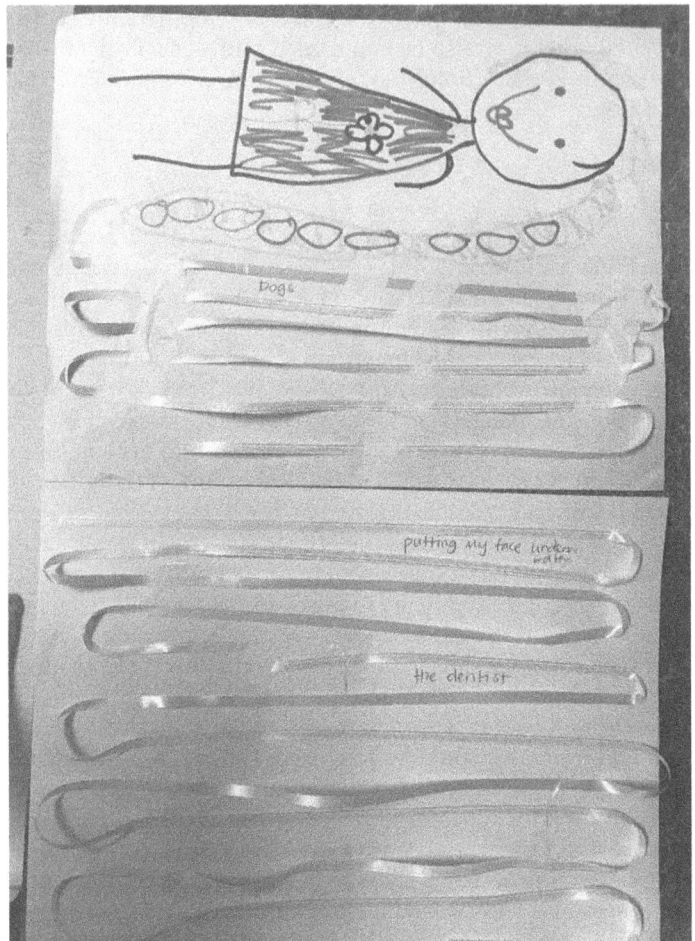

Figure 2.13 *Rapunzel's Hair Picture for Scaling Feelings*

had happened to Rapunzel and reflected much comfort in this titrated exposure to the idea of hard things and was soon able to verbalize some of her own hard things that were causing her so much upset. As she sat with the comforting image of her brave princess and the memory of hard things that had happened to her personally, Emily began to give me glimpses into her story and her emotional experience of it. As she worked with the metaphor and visual image of Rapunzel, we began using the concept of Rapunzel's "hair length" as a measuring tool for how distressing each memory felt to her. As Emily identified each traumatic memory, she took a yellow piece of string and showed me where on the string to cut in proportion to how big or small she felt that fear. After the completion of the activity, Emily was able to titrate her exposure to the difficult memories through the use of art and identify an EMDR processing sequence by reflecting an SUD for each as reflected in the scaling of various hair lengths and corresponding fears (see Figure 2.13).

ADDRESSING THE THOUGHT LIFE DURING REPROCESSING

Because children have had fewer experiences than adults and less complex memory networks, traumatic events can often be reprocessed in less time. I (Paris) had understood this theoretically but really learned it during my work with an 8-year-old boy named Eddie. He was referred for encopresis that had begun several months before the family sought help. They had tried positive reinforcement charts, habitual potty sits, and so forth. The behavior was very embarrassing to Eddie, who refused to talk with his parents about it. During the intake appointment, I asked lots of exploratory questions related to trauma but the parents seemed bewildered about how this behavior had been triggered. One of the tenets of TraumaPlay is that we bring the hard thing (often the reason for referral) into the room, particularly if there has been a taboo around the subject in the family. We do this because we believe the hard thing is already in the room and we feed it by ignoring it. If we tiptoe around it, we will be communicating that the subject is too big and scary to be held by the therapist. We also do not want the child spending any of his valuable psychic energy wondering if the therapist already knows or how the therapist might react if they do learn about the taboo thing. Within the first 10 minutes of Eddie exploring the playroom:

> Paris: *So, I know about you that you love to play baseball, you have a little sister named Sally, and that you are having poop accidents just lately.*
>
> Eddie (packing the kinetic sand into balls): *Yeah, it's kind of embarrassing.*
>
> Paris: *Yeah, I see lots of kids with poop accidents and they all say it's embarrassing.*
>
> Eddie (perking up at the idea that there are others with the same issue): *Yeah.*
>
> Paris: *Sometimes poop accidents start after something scary has happened.*
>
> Eddie (still packing sand spheres): *Well, for me it's because my colon is broken.*
>
> Paris (the parents had not mentioned this belief, so I needed a minute to absorb it): *It makes sense to me that if your colon is broken, it would be hard to control your poop. How did it break?*

He has given me the gift of his cognitive distortion. Whether it is true or not does not matter, it is the story—the blocking belief—that is creating this physical symptom. In order to be helpful, we need to first enter into the distortion and see his truth from his perspective.

> Eddie: *Well, it happened when we got in that car accident.*
>
> Paris: *Oh, your parents didn't mention a car accident. Can you tell me about it?*
>
> Eddie: *There was a truck and we were in a parking lot . . . it hit mom's side of the car, her window glass broke, and that's when my colon broke.*

Now that I understood this distortion as a target, Eddie and I went into the lobby and shared this info with mom. I explained how EMDR works using the brain that chews things up (remember Figure 2.3) and got her permission to begin right away. Eddie and I returned to the playroom, he called up a Safe Place image, and we installed it further with BLS (I just tapped alternately on his hands.) This helped acclimatize him to the methods while enhancing safety.

> Paris: *Can you draw me a picture of your broken colon?*
>
> Eddie got right to work and when he was finished, he had drawn what looked like a broken bone surrounded by muscles.
>
> Paris: *Okay. When you look at the picture and think "my colon is broken," where do you feel it in your body?*
>
> Eddie: *It's like a stabbing pain—right here* (and he gestured to his stomach).
>
> Paris: *And what feelings do you have when you think about it?*
>
> Eddie: *Scared.*
>
> Paris: *Okay. Can you keep the picture of your broken colon, that scared feeling, and the feeling of stabbing pain in mind while I tap your hands?*
>
> Eddie (closing his eyes and putting his hands on the pillow in his lap): *I see my broken colon.*
>
> Paris: *Go with that.*
>
> Eddie: *I see the muscles around my colon getting bigger.*
>
> Paris: *Go with that.*
>
> Eddie: *The muscles are popping my colon back into place!*
>
> Paris: *Go with that.*

We did a few more sets, after which he said his colon was still back in place and then we ended the session. I was skeptical as the whole process had only taken about 10 minutes, but next week mom called and said that they no longer needed to come in, because he had been pooping in the toilet ever since our appointment. I was sold on the power of EMDR and began to find it a powerful augmentation to the goal of helping shift the internal narrative that is an integral part of TraumaPlay.

Eddie's case example demonstrates an organic move in client's perceptions/beliefs about himself and his body using simply the EMDR framework. Many children have trouble identifying NCs and choosing or crafting PCs on their own. *The Thoughts Kit for Kids* (Gomez, 2008) is a useful aid in this work. As addressing the thought life is a key component of TraumaPlay, the model offers a host of play-based interventions that help children identify cognitive distortions, generate restructured cognitions, and then practice replacing one with the other. Games such as *Punching Holes in That Theory* and *Erase the Place* (Goodyear-Brown, 2005) can help clients physically dismantle the negative self-talk while practicing replacement thoughts. The *Why Wheel* helps clients deconstruct false attributions they may have about why the traumatic event happened (particularly thoughts involving self-blame) and *Thinking Caps* helps children practice quickly moving between thoughts and their resulting somatic states (Goodyear-Brown, 2005). The most popular game used during this phase of TraumaPlay is called *Lose the Bruise* (Goodyear-Brown, 2002). After a child has identified the NC and crafted a replacement thought, the therapist takes some small balls (our set has Emoji faces that are all bruised up) and asks the child to pretend that these are the NCs "coming at them." The child is given a sword and a shield and their job, after the therapist has spoken the negative thought out loud and thrown the ball, is to make sure the ball does not hit them while simultaneously verbalizing the restructured cognition. Boys and girls alike love this game as it allows for full-body kinesthetic involvement in the practice of empowering self-talk.

TITRATION AND THE DANCE TOWARD AND AWAY FROM TRAUMA CONTENT

Sometimes, children are all in, ready to reprocess the trauma, and build coherence in their life narrative. At other times, there are particular aspects of the trauma—it might be the somatic encoding or it might be the encoded visual images themselves—that are the most terrifying for the child and therefore the parts they most want to avoid. One way that we work with the approach to previously avoided images while integrating EMDR and TraumaPlay is to use a simple titration: tracing paper. Rodney was a 10-year-old boy who had witnessed his father's traumatic brain injury and then lived with dad through his recovery. When I (Paris) met Rodney, he was avoiding talking about or thinking about the way dad had looked, sounded, and so forth, but all that repression was making him sick and anxious. Rodney soon began recreating the scene of the accident in the sand tray. I asked dad to bring in pictures of himself in recovery, and Rodney and I agreed we would spend some time desensitizing him to these. They were all in a manila folder, and Rodney said, "I can't stand to look at them." I said, "It would be cool if we could look at them through a haze . . . like a fogged-up window first." Rodney thought about it and said, "Do you have any tracing paper?" I said, "Rodney, you're a genius!" I presented each picture to him underneath a sheet of tracing paper. He chose the two scariest images and decided to paint the most prominent details onto the paper. Rodney had the buzzies in his pockets the whole time, and we turned them on and off as needed. When he first identified the staples that had been put in dad's head through the paper, we spent time focusing on them with the BLS, as Rodney carefully painted each one with red paint through the paper. After we had finished this process of titrating his approach to the content, the visual memories of dad's head and face during his recovery were no longer bothersome to him (see Figure 2.14).

SOMATIC EXPERIENCING WITH TRAUMA TARGETS

Children are sometimes unable to articulate their somatic experiences verbally, particularly if the trauma has occurred prelinguistically. In TraumaPlay, we ask children to identify where emotions are activated in their bodies through the use of Band-Aids™, buttons, or felt symbols (such as a tornado). Some clients place Band-Aids on a self-portrait. Other clients prefer to use a chalk board outline of a person, a gingerbread cut-out figure, or even a baby doll. The doctored doll in Figure 2.15 was the creation of a child who had been physically restrained while being abused.

The Band-Aids on the arms and legs represent places where the restraints chafed at her skin. The three stickers around her midsection are indicators of the panic and fear she held in her abdomen. She has put the pacifier into the baby's

68   I. MODELS FOR INTEGRATION

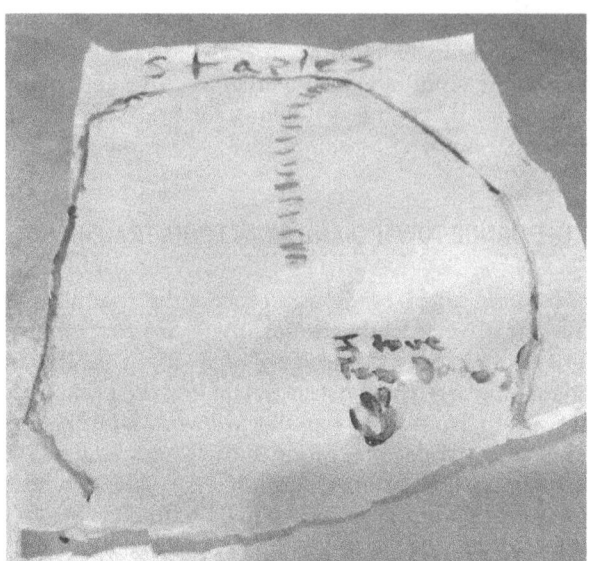

Figure 2.14 *Titrating the Trauma Content: Rodney's Trace Painting of Dad's Staples in His Head After the Accident*

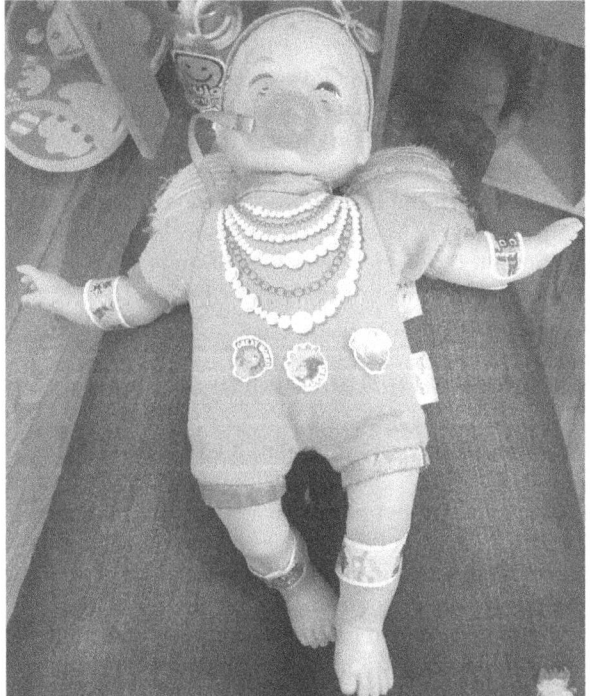

Figure 2.15 *The Doll Showing the Somatic Experiences*

mouth as she herself is beginning to experiencing soothing in those places of distressed remembrance. Starting with this concrete expression of somatic experiencing, we can incorporate BLS to move toward integration.

MAKING POSITIVE MEANING OF THE POSTTRAUMA SELF

When a crisis hits the life of a child, it can turn their world upside down, shatter their trust in what they believed to be true, and deeply change their sense of who they are. These natural responses to crisis can manifest as developmental delays in some areas while showing a profound depth of insight in others (Goodyear-Brown, 2010a), in addition to creating difficulties in learning, memory, and affect regulation. However, despite the many losses resulting from traumatic experiences, adversity can be used as an impetus for personal growth and wisdom. Research conducted by Tedeschi and Calhoun on the positive changes that individuals experience in their struggle with trauma are defined as "posttraumatic growth" (Tedeschi & Calhoun, 2004, p. 406). They describe posttraumatic growth as evidence of "improved relationships, new possibilities for one's life, a greater appreciation for life, a greater sense of personal strength, and spiritual development" (Tedeschi & Calhoun, 2004, p. 406). Their research supports the importance of using the therapeutic relationship as a vehicle for promoting growth and enhancing personal strength at a time of vulnerability. TraumaPlay therapists recognize that the relationship between the clinician, the client, and the play materials creates a unique environment for the emergence of posttraumatic growth. Many of the dysregulated children we see at Nurture House live the majority of their lives outside of their optimal arousal window. It can help to conceptualize these children as surrounded by static. Through the witness and coregulation of the TraumaPlay therapist and the vocabulary offered in the playroom, we will see moments of great clarity arise out of the chaos of their internal lives. One activity offered at this stage of TraumaPlay is called *Wisdom Feathers*. Years ago, I (Paris) created an intervention in which the child and parent are presented, during the termination phase, with a variety of feathers in different shapes and sizes. We craft a clay owl together and then plug in feathers, each one of us in turn verbalizing something that we have learned about ourselves, each other, or the process of growth over our time together. A new addition to my sand tray collection offers a new way to package this intervention. The painted owl (Figure 2.16) was a treasure found at the airport in Guangzhou, China. The owl tilts backward, opening so that a small message, the size of a fortune cookie message, can be enclosed. Lately, I have been taking just this symbol, placing it in the middle of the sand tray during the goodbye process, and having parent and child each write one message of wisdom to the other.

In a recent article in *Go With That*, EMDRIA's magazine (Goodyear-Brown, 2019a), I (Paris) describe a piece of work done by a young man and his mother in which they begin to bring coherence to the story of how mom first met him. Mom brought Johnny to treatment because his intense rage reactions were causing severe damage to his relationships. It became clear early on that he lacked a coherent narrative of his early trauma. I invited mom to set up a scene in the sand tray of the hospital room and describe in story form what had been happening medically with Johnny when she received the call that she could come and take him home.

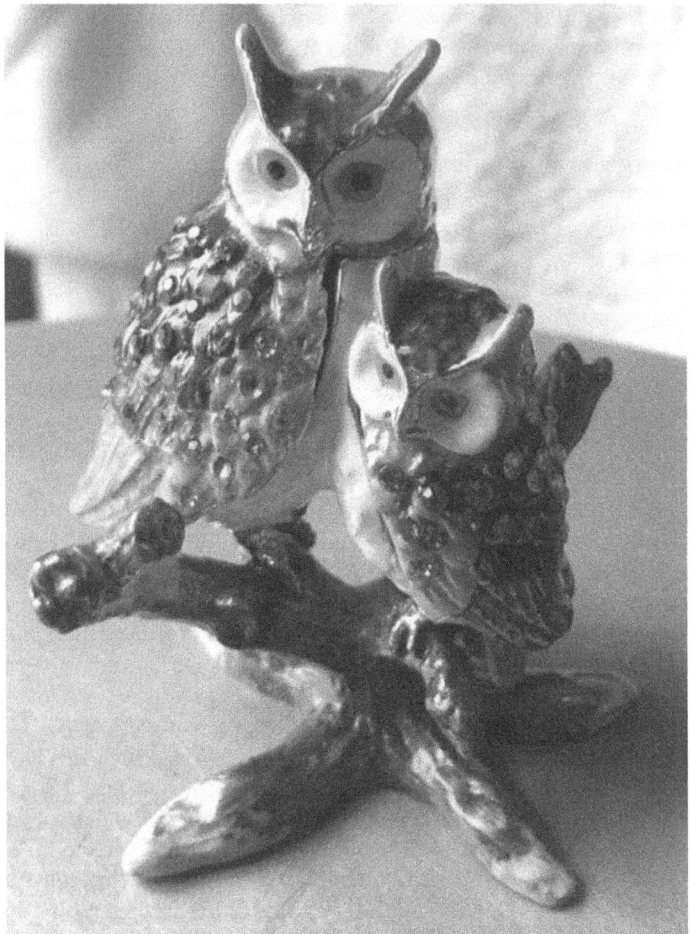

Figure 2.16 *Owl for Wisdom Feathers Closure Activity*

Johnny, who had been hiding behind an exercise ball while mom built the tray, became enamored of the story she was telling and began to bounce on the ball, inching closer and closer to the scene, eventually holding onto the sand tray for stability. The miniaturized elements enclosed within the boundaried space of the sand tray made it easier for Johnny to approach the material. Mom described (both verbally and concretely with symbols) a baby burning up with fever, surrounded by doctors, without a blanket. She described the potential somatic experience of the baby and her own desire to make him more comfortable. Mom enacted the mom figure in the tray picking up the baby off the bed, demanding more help for him, and running out of the hospital with him. Mom had also created a scene of dad at home preparing Johnny's crib, eagerly anticipating his arrival. I asked if there were any special things that the baby needed, and Johnny became involved in helping to find a baby blanket and a baby bottle to help take care of baby Johnny. Throughout all of this work, Johnny had the tappers in his socks for BLS, and I would turn them on and off at various parts of mom's story. Johnny had already begun enhancing

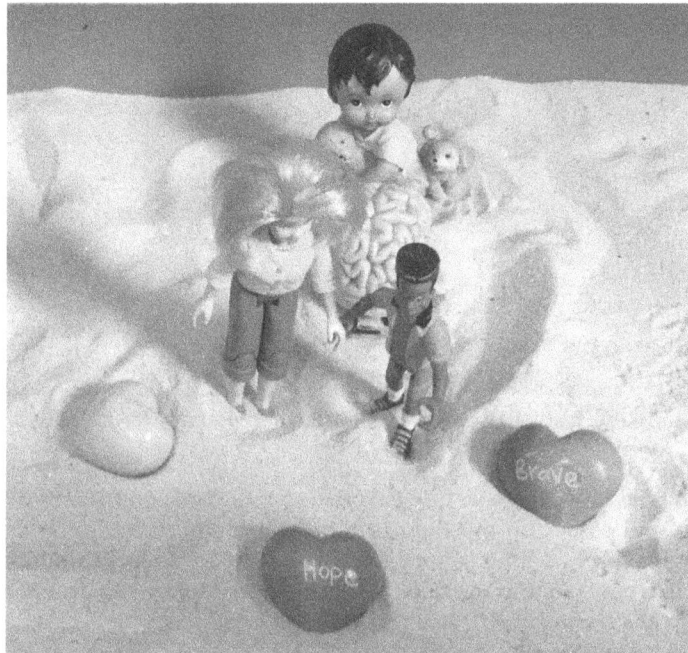

Figure 2.17 *Mom's Termination of Therapy Tray*

his neural nets surrounding enjoyable experiences with mom during earlier sessions, but this day marked a shift in his understanding of his story. After 10 to 12 minutes of reprocessing, Johnny was abruptly asked to build with blocks. This was new play for Johnny, as he had previously shied away from the blocks, believing they were too hard, that things would fall down, and that he would fail.

TraumaPlay recognizes new play patterns as potential growth or shift in internal working models. He started to build a wall of blocks and almost immediately asked mom to help him hold them up. Several months of treatment have elapsed since that article was written, and the family is in a happier, healthier place. We are in the process of saying goodbye and in TraumaPlay, some of our time spent *Making Positive Meaning of the Post-Trauma Self* is *Making a Meaningful Goodbye*. In this case, during our termination phase, I asked mom and Johnny to each create a sand tray that showed the growth/changes they could identify. The picture in Figure 2.17 is of mom's tray. She chose the same symbol for Johnny that she had put in her original sand tray—the little boy with the puppy and the teddy bear to represent Johnny when he started treatment. It cannot be seen in this image, but that figure is missing a foot and often communicates brokenness and delayed development. In her initial tray, mom had also placed a giant troll to represent her experience of Johnny when he would begin to rage. Here, she puts the walking brain in front of the baby and then has her self-symbol and a more developed, confident-looking boy holding hands. She has surrounded the dyad with three heart stones that read "peace," "hope," and "brave," respectively.

Johnny took a long time to do his sand tray . . . picking up multiple objects and putting them back down. Eventually, he picked up the bucket of remaining

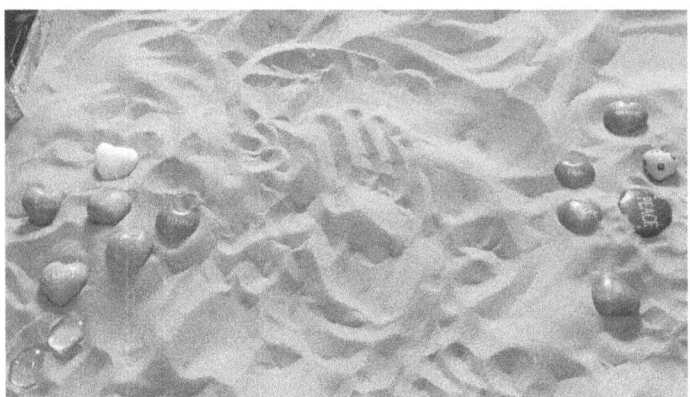

Figure 2.18 *Johnny's Termination of Therapy Tray*

heart stones and he put several hearts with hopeful words on the left to represent himself, several stones on the right to represent mom, including a large, black stone that says Peace and then after gazing at the tray for a few seconds, he quietly made his own handprint in the middle. When I asked Johnny to describe his tray, he said "I'm just a lot happier" (see Figure 2.18).

CONCLUSION

Effective trauma work with children requires clinicians to respect the dance toward and away from the trauma content, to enlist the aid of every possible mitigator of the approach to scary stuff, especially play, a deep understanding of the zone of proximal development (Vygotsky, 1967), and the power of the attachment relationships that are developed between therapist and members of the family system. TraumaPlay offers a path for this work to be accomplished through developmentally sensitive mediums while harnessing the therapeutic powers of play (Schaefer & Drewes, 2014). The AIP model that is so seminal to EMDR runs parallel to the foundational ideas in TraumaPlay work wherein we are laying down new neural wiring (positive neural networks) to aid in the leaching of toxicity out of traumatic memories, while resourcing the child both relationally and intrapersonally. As the field of trauma therapy continues to adapt, integrations of effective therapies will continue to evolve (Drewes, Bratton, & Schaefer, 2011). The integration of TraumaPlay and EMDR offers one such powerful integration.

REFERENCES

Axline, V. M. (1969). *Play therapy* (Vol. 125). New York, NY: Ballantine Books.

Baggerly, J. (2006). Preparing play therapists for disaster response: Principles and procedures. *International Journal of Play Therapy, 15*(2), 59–81. doi:10.1037/h0088915

Bartz, J. A., Zaki, J., Bolger, N., & Ochsner, K. N. (2011). Social effects of oxytocin in humans: Context and person matter. *Trends in Cognitive Sciences, 15*(7), 301–309. doi:10.1016/j.tics.2011.05.002

Baumgarten, B., & Otoshi, K. (2015). *Beautiful hands*. Novato, CA: Blue Dot Press.
Beckley-Forest, A., Goodyear-Brown, P., & Monaco, A. (2018, October). *EMDR and play therapy: A powerful combination* [Conference Session]. 23rd EMDR International Association Conference, Atlanta, GA.
Booth, P. B., & Jernberg, A. M. (2009). *Theraplay: Helping parents and children build better relationships through attachment-based play*. Somerset, NJ: Wiley.
Cicchetti, D., & Rogosch, F. A. (2001). Diverse patterns of neuroendocrine activity in maltreated children. *Development and Psychopathology, 13*, 677–694. doi:10.1017/s0954579401003145
Cicchetti, D., & Rogosch, F. A. (2009). Adaptive coping under conditions of extreme stress: Multilevel influences on the determinants of resilience in maltreated children. *New Directions for Child and Adolescent Development, 124*, 47–59. doi:10.1002/cd.242
Cohen, J. A., & Mannarino, A. P. (2008). Trauma-focused cognitive behavioural therapy for children and parents. *Child and Adolescent Mental Health, 13*(4), 158–162. doi:10.1111/j.1475-3588.2008.00502.x
Corrigan, F. M., & Hull, A. M. (2015). Recognition of the neurobiological insults imposed by complex trauma and the implications for psychotherapeutic interventions. *BJPsych Bulletin, 39*(2), 79–86. doi:10.1192/pb.bp.114.047134
Crenshaw, D. A., Kenney-Noziska, S., & Demanchick, S. P. (2014). Therapeutic presence in play therapy. *International Journal of Play Therapy, 23*(1), 31–43. doi:10.1037/a0035480
Drewes, A. A., Bratton, S. C., & Schaefer, C. E. (2011). *Integrative play therapy*. Hoboken, NJ: Wiley.
Duncan, B. L., & Moynihan, D. W. (1994). Applying outcome research: Intentional utilization of the client's frame of reference. *Psychotherapy: Theory, Research, Practice, Training, 31*(2), 294–301. doi:10.1037/h0090215
Garavan, H., Pendergrass, J. C., Ross, T. J., Stein, E. A., & Risinger, R. C. (2001). Amygdala response to both positively and negatively valenced stimuli. *NeuroReport: For Rapid Communication of Neuroscience Research, 12*(12), 2779–2783. doi:10.1097/00001756-200108280-00036
Geller, S. M., & Greenberg, L. S. (2002). Therapeutic presence: Therapists experience of presence in the psychotherapeutic encounter. *Person Centered and Experiential Psychotherapies, 1*, 71–86. doi:10.1080/14779757.2002.9688279
Gil, E. (2017). *Posttraumatic play in children: What clinicians need to know*. New York, NY: Guilford Press.
Gomez, A. M. (2008). *The thoughts kit for kids*. Board Game. Retrieved from https://www.anagomez.org/product/the-thoughts-kit-for-kids/
Gomez, A. M. (2012). *EMDR therapy and adjunct approaches with children: Complex trauma, attachment, and dissociation*. New York, NY: Springer Publishing Company.
Goodyear-Brown, P. (2002). *Digging for buried treasure: 52 prop-based play therapy interventions for treating the problems of childhood*. Franklin, TN: Self-published by Author. Retrieved from https://www.parisgoodyearbrown.com/all-products/digging-for-buried-treasure
Goodyear-Brown, P. (2005). *Digging for buried treasure 2: 52 more prop-based play therapy interventions for treating the problems of childhood*. Franklin, TN: Self-published by Author. Retrieved from https://www.parisgoodyearbrown.com/all-products/digging-for-buried-treasure-2
Goodyear-Brown, P. (2010a). *Play therapy with traumatized children: A prescriptive approach*. Hoboken, NJ: Wiley.
Goodyear-Brown, P. (2010b). *The worry wars: An anxiety workbook for kids and their helpful adults*. Franklin, TN: Self-published by Author. Retrieved from https://www.parisgoodyearbrown.com/all-products/the-worry-wars-an-anxiety-workbooks-for-kids-and-their-helpful-adults
Goodyear-Brown, P. (2019a, March). Parents as partners: Enhancing co-regulation and coherence though an integration of play therapy and EMDR. *Go With That EMDRIA*

Magazine, 28–33. Retrieved from https://issuu.com/emdriagwt/docs/emdria_march_2019_magazine__3_

Goodyear-Brown, P. (2019b). *Trauma and play therapy: helping children heal*. New York, NY: Routledge.

Goodyear-Brown, P. (in press). *Parents as partners in child therapy: A clinician's guide*. New York, NY: Guilford Press.

Jernberg, A. M., & Booth, P. B. (1999). *Theraplay: Helping parents and children build better relationships through attachment-based play*. San Francisco, CA: Jossey-Bass.

Jernberg, A. M., & Booth, P. B. (2009). *Theraplay: Helping parents and children build better relationships through attachment-based play* (3rd ed.). San Francisco, CA: Jossey-Bass.

Karst, P. (2000). *The invisible string*. Camarillo, CA: DeVorss & Company.

Malchiodi, C. (2014). *Breaking the silence: Art therapy with children from violent homes*. New York, NY: Routledge.

Malchiodi, C. A., & Crenshaw, D. A. (Eds.). (2015). *Creative arts and play therapy for attachment problems*. New York, NY: Guilford Press.

Perry, B. D., Pollard, R. A., Blakley, T. L., Baker, W. L., & Vigilante, D. (1995). Childhood trauma, the neurobiology of adaptation, and "use-dependent" development of the brain: How "states" become "traits." *Infant Maternal Health Journal, 16*(4), 271–291.

Porges, S. W. (2011). *The polyvagal theory: Neurophysiological foundations of emotions, attachment, communication and self-regulation*. New York, NY: W. W. Norton.

Sahar, T., Shalev, A. Y., & Porges, S. W. (2001). Vagal modulation of responses to mental challenge in posttraumatic stress disorder. *Society of Biological Psychiatry, 49*, 637–643. doi:10.1016/s0006-3223(00)01045-3

Schaefer, C. E., & Drewes, A. A. (2014). *The therapeutic powers of play: 20 core agents of change*. Hoboken, NJ: Wiley.

Schultz, W. (2016). Child-centered play therapy. *Reason Papers, 38*(1), 21–37.

Shapiro, F. (2017). *Eye movement desensitization and reprocessing: Basic principles, protocols and procedures* (3rd ed.). New York, NY: Guilford Press.

Shapiro, F., & Laliotis, D. (2011). EMDR and the adaptive information processing model: Integrative treatment and case conceptualization. *Clinical Social Work Journal, 39*(2), 191–200. doi:10.1007/s10615-010-0300-7

Siegel, D. J., & Bryson, T. P. (2012). *The whole-brain child: 12 revolutionary strategies to nurture your child's developing mind*. New York, NY: Bantam.

Stewart, A. L., Field, T. A., & Echterling, L. G. (2016). Neuroscience and the magic of play therapy. *International Journal of Play Therapy, 25*(1), 4–13. doi:10.1037/pla0000016

Tedeschi, R. G., & Calhoun, L. G. (2004). A clinical approach to posttraumatic growth. In P. A. Linley & S. Joseph (Eds.), *Positive psychology in practice* (pp. 405–419). Hoboken, NJ: Wiley.

Thornback, K., & Muller, R. T. (2015). Relationships among emotion regulation and symptoms during trauma-focused CBT for school-aged children. *Child Abuse & Neglect, 50*, 182–192. doi:10.1016/j.chiabu.2015.09.011

University of California Davis PCIT Training Center. (2013). *Dyadic Parent Child Interaction Coding System for traumatized children*. Retrieved from https://pcit.ucdavis.edu/wp-content/uploads/2019/10/104_DPICS-Manual.2.18.pdf

Vygotsky, L. S. (1967). Play and its role in the mental development of the child. *Soviet Psychology, 5*(3), 6–18. doi:10.2753/RPO1061-040505036

Weiner, D. A., Schneider, A., & Lyons, J. S. (2009). Evidence-based treatments for trauma among culturally diverse foster care youth: Treatment retention and outcomes. *Children and Youth Services Review, 31*(11), 1199–1205. doi:10.1016/j.childyouth.2009.08.013

Zeman, J., Shipman, K., & Suveg C. (2002). Anger and sadness regulation: Predictions to internalizing and externalizing symptoms in children. *Journal of Clinical Child and Adolescent Psychology, 31*(3), 393–398. doi:10.1207/S15374424JCCP3103_11

3

Room for Everyone: EMDR and Family-Based Play Therapy in the Sand Tray

MARSHALL LYLES

The tree gives because its nature is to nurture.
The tree protects because it is built for strength.
The tree shades because it understands rest.
Each day I borrow from the tree.
And together we offer you a nest.
—Marshall Lyles

INTRODUCTION

In the three decades since Francine Shapiro introduced the model, adaptive information processing (AIP) and eye movement desensitization and reprocessing (EMDR) have provided mental health clinicians with a method for conceptualizing clients' responses to traumas as adaptive and protective without diminishing the pain that comes from holding stored trauma. For those working with child clients, the goal of healing emotional and relational wounds becomes substantially more attainable when caregivers also come to view children's trauma responses as adaptive and protective, all the while developing increasing capacity for being with their children's woundedness. EMDR therapists who provide family-based play therapy need ways to establish and monitor safety within family systems in order for the integration of these modalities to offer their full power. This chapter aims to offer sandtray as a modality that allows for this integration.

ADAPTIVE INFORMATION PROCESSING IN A FAMILY/PLAY THERAPY CONTEXT

AIP emphasizes that memory presents as a core element in EMDR treatment (Gomez, 2013) and that traumatic memories can transform into resiliency when following EMDR's phased treatment plan (Shapiro, 2007). When working with children in a family therapy context, clinicians have the opportunity to support the creation of new memories, to reinforce past security-generating memories, and to support healing from painful memories. This occurs within the reality that multiple members of a family system may have different perceptions of the memory, different symptoms related to the traumatic memory networks, and different capacities for the healing from the effects of trauma.

The phases of an AIP-informed treatment plan emphasize the need to begin treatment with relationship-building, thorough history-taking, and installation of resources (Shapiro, 2007). Only after these have been established does an EMDR clinician assist a client in addressing their unprocessed, trauma memory networks (Shapiro, Kaslow, & Maxfield, 2007). With this sequencing, clients are more able to remain grounded in the present when healing past memories and anticipating future successes around potentially activating material. EMDR therapists are taught this standardized approach by approved trainers who provide instruction, practice, and consultation to trainees (Adler-Tapia & Settle, 2008).

There is some research support for the use of EMDR to treat children's traumatic stress symptoms (Beer, 2018; Swinden, 2018). EMDR clinicians who work with children often attend advanced training opportunities after completing all basic training requirements (Adler-Tapia & Settle, 2008). While some EMDR basic trainers include developmentally appropriate strategies for bringing EMDR to minors, there are many higher-level concepts and skills still to be learned and practiced so that this traditionally verbal modality can be utilized through play-based and expressive means. As a result, EMDR child therapists have often accrued many hours of education and consultation in order to ethically practice their craft. For those who treat children in a family context, this presses the need for even further development of skills.

Having caregivers involved in the therapeutic work incorporates the emerging, but still fragile, healing self of the child into the family context (Bardin, Comet, & Porten, 2007; Wesselmann, Schweitzer, & Armstrong, 2014). While the overwhelming majority of caregivers desire for their children to heal, not all can tolerate the shifts that healing can bring to a system. More involvement in the therapeutic process can provide scaffolding to update templates regarding needs, roles, and expectations. Without this, caregivers may sabotage the treatment process, often without conscious intention to do so because they may not yet comprehend what the healing process entails (Wesselmann, 2007). Additionally, meta-analytic reviews in the field of child psychotherapy have shown that play-therapy interventions have an overall large treatment effect size, and that involving parents can increase the effectiveness of play therapy (Lin & Bratton, 2015). In short, treating a child's trauma in a systemic manner allows for more comprehensive healing and restoration in all members of the system.

Historically, family therapy and play therapy had a common starting point, but they quickly developed differing areas of focus (Gil, 2015). Family therapy examines the system(s) of the family unit, while largely ignoring the specific needs of children. Play therapy tends to overlook systemic dynamics as the needs of children became the point of intervention. This occurs despite evidence that families seeking mental health treatment desire more comprehensive service (Cornett, 2012). There are notable exceptions to both of these dynamics, with filial therapy serving as one such example (Guerney, 1964).

One of the most steadfast and eloquent advocates of treating children's traumas in a family play context is Eliana Gil. Gil (2015) proposes that combining play therapy and family therapy magnifies the goal-meeting potential of each. Because members of a family system are constantly influencing one another, engaging in family play therapy allows this dynamic to pool resources and healing energy and not just reinforce painful patterns sometimes exaggerated by trauma. Families find their way to innovation and novelty when the power of play rises to meet the force of trauma.

As stated previously, play-therapy research suggests that involving caregivers in children's mental health treatment improves outcomes. Also, trauma-informed care, in general, often insists on impacting both children and the systems to which they belong while addressing vulnerabilities and traumas (Cutuli, Alderfer, & Marsac, 2019). Play in family therapy needs to prioritize creating experiences that are playful enough for children to feel safe while they are communicating, nonverbally and sometimes verbally, about stored aspects of previously painful experiences. "Play is a core element of attachment because it provides ample opportunities for the attunement that is necessary in developing emotional regulation and the anticipation of positive relationships" (Kestly, 2014, p. 96). When children feel safe, regulated, and connected, they can anticipate joy, which interrupts the trauma-induced tendency of vigilantly waiting for the next moment of pain and struggle. For example, when a child has experienced a traumatic loss, they are living with the pain of the loss each moment but may struggle to make sense of the experience when continually noticing the weight of grief and dysregulation of a caregiver's own pain. Bringing playful experiences to this dyad allows for coregulation and safety to return without diminishing the opportunity for introducing trauma-resolving themes into the play. Children take cues from caregivers when assigning meaning to traumatic experiences. EMDR therapists are better prepared to attend to children's healing when they carefully consider ways to involve caregivers into treatment (Bardin et al., 2007).

Play in family therapy also needs to provide opportunity for parents to understand what is occurring in play (Edwards, Sullivan, Meany-Walen, & Kantor, 2010; Higgins-Klein, 2013). When children are attempting to integrate painful memories into the rest of their system, they need to be in the presence of a loving and attuned other (Fosha as cited in Van der Kolk, 2015), which requires caregivers to be able to hold the pain; they then begin to understand and tolerate the ambiguity that comes with not yet understanding. Kestly (2014) references Panksepp and Biven as she points out that parents and children "share a joint system" at the neurobiological play level. As a result of this, caregivers and therapists need to be able to understand the processes of the children they are experiencing while staying playfully engaged (and without moving toward interpretation or agenda; Badenoch, 2008). Also, caregivers need to be able to recognize relational ruptures that will inevitably occur during the treatment process, so that repair can be prioritized. The EMDR therapist can take advantage of parent consultations to help caregivers stay grounded, moving toward increasing tolerance of the many ambiguous moments in play-based healing.

> By engaging in play together, not only can the child develop deeper meaning, understanding, and insight, but the parent is able to take a

walk in their child's shoes and see the world from their perspective. This offers a chance to the parent and child to develop stronger skills in attunement, compassion, and attachment. (Mellenthin, 2019, p. 169)

The *family play EMDR therapist* accepts responsibility that comes with a system, not just an individual being the client. While this approach can multiply complexities, it can also magnify healing potential and establish shared resilience for managing future stresses. Later sections of this chapter systematically address the involvement of caregivers in children's trauma healing throughout each of the EMDR phases, using sandtray therapy as the intergenerational play-based communication tool.

SANDTRAY AS THE MODALITY

Sandtray is one expressive modality for bringing EMDR to family therapy. Sandtray provides a play-based tool that transcends age and, as a result, can be used during child sessions, parent consultations, and family play therapy. The consistency of focusing on this one tool may help all members of the system to internalize a felt sense of comfort and mastery while offering all a common "language" by which to communicate. When caregivers can be fully present with their children's developmental need to communicate through play, all members of the system can fully engage in the sandtray while still working through trauma. Sandtray can offer an empowering method for supporting clients' integration of their emerging material through the stages of EMDR therapy (Gomez, 2013). With that being said, using sand tray with children at a developmental age of 6 and younger (to age 3) may be more akin to a traditional play session as young children tend to play dynamically rather than creating a static scene for processing (Homeyer & Sweeney, 2017). Some theorists believe that creations of scenes in the sand offer the therapist more information about a client's internal world than other play-based modalities (Norton & Norton, 1997). For the purposes set forth in this chapter, the family play techniques integrating sandtray and EMDR focus on slightly older children and adolescents, who are often more capable of traditional sandtray therapy processing.

"Sandtray therapy is an expressive and projective mode of psychotherapy of involving the unfolding and processing of intra- and inter-personal issues through the use of specific sandtray materials as a nonverbal medium of communication" (Homeyer & Sweeney, 2017, p. 5). Margaret Lowenfeld brought sandtray therapy into the mental health landscape through creation of the World Technique (Lowenfeld, 1999). This technique makes use of trays of sand and small figurines, often called miniatures. Clients are invited to create worlds in the sand, and then trained therapists assist clients in the processing of the completed sand worlds.

Lowenfeld (1999) was attempting "to find a medium which would in itself be instantly attractive to children and which would give them and the observer a language, as it were, through which communication could be established" (p. 281) so that children "would find their way to communication of their interior experience" (p. 281). Having witnessed children in the throes of trauma, Lowenfeld sought to find a tool that allowed children to communicate in their native language of play while feeling contained and understood. She wanted this tool to be separate from any specific clinical theory so that any trained clinician could participate in meaning-making with the client.

Sandtray therapy has not been universally standardized, but practicing therapists are served by access to quality training and being deliberate about organizing their thoughts on best practices and processes congruent with the clinician's theory of choice. One set of sandtray session-organizing principles was put forth by Homeyer and Sweeney. According to Homeyer and Sweeney (2017), the sandtray session process includes six distinct steps, each executed to be congruent with the therapist's clinical theory:

1. Preparation of the sandtray setting
2. Introduction of the process to the client
3. Creation of the sandtray
4. Postcreation phase
5. Sand tray cleanup
6. Documentation of the session

The following sections speak briefly of some pertinent concepts belonging to each step. However, if a clinician desires mastery of skills related to the use of sandtray therapy, further training in sandtray materials, processing, and theory integration would be beneficial. Furthermore, due to the expressive and projective potential with this modality, particularly when paired with EMDR, seeking consultation in addition to training would be prudent.

STEP 1: PREPARATION OF THE SANDTRAY SETTING

"The tools of the sandtray therapist are simple: *sand and water*, which are basic elements of the Earth; a *tray*, in which to contain the work; and a *collection of miniatures*, which serve as a universe of symbols and images" (Homeyer & Sweeney, 2013, p. 162). These simple tools can become powerful when treated with respect and understanding. This process begins before a client even enters the therapy room.

As a material-heavy modality, sand therapy practitioners bear the responsibility of maintaining these tools in an orderly and inviting manner. Returning the space to its predictable form and settling the person-of-the-therapist (De Little, 2019) make up the preparation step. The sand tray itself, typically a rectangle large enough for exploring complex worlds while still being able to be viewed in a glance, needs to be easily accessible to all clients (Homeyer & Sweeney, 2017). Other shapes of trays, such as circles and hexagons or octagons, are available choices for the sandtray therapist to have as options. These choices are made with awareness that it can be useful to have one "dry" tray and one "wet" tray as water presents its own healing potential in sandtray work (Homeyer & Sweeney, 2017).

All of these elements serve clients best when they exist in the same location from session to session. This facilitates easier decision-making and allows clients to focus on their inner worlds (not on looking for materials).

Sand (and water) presents sensory elements that aid clients in staying connected to and being aware of their bodies (Lowenfeld, 1991). In addition to its kinesthetic appeal, encountering sand in an indoor setting can be experienced as novel and inviting to children (Oaklander, 1988). As part of the preparation step in the sandtray therapy process, the therapist smoothes the sand, checking for leftover artifacts, and refreshes the water supply, which can be controlled, if needed, by having a limited amount of water in a spray bottle.

The remaining materials are the sand tray figures or miniatures. These serve as symbols, even when used more concretely, as children select and arrange them in the tray of sand to create scenes (often called worlds). Some sand practitioners have no set rules about miniature selection for their offices other than having a properly diverse collection (Rae, 2013). Other sandtray therapists select and arrange miniatures according to categories: people, animals, vegetation, buildings, vehicles, fences and signs, natural items, fantasy, spiritual/mystical, landscaping, and household (Homeyer & Sweeney, 2017). As miniatures represent the words clients will use to express their inner worlds (Rae, 2013), these figures need to be plentiful enough to facilitate a strong voice, but not so many that the selection overwhelms the voice. Also, the miniatures need to be placed in their typical locations before clients enter the therapy room.

STEP 2: INTRODUCTION OF THE PROCESS TO THE CLIENT

The second step, when the process is introduced to the client, features the delivery of the *prompt*. The prompt provides the concept to which clients will respond when choosing miniatures and creating a scene in the sand (Homeyer & Sweeney, 2017). Prompts can range from nondirective ("create a world in the sand") to any of a multitude of directive options (Day & Day, 2012; Garrett, 2014). Choosing a prompt requires holding in mind the client's developmental abilities, the therapist's clinical point of view, and the client's current stage in the treatment plan. Prompts are delivered clearly and succinctly so as not to confuse the client's creation stage. As the choice of prompts is shaped by clinical theory, this chapter discusses potential prompts relevant to the different phases of the EMDR treatment plan. Examples for the wording of prompts are provided with each EMDR phase.

STEP 3: CREATION OF THE SANDTRAY

Being with a client who is creating a world in the sand tray requires attention to both process and product (Homeyer & Sweeney, 2013). The creation step embraces a quieter and more contemplative stance (Armstrong, 2008) than traditional play therapy as space is given for the client to make contact with the self and find their way to expression. Even in (and perhaps especially in) the quiet, the sandtray therapist stays attuned and connected to the client (Armstrong, 2008; Homeyer & Sweeney, 2017; Rae, 2013). Clients will need this felt connection as they make contact with symbols and allow the awakening of deep right brain processing (Badenoch, 2008). The creation phase can be grounding, cathartic, or even flooding, so careful attention must be given to the creator and not just the creation so as to facilitate a gentle transition to the next step.

STEP 4: POSTCREATION

Step four in the sandtray process highlights how a sandtray therapist engages a client after the sandtray world has been created. In general, Homeyer and Sweeney (2017) recommend moving a client from global awareness of the sand scene to discussion about specific elements in the finished world. Sandtray therapists may begin the processing by asking for a general emotion or a title for the world. Then, as the client views and discusses the scene, the therapist helps to enlarge awareness and explore meaning of the various metaphors, while not taking away the safety and distance the metaphor allows before the client is ready (if the client ever needs to move beyond the symbolic). As mentioned previously, therapists need adequate training and supervision in sandtray therapy in order to appropriately handle the sacred aspects of the process.

Lowenfeld poetically reflects that "the subjective experience therefore of an individual making a World is of meeting a slice of reality; almost as if meeting oneself in a mirror" (Lowenfeld, 1999, p. 270). Sandtray therapists who wish to work with children on their traumas must keep in mind the intensity of looking at these moments in such a mirror during the postcreation step. When handled with care, work in the sand tray "has the effect . . . of enlarging the boundaries of one's comprehension of self, and in patients of giving them a tool of expression which can present . . . aspects and subtleties of feeling and thought which both speech and gesture fail to present" (Lowenfeld, 1999, p. 270).

As trauma can often be stored in memory networks that have not yet connected to speech (Van der Kolk, 1998), sandtray therapy offers a healing advantage as speech is not the primary tool for expression. Even during the postcreation (or processing step), the client says as little or as much as they need (or are capable of) in order to feel seen and understood. Armstrong (2008) discusses that clients can shift awareness back-and-forth from the tray during the processing step as they move toward "exploration, expression, awareness, and discovery" (p. 67).

While there is need for more empirical support for the notion, the aforementioned aspects of sandtray therapy's postcreation processing seem congruent with trauma-sensitive concepts. Wheeler and Dillman Taylor (2016) have written on how play therapy impacts the domains of interpersonal neurobiology integration (see Table 3.1). Noticing the column that highlights the play-therapy skills and techniques, sandtray therapy holds many, if not all, of the same components as general play therapy. This becomes particularly salient as one considers the impact of continued integration practice and embracing an unfolding narrative meaning-making process on the healing of a traumatized mind (Badenoch, 2008). Gaining mastery over previously nonintegrated memories, through neural integration and

Table 3.1 *Interpersonal Neurobiology Domains of Integration and Play-Therapy Approaches*

Domains of Integration	Domain Summary	Play Therapy Skill/Technique
Consciousness	Awareness of the here-and-now and mindful acceptance of experiences in the moment	Playroom design Therapeutic relationship Activity or reflection to engage all senses Brain in the palm of your hand model
Bilateral	Connection between the left and right hemispheres	Connect to redirect "Be with" attitude Reflection of feeling Name it to tame it
Vertical (integrating upstairs and downstairs brain)	Connection between "top" and "bottom" regions of the brain (residing throughout the body) that allows for receptivity of internal experiences and higher-order thinking	Engage, do not enrage Rule of thumb: Say it in 10 words Reflection of feelings Encouragement Limit setting Use it or lose it
Memory	Differentiation between implicit and explicit memories that allows the past to be experienced as the past	Use the remote of the mind Meta communications Remember to remember
Narrative	Meaning made of our experiences through the story we keep and share	Retelling of stories (e.g., puppetry, dance, art, music, sandtray, or free play) Externalization of problems
State	Resolution between different and sometimes conflicting parts of ourselves and personality	Let the clouds of emotion roll by SIFT Exercise mindsight Focus on the breath
Interpersonal	Connection between two individuals when we resonate with one another	Increase the family fun factor Facilitative responses Connect through conflict

(continued)

Table 3.1 *Interpersonal Neurobiology Domains of Integration and Play-Therapy Approaches (continued)*

Domains of Integration	Domain Summary	Play Therapy Skill/Technique
Temporal	Organization of time (past, present, and future); existential questions purpose/finality of life	Facilitative responses Process and integrate events into life story
Transpirational	A perceived interconnection to the whole of time, place, and people	Not developed until adolescence

Note: SIFT, sensations, images, feelings, and thoughts.
Source: Reproduced with permission from Wheeler, N., & Dillman Taylor, D. (2016). Integrating interpersonal neurobiology with play therapy. *International Journal of Play Therapy, 25*(1), 24–34. doi:10.1037/pla0000018

narrative coherence, allows for past elements of a child's story to feel as if they are indeed in the past. Working with miniatures in a contained tray of sand seems to allow for such opportunities to be practiced with safety. "Grounded in the body, sandplay unfolds through the limbic region and cortex, and spans both hemispheres as the symbolic unfolds into words" (Badenoch, 2008, p. 220).

STEP 5: SANDTRAY CLEANUP

Typically, clients are invited to leave their completed worlds intact in the sand. This allows clients to experience the therapist as holding their expressed material. Once a sandtray therapy session has ended and the client has left the room, the therapist returns the miniatures to their respective, consistent locations. The sand is smoothed as there is a final check for buried items. If water has been used, then the bottle is refilled and the sand is thoroughly combed to incorporate the water into all of the sand to aid in drying.

Some clients may need to participate in the putting away of their own miniatures. This could be a function of reducing time spent noticing painful material or due to a number of other reasons. Sandtray therapists may want to reassure clients that they do not bear responsibility for cleanup, while still providing freedom for clients to advocate for their needs.

STEP 6: DOCUMENTATION OF THE SESSION

Sandtray-session documentation requires capturing the prompt given, commenting on the client's process and noting the significant content information during processing of the completed world. Ideally, pictures of the completed world are taken and kept with each session note, though special permissions may be needed for this step. When integrating EMDR into the sandtray process, specific information relevant to the phase of EMDR also needs to be documented. See the example in the text box that follows.

EMDR Sandtray-Session Summary

Client name: _____ Session #: _____

EMDR phase(s) covered: 1 2 3 4 5 6 7 8 Type of BLS/DAS used: _____

Sandtray prompt: _____

If EMDR target set up, then complete the following:

    Representative image for memory: _____

    NC: _____

    PC: _____

    VoC: _____ Emotion(s): _____

    SUDS: _____ Body sensations: _____

Prominent miniatures: _____

Title of tray (if given): _____

Process notes (observations during creation and significant content during processing):_____

    Closing SUDS: _____ Ending containment/grounding: _____

Caregiver involvement: _____

Insert picture of tray:

Plan for upcoming session: _____

BLS, bilateral stimulation; DAS, ; EMDR, eye movement desensitization and reprocessing; NC, negative cognition; PC, positive cognition; SUDS, Subjective Units of Disturbance Scale; VoC, Validity of Cognition

---

WEAVING EMDR, SANDTRAY, AND FAMILY PLAY THERAPIES

EMDR therapy, as "a comprehensive method of psychotherapy addressing problems that are based on earlier life experiences" (Shapiro as cited in Lovett, 1999, p. xi), has been effectively paired with multiple types of expressive modalities, such as bibliotherapy and storytelling (Wohl & Kirschen, 2019), game play (Courtney, 2016), and art materials (Banbury, 2016). Sandtray therapy presents as another option for integrating a creative and play-based approach with each of the EMDR phases (Gomez, 2013); it does offer its own unique healing opportunities that highlight family involvement and safety gained through externalizing metaphors (Kosanke, 2013) and ease of change with those expressed metaphors. The rest of this chapter outlines methods for executing this integration, while illustrating the concepts with a case study (a fictitious family, to protect confidentiality, based on combined traits and processes existing in dozens of cases from the author's years of practice).

Some therapists integrate EMDR and play therapy sequentially, seeing these as two separate modalities that can be accessed separately through the client's treatment (May, 2019). Others see these as approaches that can be integrated into one approach (McGuinness, 2011; Sullivan & Thompson, 2016). The same is true for therapists attempting to create an integrative treatment plan that includes traditional family therapy and EMDR (Maxfield, Kaslow, & Shapiro, 2007). This chapter presents a case for using sandtray processing to integrate EMDR and family-based play therapy into a single treatment approach; this is primarily informed by the rhythm of play that sandtray already inherently offers.

PHASE 1: HISTORY AND TREATMENT PLANNING

As with all therapeutic frameworks, EMDR treatment needs to have as its foundation proper informed consent, strong relational connections, and an articulated treatment plan. These tasks are central to EMDR's Phase 1. As EMDR primarily focuses on treating trauma, there is special emphasis on attending to felt safety from first contact with the client(s), always remembering to privilege attunement over information gathering (Parnell, 2013) because all successful treatment is built on safety (Badenoch, 2017).

When a child's trauma is to be treated in a family context, the EMDR therapist must be on solid relational footing with each member (Wesselmann, 2007). Struggles and goals should be heard from the perspective of all who will be involved in therapy (Wesselmann, 2007). This may require multiple appointments, but the time spent accomplishing these initial goals will pay off in later phases. While not all of these beginning tasks will feature use of the sand tray, there will be references to its use with some specific early interventions. The first step requires being able to gain proper informed consent by explaining the processes involved in EMDR and sandtray therapies in simple language to all ages of clients. The following text provides examples of accomplishing this.

Informed Consent Language for Clients

> **Informed Consent Language for Sandtray**
> *A tool I frequently use in therapy is called sandtray. Sandtray therapy prompts you, as the client, to use as few or as many objects as needed to create a symbolic "world" in the sand. This allows for therapy to occur in a way that feels safe because the client takes the lead in making meaning, but it also allows for therapy to go more deeply into places where we may not always have words to describe our experiences.*
>
> *Because sandtray is a visual medium, I will take photos of completed scenes that will be part of the counseling file. If you are uncomfortable with this, let me*

(continued)

> *Informed Consent Language for Clients of All Ages (continued)*
>
> know. If you have discomfort in touching sand, let me know and I can accommodate to meet your needs. You can always ask questions or advocate for yourself during any part of our work together.
>
> **Informed Consent Language for EMDR**
> When certain kinds of stress (like hard events or big forms of fear and worry) start to affect how the brain works, then the brain may need specific kinds of help. EMDR allows kids to play and talk about big feelings while adding back-and-forth sights, sounds, and sensations. This helps to tell the brain it is safe to let go of the big feelings that had been doing the protecting. The process of EMDR starts with working on feeling safe before moving to working on the harder feelings. It doesn't erase memories, but it can help with the feelings and thoughts about the hard memories. EMDR isn't right for everyone, so the therapist, parent, and child all need to agree before moving forward. Plus, the therapist will need to do some specific assessments before beginning EMDR. Sometimes, things start to feel harder before they feel easier, especially when new to learning how to think about difficult memories. If anyone feels uncomfortable with EMDR after it has begun or if new problems show up, it should be talked about soon (even though it may take a little time before things get better or before EMDR could easily be ended).

ASSESSING PARENTS

Similar to most child and family play therapies (McGuinness, 2011), sandtray-based EMDR is best served by meeting with the caregivers before meeting with the child. This helps to elicit treatment cooperation from caregivers and alleviate caregivers' concerns. Schottelkorb, Swan, and Ogawa (2015) discuss the necessary therapist attitudes for effectively connecting with parents as showing respect for the parents' role and knowledge, communicating care for the parent, maintaining focus on the child, and the ability to present self (therapist) as an expert. When caregivers feel respected and heard, they will be in a better position to help build trust between their child and the therapist.

For the purposes of efficiency in later treatment, EMDR and family play therapists need tools for gathering significant aspects of family history relatively quickly. Intake forms and interviews need to solicit information about family medical and mental health history, attachment history, including relevant data regarding pregnancy, delivery, postpartum issues, early caregiving patterns, and/or adoption (Wesselmann, 2007), physical health and developmental history (Bardin et al., 2007), previous counseling experience, beliefs about play, family changes (including deaths and divorces), known and/or suspected traumas, family and child strengths, desired positive cognitions (Wesselmann et al., 2014), academic performance, and so forth. Therapists often benefit by having assessment instruments as part of the intake process. Beer (2018), in a review of EMDR literature on its use with children, listed the measures used in recently published studies. See the text box that follows for a complete list of instruments that could be helpful in this phase of treatment.

Measures Used in the EMDR Studies With Children and Adolescents

1. Anxiety and Related Disorders Interview Schedule (ADIS for *DSM-IV*; Albano & Silverman, 1996)
2. Center for Epidemiologic Studies Depression Scale (CES-D; Radloff, 1977)
3. Child Behavior Checklist (CBCL; Achenbach, 1991)
4. Children's Depression Inventory (CDI; Kovacs, 1992)
5. Child Post Traumatic Stress Reaction Index (Frederick, Pynoos, & Nader, 1992)
6. Child Post Traumatic Stress Reaction Index: Parent Questionnaire (Parent PTS-RI; Nader, 1994)
7. Child Report of Post-Traumatic Symptoms (CROPS; Greenwald & Rubin, 1999)
8. Child Reaction Index (CRI; Pynoos et al., 1987)
9. Child Somatization Inventory, Child and Parent Version (CSI-C/P; Meesters, Muris, Ghys, Reumerman, & Rooijmans, 2003)
10. Children's Attributional Style Questionnaire-Revised (CASQ-R; Thompson, Kaslow, Weiss, & Nolen-Hoeksema, 1998)
11. Children's Depression Scale (CDS; Lang & Tisher, 1983)
12. Children's Post Traumatic Cognitions Inventory (C-PTCI; Meiser-Stedman et al., 2009)
13. Children's Revised Impact of Event Scale (CRIES; Dyregov & Yule, 1995)
14. Clinician-Administered PTSD Scale for Children and Adolescents (CAPS-CA; Nader, Kriegler, Blake, Pynoos, & E., 1996)
15. Depression Questionnaire for Children (DQ-C; de Wit, 1987)
16. Depression Self Rating Scale (DSRS; Birleson, 1981)
17. General Functioning Scale (GFS derived from Family Assessment Device; Epstein, Baldwin, & Bishop, 1983)
18. General Health Questionnaire-12 (GHQ-12; Goldberg, 1978)
19. Impact of Event Scale (IES; Horowitz, Wilner, & Alvarez, 1979)
20. Inventory of Prolonged Grief for Children and Adolescents (IPG; Spuij et al., 2012)
21. Kidscreen-27, Child and Parent Version (Ravens-Sieberer et al., 2007)
22. Multidimensional Anxiety Scale for Children (MASC; March, Parker, Sullivan, Stallings, & Conners, 1997)
23. Negative Affect Self-Statement Questionnaire (NASSQ-A; Ronan, Kendall, Rowe, & Rowe, 1994)
24. Parent Report of Post-Traumatic Symptoms (PROPS; Greenwald & Rubin, 1999)

(continued)

Measures Used in the EMDR Studies With Children and Adolescents (continued)

25. Parenting Stress Index (PSI; Abidin, 1983)
26. Positive and Negative Affect Self-Statement Questionnaire for Children (PNG-C; Bracke & Braet, 2000)
27. Post-Traumatic Stress Symptom Scale for Children (PTSS C; Ahmad, Sundelin-Wahlsten, Sofi, Qahar, & von Knorring, 2000)
28. Revised Child Anxiety and Depression Scale (RCADS; Chorpita, Yim, Moffitt, Umemoto, & Francis, 2000)
29. Revised Children's Manifest Anxiety Scale (RCMAS; Reynolds & Richmond, 1978)
30. Revised Children's Responses to Trauma Inventory (CRTI; Alisic & Kleber, 2010)
31. Rutter Teacher Scale (Kresanov, Tuominen, Piha, & Almqvist, 1998)
32. Self-Perception Profile for Children (SPCC; Harter, 1985)
33. State Trait Anxiety Inventory for Children (STAIC; Spielberger, 1979)
34. Strength and Difficulties Questionnaire (SDQ; Goodman, 2001)
35. UCLA PTSD Index (Rodriguez, Steinberg, & Pynoos, 1998); UCLA PTSD Reaction Index (PTSD-RI) for *DSM-IV* (Steinberg, Brymer, Decker, & Pynoos, 2004)

Source: Beer, R. (2018). Efficacy of EMDR therapy for children with PTSD: A review of the literature. *Journal of EMDR Practice and Research, 12*(4), 177–195. doi:10.1891/1933-3196.12.4.177

Aside from raw data, it can be useful to develop skills in assessing caregivers' capabilities and limitations. While more specific data will be gathered when observing caregivers and children together, therapists can get a sense of the presence of collaborative skills caregivers need to possess in order to be a safe part of the treatment team. When asking about the many intake topics mentioned earlier, notice the presence or absence of caregiver traits such as:

- Ability to know child's needs and emotions
- Skills for noticing and repairing ruptures
- Capability to recognize themes across seasons (and not hyperfocus on behaviors)
- Ability to maintain an accepting tone
- Regulation skills

For the sake of all involved, caregivers need to be assessed in this manner before being included in family work. Without hesitation, compassionately refer parents for their own EMDR therapy when needed (Wesselmann, 2007). When parents can be effective partners in these consultations, it increases caregiver satisfaction with services, leads to better clinical outcomes, decreases reports of problem behaviors, and helps with understanding and cooperation in the play-therapy process (Bornsheuer & Watts, 2012).

Regarding the work that will feature in sandtray, communicate expectations to caregivers about their role in the therapy sessions, allowing frequent enough consultations that roles can be updated as needed. This will provide the EMDR play therapist with chances to model acceptance that the child will need. Caregivers who feel judged by the therapist will struggle to maintain an atmosphere of acceptance with the child.

It can be helpful to explain to parents that they will follow the lead of the therapist in EMDR and sand tray elements (with less dependency on therapist's leadership later on in the treatment plan). The more caregivers understand what EMDR and sandtray therapy will look and sound like (Tinker & Wilson, 1999), the better prepared they will be to participate in a helpful manner. Help caregivers specifically understand that silence will exist for long moments during sand tray creation stages and certain EMDR moments but that offers prime attunement practice. Exhibit 3.1 features a worksheet that can be used to help parents understand what they are being asked to notice in quiet moments. The EMDR sandtray therapist can cover the concepts listed on the worksheet in a parent consultation, which can help parents to understand how to focus on the process and not the product. If a one-way mirror or video monitoring of live sessions is an option, parents can also work through the lists as they observe a sandtray therapy session. They would not be able to actually comment on the parent part of the sheet as they would not be in the room responding but could be coached to notice their instincts of what they might do if they were in the room or even track the therapist's skills. A final option could exist by having the caregiver to complete the self-reflection form after a family session and then debrief with the therapist.

During processing of trays, prepare caregivers that they may be prompted by the therapist using sentence starters like, "Mom. . . I wonder what your eyes notice in this corner?" and "Dad . . . I wonder what feeling you heard from that figure?" This could be useful in moments of needed interweaves (Gomez, 2013). Additionally, if a caregiver might be used in the administering of bilateral stimulation (BLS), then careful practice should occur before involving the child.

In short, the EMDR therapist remains watchful in early interactions with parents to determine if there are sufficient security-producing behaviors to communicate safety, which Brabender and Fallon (2013) describe as featuring flexibility, balance, and integration. In the absence of these, insecurity-producing behaviors like repression and denial of bonding's importance, cognitive disconnection (such as in excessive guilt), and unresolved trauma (Brabender & Fallon, 2013) will be noticeable. Caregivers do not need perfect parenting competency, which is unattainable, but do need to be capable of engaging with the therapist when struggles appear in the sand tray room. As a sandtray therapist, if there is doubt about the caregivers' abilities to participate in the work, inviting them to do a tray can bring more tangible evidence into the treatment space. Also, parents who resolve their own traumas through EMDR benefit from an improved relationship with their children and a clearer mind (Zaccagnino & Cussino, 2013).

Finally, ahead of meeting with the child client, it is useful to have a coherent sense of the child's history in mind. It is the recommendation of the author to save structured timeline work involving the child client until after resources have been assessed, strengthened, and/or created. However, the EMDR therapist needs to know if the caregiver has a cohesive sense of the child's timeline that features both positive and negative memories (Hofmann & Luber, 2009). This will lay the groundwork for all upcoming phases.

Exhibit 3.1 *Attunement Worksheet for Parents in Sandtray Sessions*

Structuring Attunement:
Knowing What to Notice During Sandtray Sessions

As attunement requires noticing your child's inner world while monitoring your own internal states, many things can get in the way of privileging relational curiosity above all else. This sheet will aid you in organizing your observations in a manner that encourages attunement. Remember to focus on developing curiosity and not reaching for interpretations. Sandtray works best when you structure your observations into what you see in the creator and what you hear in the narrative. The creator is always more important than the creation.

Observations about the sandtray creator	
Body language	
Facial expression	
Voice	
Needs expressed	
Emotions	
Beliefs about self	
Beliefs about world	
Problem-solving	
Humor/playfulness	
Interactions	
Response flexibility	
Observations about self	
Body language	
Facial expression	
Voice	
Needs	
Emotions	
Thoughts about self	
Thoughts about child	

(continued)

Exhibit 3.1 *Attunement Worksheet for Parents in Sandtray Sessions (continued)*

Am I communicating (through presence)...?	
Interest/responsiveness	
Playfulness/delight	
Flexibility	
Care	
Acceptance	
Curiosity	
Empathy	

CASE EXAMPLE: MEET THE SMITHS*

Mike and Kate Smith, both 36 years old and Caucasian, are parents of 11-year-old James. The Smiths report that James began to demonstrate signs of anxiety after seeing a fatality resulting from a car accident. The Smiths were not involved in the accident, but, due to stopped traffic, were in full view of the wreckage and first responders for several minutes. Since the accident, James has become preoccupied with even minor somatic issues and is frequently retelling the story of the tragedy. Assessment tools show the presence of traumatic stress and panic as well as decreased parenting satisfaction. This is the first marriage for both Mike and Kate, and there are no other children in the family. After several years of fertility complications, including multiple miscarriages, Kate became pregnant with James and carried him to full term, while being closely monitored and was on bed rest for her final trimester. Delivery occurred without incident, and James hit all developmental milestones on target. He is academically gifted and has a small peer group, which parents believe is a result of his introversion. Kate reports feeling increased anxiety of her own in response to James's struggles, and Mike describes that he has not been as attentive as he would like to due to work demands. The therapist was chosen specifically for EMDR, but Mike and Kate were unfamiliar with sandtray therapy. After explaining the modality, the therapist invited the parents to work together to create a world in the sand. Kate took the lead as they created a world titled "Lurking around the corner" (see Figure 3.1). The therapist processed

---

*Note: This case study features a fictional client. While the details do not exactly match those of an actual client, the information is consistent with clinical work typically performed by the author. All of the sand tray worlds shown in the photographs were created by the author but inspired by previous sessions typical to the presenting issue. This has been done so that the teaching tool does not compromise the privacy of any client.

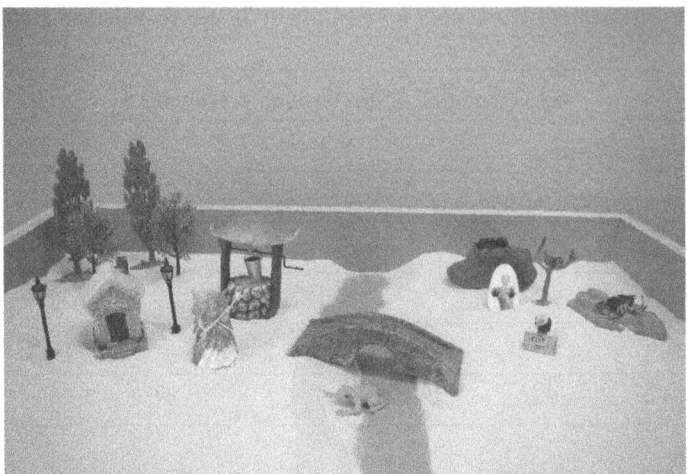

Figure 3.1 *Phase 1—Parents' Assessment Sand Tray*
Photo credit: Caleb Matthews

the tray with the couple, who became tearful as they focused on a theme of powerlessness. This theme was mostly evident in reference to not being able to "rest" in peaceful moments for fear that the dark side will intrude without warning. The couple showed congruent affect with one another and the unfolding thematic content. They were able to be comforting to one another and find resolution of the world by discussing hope that comes from their spiritual beliefs. The therapist recommended to Kate that she might benefit from her own EMDR for the fertility losses and encouraged her to prioritize self-care.

ASSESSING CHILDREN

As the goal of this chapter primarily involves treating children's traumas in a family context, there will not be much information presented on assessing children outside of the family sessions. However, the most common approach this author takes to EMDR Phase 1 work when meeting alone with children is to prompt nondirective sand tray worlds with the aim of creating comfort with the therapist, the office, and the modality. After orienting the child to the available sand tray materials, often inviting them to place their hands in the sand, the child is simply prompted to "create a world in the sand using as few or as many sand tray figures as needed."

While there are not adequate empirical data for sandtray as a formal assessment tool (Homeyer & Sweeney, 2017), Koehler, Wilson, and Baggerly (2015) do point out that play is known to be effective for assessment purposes when treating children. Playful assessment for family therapy strengthens relationships between the child and the parents as well as the child and the therapist (Willis, Walters, & Crane, 2014). The EMDR sandtray therapist can assess the client's comfort with the materials, ability to verbally reflect on their creation, presence of affect and physical activation, and interact with both boundaries and resources that arise during the process.

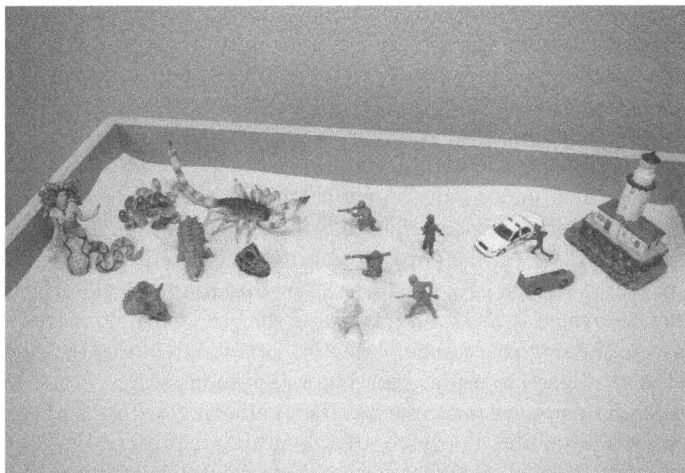

Figure 3.2 *Phase 1—Nondirective Assessment Sand Tray With Child*
Photo credit: Caleb Matthews

CASE EXAMPLE CONTINUED: MEET JAMES

After discussion with Mike and Kate, all agreed that James would do an assessment session alone with the therapist in order for him to explore the space without feeling "pressured to talk about the accident." James was initially reserved but showed curiosity toward the sand and the sand tray miniatures. James was invited "to create a world in the sand," and he made a scene featuring a battle (see Figure 3.2). In the battle, first responders were fighting against "evil" creatures who routinely hurt the bodies of innocent people. James stayed in the metaphor of the scene and did not reveal any details of his own story. The therapist prompted James through processing of the world, leading to a message the evil creatures had for the innocent people being protected by the first responders. They said, "You never know when we might show up, and we're more powerful than you know." James was animated throughout processing but remained regulated (though increasing in hyperarousal). The story ended with a "to be continued" and a containment activity. James asked to return for another sand session and the therapist asked if parents could join next time.

ASSESSING FAMILIES

Many times, as families come together for their first conjoint sandtray EMDR sessions, it can be helpful to make the first directive prompts about intergenerational dynamics. Not only is this helpful contextual information for the therapist as understanding a family's culture and shared belief system is imperative (Bardin et al., 2007), but it also serves to pull pressure off the focus on the child's traumas. This can allow the therapeutic relationship time to develop so that coregulation feels more possible when the activating elements of a trauma narrative come forward.

One method for getting intergenerational information in the sand is the genogram. Genograms provide the aforementioned cultural context (Gil, 2015), while also allowing the therapist to witness family members' perceptions and relational dynamics. A genogram can be done with all members present (Gil, 2015; Higgins-Klein, 2013; Shellenberger, 2007; Wesselmann, 2007) and requires little leadership from the therapist after the structure is initiated. Some sandtray therapists prompt families to create their genograms on paper, showing the basic family tree structure and needed symbols for creation, and then have the members choose sand tray miniatures to place on the paper to represent different people and relationships. The author prefers to give families square and round blocks. The genogram structure can be created in the sand tray, using the blocks to hold places for people in the sand, and then figures can be placed on top of each block. This leaves room directly in the sand itself to represent relational dynamics.

Even though this phase is primarily about gathering history and establishing relationships, the possibility for dysregulation is always present. EMDR therapists need several containment strategies for managing overwhelming feelings. Many authors have written about helpful containment techniques to use with children and families (Goodyear-Brown, 2019), but one containment option is always available to the EMDR sandtray therapist. The tray of sand itself is a container, and families can always be invited to move awareness from the created world to the walls of the tray. As fingers and eyes trace the edges of the container, breathwork can be modeled and permission given to notice the container more prominently than the contents.

When possible, the author finds it helpful to invite the family to create another nondirectively prompted world. Especially after witnessing a parent tray and a child tray, this prompt presents an opportunity to witness how dynamics shift when all are in the room.

CASE EXAMPLE CONTINUED: ROOM FOR EVERYONE

As the family gathered for the first time all together in the therapist's office, James sat with his mother near the sand tray and Mike sat alone in a chair. James initially presented as shyer than in his first appointment but returned to form as the therapist invited them all to "work together to create a world in the sand." Kate attempted to organize the family to get a concept and plan, but James quickly chose a baby to be guarded by two knights (see Figure 3.3). Mike and Kate each tried to get James to talk about his intentions, but he became slightly frustrated at their attempts. Kate added a swan caring for its young ones, and Mike added doctors seeing over the world. The disconnection culminated with James choosing a shadowy figure and placing it behind a locked door. He declared the world finished. The therapist modeled staying in metaphor for Mike and Kate, and all were quickly able to find their way to group processing for the world they agreed to title "Protection." The therapist closed the session with a containment activity. Before the next appointment, the therapist did a phone consultation with Mike and Kate to debrief the appointment. They were open to coaching about relaxing their focus around their agenda of moving so quickly toward meaning-making

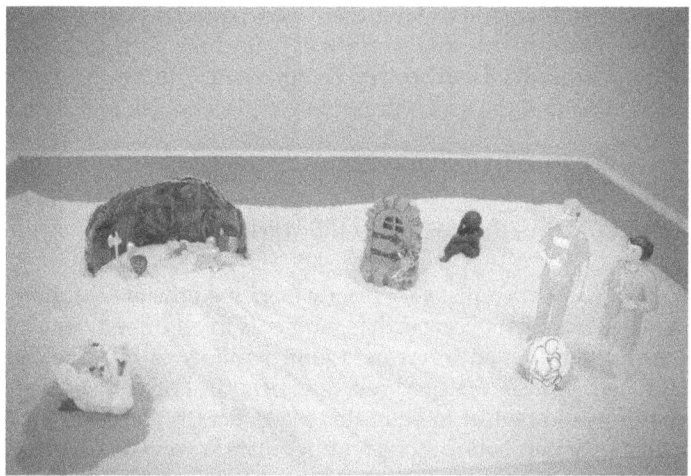

Figure 3.3 *Phase 1—Family Assessment Sand Tray*
Photo credit: Caleb Matthews

and expressed they saw a difference in James's countenance when they focused on staying regulated instead of just trying "to fix him."

PHASE 2: PREPARATION

As mentioned earlier, safety should be prioritized from the first moments of EMDR treatment, but it is formally addressed during this phase (Wesselmann, 2007). When parents have been asked to brainstorm child and family strengths in Phase 1 (Bardin et al., 2007), this list can become a foundation for knowing what resources are already inherently available so the therapist can deepen them and offer potential methods for increasing intrapersonal and interpersonal safety (Wesselmann, 2007). Also, the nondirectively prompted sand trays have given the therapist a sense of what traits the family can access even if outside of their awareness and has shown both the child's sense of felt safety alone in therapy and of being vulnerable in front of parents (Wesselmann, 2007).

The preparation phase can feature moments of psychoeducation about resources and BLS-enhanced accessing of personal resources. All of this can be done in the sand. One psychoeducation possibility for Phase 2 is teaching about the window of tolerance (Siegel, 1999). The window of tolerance brings awareness—somatically, emotionally, and cognitively—to the nervous system's response to the perception of too much stress. Every person has a zone of regulation and the capacity to move to hyperarousal or hypoarousal. These shifts can be taught and illustrated in the sand or turned into a prompt for the family. If prompting a family to create a window of tolerance in the sand, the EMDR sandtray therapist should prepare caregivers to be supportive, but not leading, so that gentle awareness can be discovered by their child and caregivers can be coached to model vulnerability about their own patterns (with age-appropriate disclosure). Also, because the sand world will have three parts (regulated, hyperarousal, and hypoarousal), it can become complicated. The family can choose one figure for each zone to serve as a representative placeholder, and then the world can be expanded.

CASE EXAMPLE CONTINUED: JAMES AND HIS WINDOW

At the next session, the therapist very briefly described the idea of the window of tolerance, normalizing that everyone has moments in all three zones. Mike, Kate, and James were then invited to create a joint window of tolerance (see Figure 3.4). The regulated window featured relaxing, beautiful objects, and all practiced noticing what it would be like to be in this place. Breath and body focusing was reinforced whenever new connections with regulation were discovered. Next, the hyperarousal section was processed as all described symptoms related to anxiety and agitation were explored, paying attention to the dragons. Before moving on, the therapist led the family to notice what would be needed to move from hyperarousal to regulation. Finally, the hypoarousal section was noticed and described, noticing the turtles. This led to "confused" and "tired" feelings. All again practiced returning to regulation. The therapist gained family permission to notice and bring to their attention if "dragons" or "turtles" showed up in therapy.

Creating moments of playful regulation practice can change the everyday lived experiences of families, while also providing a solid ground from which to explore painful, unprocessed memories. Regarding "implicit memories of dyadic play in attachment," Kestly (2014) points out that "positive dyadic play creates a life-long template for emotional regulation so that our social relationships can blossom" (p. 96). Regulation becomes a power source for safe meaning-making.

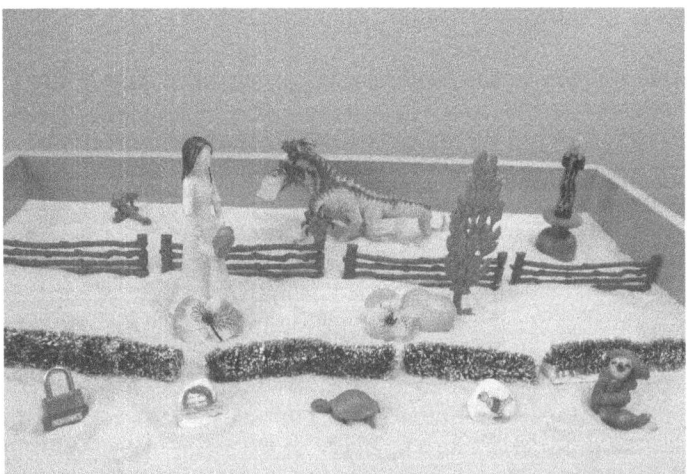

Figure 3.4 *Phase 2—Preparation Phase Window of Tolerance Sand Tray*
Photo credit: Caleb Matthews

A prominent Phase 2 technique along these lines features the creation of a Safe Place. While the word "safe" may be difficult for some children (Wesselmann et al., 2014), *comfortable* or *calm* places can be installed in the same manner. Safe Place works well in the sand tray (Lovett, 1999), requiring few, if any, modifications from the adult script. Safe Place is often a client's first experience with BLS; giving a child some control over the type of BLS and parental involvement can be beneficial (Lovett, 1999). Frequently, unwanted and dysregulating material, called contaminants, can show up in Safe Place. In the sand tray, this can be easily addressed by empowering the client to decide how to facilitate removal, because practice with symbolic containment can be quite effective (Goodyear-Brown, 2019). The child EMDR client should stay in resourcing (Phase 2) until they can return to regulation with the support of the caregiver (Marks, 2017).

CASE EXAMPLE CONTINUED: SAFE PLACE PRACTICE

At the next session, James and Mike came without Kate. The therapist introduced the prompt to create a safe, comfortable place in the sand tray. James quickly created a world full of play, favorite foods, a friend, and himself as ruler. As James processed his Safe Place (and before the BLS), he added a last-minute question mark figure to the tray (see Figure 3.5). Upon questioning, he stated that "you never know what else might show up." As a potential contamination, the therapist coached James through sealing off this possible danger, so he could feel completely comfortable in his world. He changed the figure to a warning light and titled his world "Comfortable Place." Having chosen the light bar for BLS, James and Mike sat near one another and Mike was prepared to follow the therapist's cue of providing BLS through shoulder tapping if a transition was needed. James was told to try and not move his head while his eyes watched the lights move

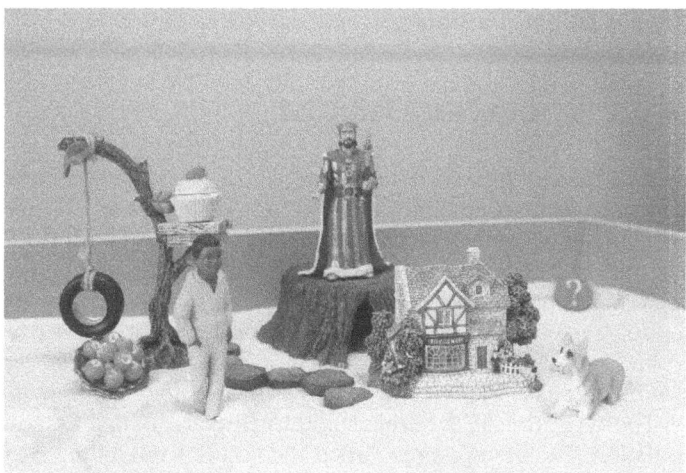

Figure 3.5 *Safe Place Sand Tray With Possible Contaminant*
Photo credit: Caleb Matthews

98 I. MODELS FOR INTEGRATION

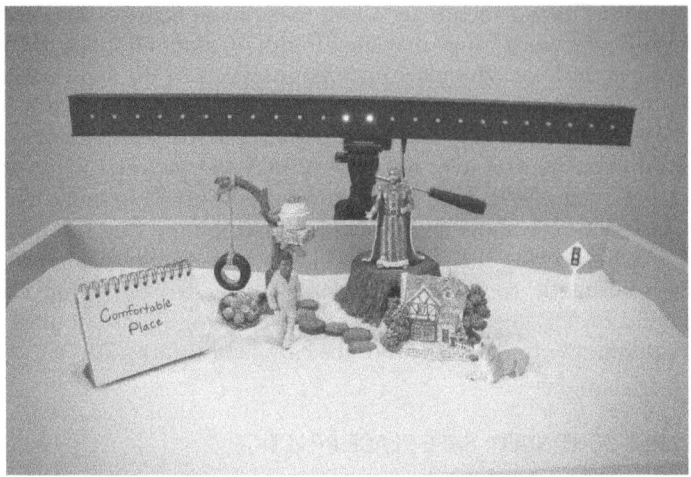

Figure 3.6 *Safe Place Sand Tray With Contaminant Contained, With Addition of Cue Phrase and Light Bar*
Photo credit: Caleb Matthews

back-and-forth over his Safe Place world. This happened in short sets, consistent with EMDR resourcing steps. BLS went on successfully and James reported a deep sense of calm (see Figure 3.6).

A final goal of Phase 2 involves moving to explicit timeline work. As caregivers have already given background, this primarily means that the child gets the benefit of helping to select their own important life moments and to witness the relationship between these without falling into dysregulation or premature processing. There are many ways clients choose to represent a timeline in the sand, and the EMDR sandtray therapist is served by giving the client space to determine that on their own. Each memory or life event can be represented by one figure, and these figures become the prompts for later reprocessing trays.

CASE EXAMPLE CONTINUED: JAMES'S TIMELINE

James arrived for his session with both parents, and all began with practice accessing the previously established Safe Place through visualization. After determining it was still effective, James was prompted, with his parents' support, to create a timeline of important life events. The containment provided by sand tray walls was reviewed. James created a timeline that showed him as a happy baby, a cop car representing a memory of his dad getting a ticket, a favorite tree from his former house's backyard, his family's move to a new house, and the fatal car accident his family witnessed (see Figure 3.7). As James showed signs of moving toward hyperarousal or hypoarousal, the dragon and turtle were invited to show the way back to regulation. The therapist restrained the family from telling stories about the memories. The parents just restated James's words, and all practiced staying contained. James asked to cover up the last figure before leaving. He chose a

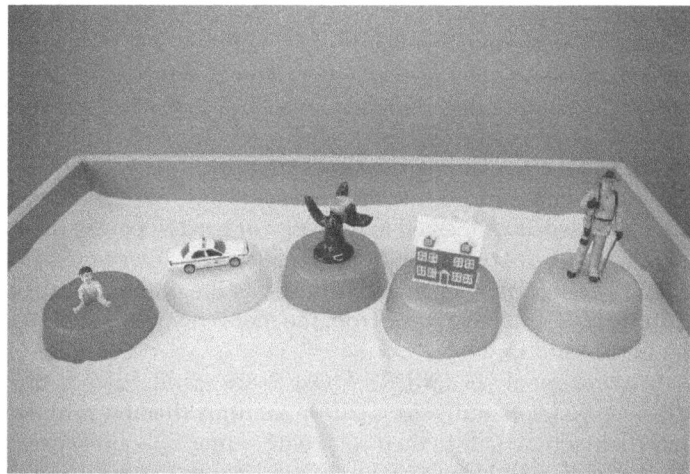

Figure 3.7 *Phase 2—Timeline Sand Tray*
Photo credit: Caleb Matthews

handkerchief and covered the fireman, with the therapist reinforcing his ability to stay regulated.

PHASE 3: ASSESSMENT

In EMDR, the third phase features the establishment of specific targets. The protocol allows the therapist and client to begin to access components of the trauma memory and to establish measures for monitoring changes as the memory is engaged (Leeds, 2009). Clients have varying capacities to picture memories, especially when implicit components are being targeted or activated, so the images for memories can be representational (Wesselmann, 2007).

Target assessment occurs as clients are invited to share whatever they would like for the therapist to know about the memory (Shapiro, 2001). It is not necessary for the therapist to know the details of the memory in order for EMDR to be successful (Shapiro, 2001). For the sandtray therapist, this is good news as much of the target construction is nonverbal. Assuming a timeline occurred in the sand, the therapist only needs to bring to the client's mind the figure chosen to represent the memory, check to see if it is still the client's choice for a representative figure, and prompt the client to *create a world about or for that figure*.

When the creation is complete, the client can share as much or as little as they desire, tracking with the typical sandtray postcreation stage. The additional material for this phase, however, comes when the therapist transitions to asking the client about EMDR target components present in the sand world, which can be directed to a chosen figure in the sand who can act as spokesperson (Gomez, 2013). The therapist may ask, "What in this world shows the worst or hardest part of the scene?" Then the therapist works with the client to identify the negative cognition (NC) and positive cognition (PC) connected to that part of the world.

Similar to the drawing protocol for adults (Carvalho, 2009), a separate world could be created for the PC if needed. The Validity of Cognition (VoC) Scale can be asked directly, can feature the use of a printed (often more playful) scale, or can even be a number added to the tray itself (written on a card, in the form of dice or playing cards, or scaled using seven increasingly bigger animals). Tinker and Wilson (1999) wrote that children can begin to use standard EMDR scaling by age 9 or so, but the therapist may still want to make the scales visual. Emotions and body sensations are assessed as connected to the worst or hardest part of the world, and the Subjective Units of Disturbance (SUD) Scale can be ascertained in the manner of the VoC. These components are the same as the ones used in EMDR talk therapy (Shapiro, 2001) but have come from the more concrete, constructed image now present in the sand tray.

While the components of EMDR's Phase 3 are standardized, the therapist should not disengage relationally. As is true in sandtray therapy, resonance allows therapist and client to stay within their roles while entering a joint space of deeper knowing. Gallerani and Dybicz (2011) say of sandtray specifically that "the therapist takes on the role of editor, which allows for reflection and reaction, while the clients remain authors of their lives" (p. 176). The EMDR sandtray therapist gets to serve in a similar function. Always more important than any technique is the resonance created through safe, therapeutic relationship, because "the trust generated in the context of attunement appears to allow our minds to be open to what we might otherwise reject" (Cozolino, 2017, p. 424).

CASE EXAMPLE CONTINUED: TARGET SETUP

When James and his parents presented for the next session (and first EMDR target session), Mike and Kate were surprised that James rated the memory of his father getting a speeding ticket as more disturbing than the recently observed car accident. James was clear in his convictions and recalled he had chosen the police car to represent the memory. James worked silently and intensely but stayed regulated as he created a world he eventually titled as "Saying bye to the dad" (see Figure 3.8). James described the scene as the father goose being taken away from his family for making a mistake. His family had no power to save him. The police took him to a scary world run by an evil character who made the father goose forget about his family. He now had to live with other animals who were also in captivity.

The therapist asked James to notice the hardest part of the world, and he answered it was the father goose on the police car. James answered the NC and PC directly (instead of having a proxy figure in the world). The NC was "I'm powerless" and the PC was "There are things I can control" with a VoC of 3. Emotions of fear and sadness were reported, specifically noticing them in his stomach. The SUD scale was at an 8.

Despite being initially surprised by the power of the chosen memory, Mike and Kate were very connected to James, seeming to quickly understand that James had been living with an unknown fear that was activated by recent events. They were affectionate, but not intrusive, providing a secure base for James as he explored his inner world.

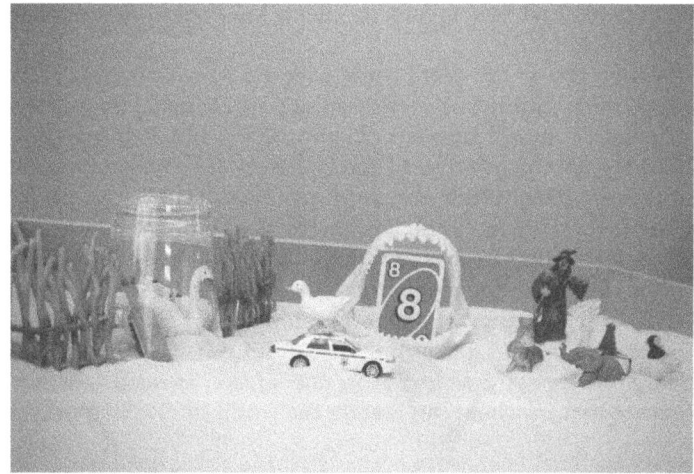

Figure 3.8 *Phase 3—Target Setup Sand Tray With Subjective Units of Disturbance*
Photo credit: Caleb Matthews

PHASES 4 TO 7: DENSENSITIZATION, BODY SCAN, INSTALLATION, AND CLOSURE

EMDR Phases 4 through 7 are comprised of desensitization (4), installation (5), body scan (6), and closure (7; Shapiro, 2001). Phases 4 to 6 are related to the work of reprocessing the trauma memory, while Phase 7 involves preparing the client to transition well out of the session (Shapiro, 2001). Desensitization is started when the therapist repeats the client's reported material from the target assessment (Adler-Tapia & Settle, 2008), initiates the chosen BLS, and intermittently checks in for what the client is noticing. This should follow basic EMDR protocol.

The client will move through associated channels of the memory with the therapist monitoring verbal and nonverbal elements that indicate if the client is remaining regulated (Adler-Tapia & Settle, 2008). If the client begins to leave their window of tolerance, as potentially indicated by looping or blocked processing where "distress remains high for numerous consecutive sets" (Litt, 2007, p. 313), then the therapist provides interweaves to support the client's return to regulated noticing of self (Gomez, 2013). Many types of interweaves are available to the EMDR therapist, including some specific use of parents in a child's session (Wesselmann, 2007) and metaphorical, story, or fable-based interweaves (Leeds, 2009), but the therapist should only intervene if the client is not returning to regulation on their own (Gomez, 2013). Clients who can hold distressing emotion, remaining safely connected to therapist and caregivers while moving through the memory, get the benefit of reprocessing a painful memory without potentially complicating factors introduced by another's point of view.

As clients reach the ends of associated channels and stop noticing any new distressing material, the EMDR therapist can check the SUD scale again to determine if the disturbance is gone. If so, the process moves forward to installation. If not, reprocessing continues. For the EMDR sandtray therapist, this material can be provided verbally and nonverbally as clients have the option of changing the sand tray world as needed.

At installation phase, the client could link the new awareness related to the reprocessed memory with the self-referencing positive belief (PC), after confirming if the original PC is still relevant (Shapiro, 2001). BLS helps deepen the connection with this growing belief until the VoC rests at 7 and positive effects have generalized (Leeds, 2009). While the sandtray client has been given freedom to change the sand world at any point, it often becomes more dynamic at this phase as the client sees the world from a new, more integrated point of view. Assuming that the body scan phase does not reveal any somatically held, leftover disturbance (Leeds, 2009), the therapist moves to intentionally closing the session with the client's containment and grounding in mind (Leeds, 2009). This is especially true if the target does not get cleared in one session as sufficient time will be needed to ensure that the client can reenter the world safely (Shapiro, 2001).

CASE EXAMPLE CONTINUED: RESOLVING THE TARGETED MEMORY

James settled into a comfortable spot between his parents where he had the sand world and the light bar in view (see Figure 3.9). In between the now longer sets of BLS, he commented on channels related to feeling nervous when he saw police cars, feeling uncomfortable when separated from his parents, feeling a nervous stomach, and being mad that kids were sometimes separated from their parents. While James knew he could change the sand world at any time, he chose to leave it alone but did eventually describe a change he would like to imagine. He said he wanted proof that the police were actually protecting kids and not working for an evil character, so he directed one of the little birds to directly ask a policeman

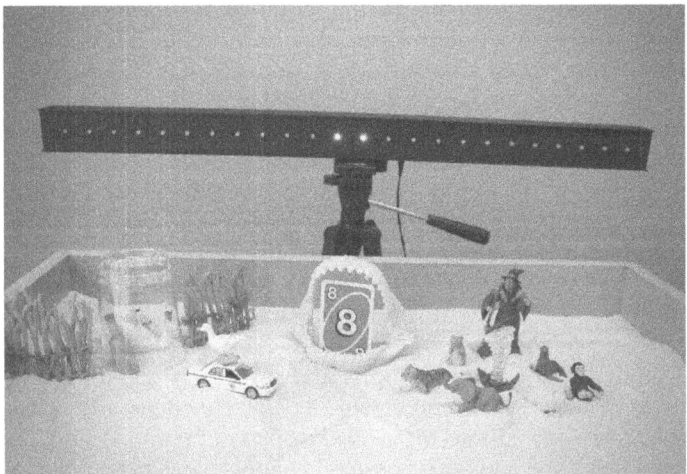

Figure 3.9 *Phase 4—Desensitization Phase With Light Bar for Bilateral Stimulation*
Photo credit: Caleb Matthews

about his intent. The policeman answered with care and reassurance, which began a sequence of increasingly positive somatic and emotional changes.

Mike and Kate remained connected, somewhat tearful at times, but regulated. When James orchestrated the confrontation between the little bird and the policeman, he solicited his dad's help. Taking a visual cue from the therapist, Mike offered a succinct comment about how important it is to feel safe and that asking safety questions is always okay. The therapist cued all family members to take a breath, and processing continued to clearance. The SUD moved to 0 after several sets of BLS. James felt the PC of "there are things I can control" still fit, and the VoC quickly moved to 7. With a clear body scan and review of containment, the session came to an end. When invited to make any final changes to the world, James stated, "They all know what's real now" and left the tray intact.

PHASE 8: REEVALUATION

Reevaluation prompts the EMDR therapist to check for a final time to see if a target has stayed resolved, if any related material has been activated, and if the new sense of self has been integrated into the client's outside world (Shapiro, 2001). At the macro level, reevaluation monitors the parts of the previously established treatment plan; at the micro level, this phase checks in with the specific and recently cleared memory (Leeds, 2009). The EMDR treatment plan is comprised of three prongs: past, present, and future (Shapiro, 2001). When past memories feel resolved and present activation has subsided, planning for a more empowered future awaits (Wesselmann et al., 2014). In the sandtray, reevaluation can be as straightforward as prompting the client to create a new world and process whether there are remaining struggles to address or to move forward. Present and future prongs are equally as direct in the sand, and the imagined future should not be neglected as it offers clients a final opportunity to address remaining fears while reinforcing new and stronger elements of self (Shapiro, 2007).

CASE EXAMPLE CONCLUDED: REEVALUATION AND FUTURE TEMPLATE

As James and his parents continued in treatment, Mike and Kate, whose countenance had also improved, reported that the previously identified struggles had significantly decreased and that James was even more engaged with his peers. After successfully clearing the original target and with the reevaluation showing no remaining distress, James moved through reprocessing of the more recent issue involving the witnessed accident with relative ease. His final session allowed him to anticipate a time in the future when he might have some fears akin to those in the past. The sandtray prompt was *"to create a world showing a future moment when his new skills might be needed."*

James created a scene where a neighborhood fireman might be seen working near a small child. James stated that the child felt safe knowing the fireman was around to watch for danger. James showed a path for the small child to mature into a strong and happy teenager. James spontaneously prompted his parents to

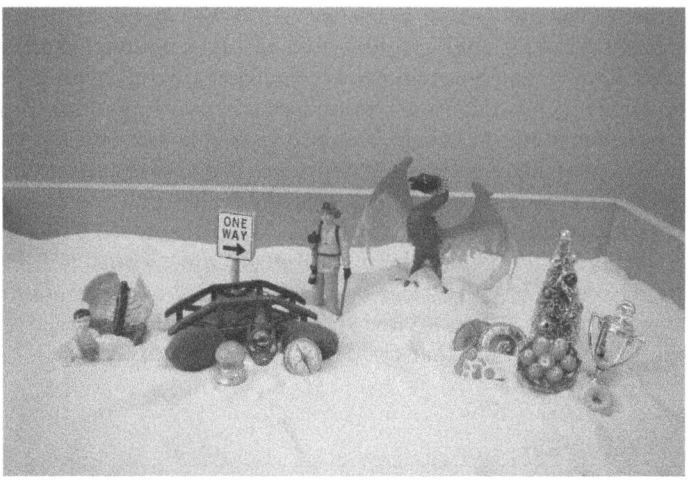

Figure 3.10 *Phase 8—Reevaluation Phase Sand Tray*
Photo credit: Caleb Matthews

add to the tray. Mike chose a phoenix rising from the ashes, and Kate placed a butterfly in the world (see Figure 3.10). The theme of transformation was celebrated by all.

CONCLUSION

Changes made by an individual during EMDR treatment impact the entire "family structure and functioning" (Tinker & Wilson, 1999, p. 7), so it seems fitting that all members of a family who are able should be involved in some way for their sake and for support of the child. Sandtray offers a common language for all who engage. While these possibilities vary from case to case, the EMDR sandtray therapist need not shy away from incorporating caregivers into treatment. This can happen through parent consultations as well as family therapy. Being prepared to properly assess and educate parents about play, sandtray, and EMDR will empower the therapist to look for inclusion opportunities. When a family has shared a wound and finds their way to sharing healing, new possibilities for dynamic change emerge. "On such patches of quicksand made solid, a life of balance and wholeness is emerging" (Badenoch, 2008, p. 241).

REFERENCES

Adler-Tapia, R. L., & Settle, C. S. (2008). *EMDR and the art of psychotherapy with children*. New York, NY: Springer Publishing Company.
Armstrong, S. A. (2008). *Sandtray therapy: A humanistic approach*. Dallas, TX: Ludic Press.
Badenoch, B. (2008). *Being a brain-wise therapist: A practical guide to interpersonal neurobiology (Norton Series on Interpersonal Neurobiology)*. New York, NY: W. W. Norton.

Badenoch, B. (2017). *The heart of trauma: Healing the embodied brain in the context of relationships*. New York, NY: W. W. Norton.

Banbury, N. M. (2016). Case study: Play therapy and eye movement desensitization and reprocessing for pediatric single incident posttraumatic stress disorder and developmental regression. *International Journal of Play Therapy, 25*(3), 166–174. doi:10.1037/pla0000026

Bardin, A., Comet, J., & Porten, D. (2007). Integrating EMDR and family therapy: Treating the traumatized child. In F. Shapiro, F. W. Kaslow, & L. Maxfield (Eds.), *Handbook of EMDR and family therapy processes* (pp. 325–343). Hoboken, NJ: Wiley.

Beer, R. (2018). Efficacy of EMDR therapy for children with PTSD: A review of the literature. *Journal of EMDR Practice and Research, 12*(4), 177–195. doi:10.1891/1933-3196.12.4.177

Bornsheuer, J. N., & Watts, R. E. (2012). *Play therapy and parent consultation: A review of best practices*. Alexandria, VA: ACA Vistas.

Brabender, V. M., & Fallon, A. E. (2013). *Working with adoptive parents: Research, theory, and therapeutic interventions*. Hoboken, NJ: Wiley.

Carvalho, E. R. (2009). The EMDR drawing protocol for adults. In M. Luber (Ed.), *Eye movement desensitization and reprocessing (EMDR) scripted protocols: Basics and special situations* (pp. 107–110). New York, NY: Springer Publishing Company.

Cornett, N. (2012). A filial therapy model through a family therapy lens: See the possibilities. *Family Journal, 20*(3), 274–282. doi:10.1177/1066480712449128

Courtney, D. M. (2016). EMDR to treat children and adolescents: Clinicians' experiences using the EMDR journey game. *Journal of EMDR Practice and Research, 10*(4), 245–255. doi:10.1891/1933-3196.10.4.245

Cozolino, L. (2017). *The neuroscience of psychotherapy: Healing the social brain*. New York, NY: W. W. Norton.

Cutuli, J. J., Alderfer, M. A., & Marsac, M. L. (2019). Introduction to the special issue: Trauma-informed care for children and families. *Psychological Services, 16*(1), 1–6. doi:10.1037/ser0000330

Day, R., & Day, C. (2012). *Creative therapy in the sand*. Rugby, UK: Brook Creative Therapy.

De Little, M. M. (2019). *Where words can't reach: Neuroscience and the Satir model in the sand tray*. Calgary, AB, Canada: Friesens.

Edwards, N. A., Sullivan, J. M., Meany-Walen, K., & Kantor, K. R. (2010). Child parent relationship training: Parents' perceptions of process and outcome. *International Journal of Play Therapy, 19*(3), 159–173. doi:10.1037/a0019409

Gallerani, T., & Dybicz, P. (2011). Postmodern sandplay: An introduction for play therapists. *International Journal of Play Therapy, 20*(3), 165–177. doi:10.1037/a0023440

Garrett, M. (2014). Beyond play therapy: Using the sandtray as an expressive arts intervention in counselling adult clients. *Asia Pacific Journal of Counselling and Psychotherapy, 5*(1), 99–105. doi:10.1080/21507686.2013.864319

Gil, E. (2015). *Play in family therapy* (2nd ed.). New York, NY: Guilford Press. [Kindle Edition].

Gomez, A. M. (2013). *EMDR therapy and adjunct approaches with children: Complex trauma, attachment, and dissociation*. New York, NY: Springer Publishing Company.

Goodyear-Brown, P. (2019). *Trauma and play therapy: Helping children heal*. London, UK: Routledge.

Guerney, B., Jr. (1964). Filial therapy: Description and rationale. *Journal of Consulting Psychology, 28*(4), 304–310. doi:10.1037/h0041340

Higgins-Klein, D. (2013). *Mindfulness-based play-family therapy: Theory and practice*. New York, NY: W. W. Norton.

Hofmann, A., & Luber, M. (2009). History taking: The time line. In M. Luber (Ed.), *Eye movement desensitization and reprocessing (EMDR) scripted protocols: Basics and special situations* (pp. 5–10). New York, NY: Springer Publishing Company.

Homeyer, L. E., & Sweeney, D. S. (2013). Sandtray therapy. In C. A. Malchiodi (Ed.), *Expressive therapies*. New York, NY: Guilford Press.

Homeyer, L. E., & Sweeney, D. S. (2017). *Sandtray: A practical manual*. New York, NY and London, UK: Routledge.

Kestly, T. A. (2014). *The interpersonal neurobiology of play: Brain-building interventions for emotional well-being*. New York, NY: W. W. Norton.

Koehler, C. M., Wilson, B., & Baggerly, J. (2015). Play-based family assessment and treatment planning. In E. Green, J. Baggerly, & A. Myrick (Eds.), *Counseling families: Play-based treatment* (pp. 91–105). Lanham, MD: Rowman & Littlefield.

Kosanke, G. C. (2013). *The use of sandtray approaches in psycho-therapeutic work with adult trauma survivors: A thematic analysis* (Doctoral dissertation, Auckland University of Technology).

Leeds, A. M. (2009). *A guide to the standard EMDR protocols for clinicians, supervisors, and consultants*. New York, NY: Springer Publishing Company.

Lin, Y. W., & Bratton, S. C. (2015). A meta-analytic review of child-centered play therapy approaches. *Journal of Counseling and Development, 93*(1), 45–58. doi:10.1002/j.1556-6676.2015.00180.x

Litt, B. (2007). The child as identified patient. In F. Shapiro, F.W. Kaslow, & L. Maxfield (Eds.), *Handbook of EMDR and family therapy processes* (pp. 306–324). Hoboken, NJ: Wiley.

Lovett, J. (1999). *Small wonders: Healing childhood trauma with EMDR*. New York, NY: Simon & Schuster.

Lowenfeld, M. (1991). *Play in childhood*. Cambridge, UK: Cambridge University Press.

Lowenfeld, M. (1999). *Understanding children's sandplay: Lowenfeld's world technique* (reprinted). Chippenham, UK: Antony Rowe Ltd.

Marks, R. P. (2017). When play therapy is not enough: Using eye movement desensitization and reprocessing/bilateral stimulation in combination with play therapy for the child with complex trauma. In A. Hendry & J. Hasler (Eds.), *Creative therapies for complex trauma: Helping children and families in foster care, kinship care or adoption* (pp. 164–180). London, UK: Jessica Kingsley Publishers.

Maxfield, L., Kaslow, F. W., & Shapiro, F. (2007). The integration of EMDR and family systems therapies. In F. Shapiro, F. W. Kaslow, & L. Maxfield (Eds.), *Handbook of EMDR and family therapy processes* (pp. 407–422). Hoboken, NJ: Wiley.

May, D. (2019). Working with child trauma through EMDR and play therapy. In P. Ayling, H. Armstrong, & L. G. Clark (Eds.), *Becoming and being a play therapist: Play therapy in practice* (pp. 247–260). London, UK: Routledge.

McGuinness, V. A. (2011). Integrating play therapy and EMDR with children: A post-trauma intervention. In A. A. Drewes, S. C. Bratton, & C. E. Schaefer (Eds.), *Integrative play therapy* (pp. 195–206). Hoboken, NJ: Wiley.

Mellenthin, C. (2019). *Attachment centered play therapy*. London, UK: Routledge.

Norton, C. C., & Norton, B. E. (1997). *Reaching children through play therapy: An experiential approach*. Denver, CO: Publishing Cooperative.

Oaklander, V. (1988). *Windows to our children: A Gestalt therapy approach to children and adolescents*. Highland, NY: Center for Gestalt Development.

Parnell, L. (2013). *Attachment-focused EMDR: Healing relational trauma*. New York, NY: W. W. Norton.

Rae, R. (2013). *Sandtray: Playing to heal, recover, and grow*. Lanham, MD: Rowman & Littlefield.

Schottelkorb, A. A., Swan, K. L., & Ogawa, Y. (2015). Parent consultation in child-centered play therapy: A model for research and practice. *International Journal of Play Therapy, 24*(4), 221–233. doi:10.1037/a0039609

Shapiro, F. (2001). *Eye movement desensitization and reprocessing (EMDR): Basic principles, protocols, and procedures.* New York, NY: Guilford Press.
Shapiro, F. (2007). EMDR and case conceptualization from an adaptive information processing perspective. In F. Shapiro, F. W. Kaslow, & L. Maxfield (Eds.), *Handbook of EMDR and family therapy processes* (pp. 325–343). Hoboken, NJ: Wiley.
Shapiro, F., Kaslow, F. W., & Maxfield, L. (Eds.). (2007). *Handbook of EMDR and family therapy processes.* Hoboken, NJ: Wiley.
Shellenberger, S. (2007). Use of the genogram with families for assessment and treatment. In F. Shapiro, F. W. Kaslow, & L. Maxfield (Eds.), *Handbook of EMDR and family therapy processes* (pp. 76–94). Hoboken, NJ: Wiley.
Siegel, D. (1999). *The developing mind: How relationship and the brain interact to shape who we are.* New York, NY: Guilford Press.
Sullivan, K., & Thompson, G. (2016). Eye movement desensitization and reprocessing and play therapy. In E. S. Leggett & J. N. Boswell (Eds.), *Directive play therapy: Theories and techniques* (pp. 81–104). New York, NY: Springer Publishing Company.
Swinden, C. (2018). The Child-Centered EMDR approach: A case study investigating a young girl's treatment for sexual abuse. *Journal of EMDR Practice and Research, 12*(4), 282–296. doi:10.1891/1933-3196.12.4.282
Tinker, R. H., & Wilson, S. A. (1999). *Through the eyes of a child: EMDR with children.* New York, NY: W. W. Norton.
Van der Kolk, B. A. (1998). Trauma and memory. *Psychiatry and Clinical Neurosciences, 52*(1), 52–64. doi:10.1046/j.1440-1819.1998.0520s5S97.x
Van der Kolk, B. A. (2015). *The body keeps the score: Brain, mind, and body in the healing of trauma.* London, UK: Penguin Books.
Wesselmann, D. (2007). Treating attachment issues through EMDR and a family systems approach. In F. Shapiro, F. W. Kaslow, & L. Maxfield (Eds.), *Handbook of EMDR and family therapy processes* (pp. 113–130). Hoboken, NJ: Wiley.
Wesselmann, D., Schweitzer, C., & Armstrong, S. (2014). *Integrative team treatment for attachment trauma in children: Family therapy and EMDR.* New York, NY: W. W. Norton.
Wheeler, N., & Dillman Taylor, D. (2016). Integrating interpersonal neurobiology with play therapy. *International Journal of Play Therapy, 25*(1), 24–34. doi:10.1037/pla0000018
Willis, A. B., Walters, L. H., & Crane, D. R. (2014). Assessing play-based activities, child talk, and single session outcome in family therapy with young children. *Journal of Marital and Family Therapy, 40*(3), 287–301. doi:10.1111/jmft.12048
Wohl, A., & Kirschen, G. W. (2019). Reading the child within: How bibliotherapy can help the victim of child sexual abuse. *Journal of Child Sexual Abuse,* 1–9. doi:10.1080/10538712.2019.1630882
Zaccagnino, M., & Cussino, M. (2013). EMDR and parenting: A clinical case. *Journal of EMDR Practice and Research, 7*(3), 154–166. doi:10.1891/1933-3196.7.3.154

4

Synergetic Play Therapy Combined With EMDR Therapy

JAN SCHAAD AND LISA DION

INTRODUCTION

This chapter addresses combining synergetic play therapy (SPT) with eye movement desensitization and reprocessing (EMDR) while maintaining fidelity to both therapies. This combined process of therapy is *synergetic* and relies heavily on theories and research regarding the storage of memory, the mirror neuron system, neurobiology of the brain, interpersonal neurobiology and coregulation, and the innate states of nervous system activation.

This chapter expands on these key concepts: understanding the neurobiology of coregulation as it relates to EMDR therapy and synergetic play through the lens of SPT; the importance of therapist regulation while facilitating EMDR in the playroom using SPT theory and its base in neuroscience; the stages of EMDR therapy with SPT and EMDR combined; and the use of EMDR as a directive and nondirective process in play therapy. We want to be the voice for EMDR being a nondirective therapy!

SPT AND EMDR: LONG-LOST BEST FRIENDS

Synergetics, a term coined by physicist Buckminster Fuller, is the study of systems in transformation, with an emphasis on total system behavior unpredicted by the behavior of any isolated components (Fuller & Applewhite, 1975). The word itself is also reflective of what is happening in the playroom and how integration and healing occur. As the therapist attunes to their own internal systems and then attunes to the internal systems of the child, a union of systems occurs. In this union, a synergy forms, allowing for coregulation to emerge. The coregulation supports both the therapist and the child in their ability to move toward the uncomfortable thoughts, feelings, and body sensations that they would not have been able to move toward as easily on their own. During this "synergy of systems," therapist and child enter something akin to a "synergetic field" where right-hemisphere-to-right-hemisphere communication emerges, allowing for integration and transformation. As a model of play therapy, SPT honors the therapeutic powers of play, the science that governs a relationship, and the development of the therapist, while recognizing that it is ultimately the interplay among these three systems that supports deep transformation for both therapist and child. Its philosophy brings an understanding of nervous system regulation, interpersonal neurobiology, physics, attachment theory, mindfulness, and therapist authenticity into the playroom. Developed in 2008, its primary play therapy influences are child-centered, experiential, and Gestalt theory based. Although SPT is a model of play therapy, it is often referred to as a way of being in relationship with the self and others. The model's philosophy is an all-encompassing paradigm that can be applied to any model of play therapy; subsequently, any model of play therapy can be applied to it. As a model, SPT is both nondirective and directive in its application (Dion, 2018).

Both SPT and EMDR are informed by the adaptive information processing (AIP) model as developed by Francine Shapiro in 1987. Both therapies view the overall client picture and synergy of systems to understand the past events and perceptions that contribute to the present dysfunction. The AIP model posits the existence of an information processing system that assimilates new experiences into memory networks in the brain. These memory networks are the basis of perception, attitude and behavior, and of health or pathology based on the resolution, or the lack thereof, of stored information about life experiences (Shapiro, 2001). Dr. Shapiro has said that EMDR has evolved since its inception in 1987 and has developed into a synthesis of therapies where all therapies used are credited in the healing process (Shapiro, 2002). Those of us who utilize EMDR as the foundation of our therapy refer to it as the "therapy that plays well with others." The underpinnings of SPT and EMDR are so similar in their understanding of how integration occurs (and both theories are so rooted in neuroscience and nervous system regulation) that many students have gone so far as to refer to SPT and EMDR as "long-lost best friends." As a note, therapists do not need to be trained in SPT to benefit from the content in this chapter because the philosophy of SPT is easily incorporated into other play therapy theories and ultimately to the application of EMDR.

Therapists who specialize in working with children often struggle to implement EMDR following the introductory course. As with all learning of new conceptual material, the process of navigating the path from concept to practice has a learning curve. Language used in the introductory course is presented in a linear fashion and in adult terms. While this is useful for learning, clinicians must take advanced training to adapt the language and procedural steps of EMDR with fidelity to the model and also learn how to infuse different therapeutic modalities and approaches together with EMDR for all variations of nuances in client populations.

As such, blending EMDR with play therapy can be confusing. It takes creativity to adapt EMDR protocols to the developmental stages of child clients and to the setting of play therapy. In general, EMDR phases need to be flexibly used to address the client's neurological state and the brain's current focus. Working with children requires practitioners to learn how to adapt the protocol to the child rather than expecting the child to adapt to the protocol. How to do this and have fidelity to the model is the challenge!

It is also important for us to teach therapists how to blend the protocols while maintaining the integrity of the therapies. Sometimes, it is useful to use EMDR and SPT separately, but they do not actually need to be split as they beautifully coexist. Learning to flow back and forth from directive application to nondirective application, depending on what is required, is an important part of being able to apply the EMDR protocol with children. Doing so allows the therapist to attune and be responsive to what the child is needing. Synergy is what this chapter focuses on, as these therapies come together to create transformation.

THE FOUNDATION

Before discovering how to effectively combine SPT and EMDR into a play process, an understanding of how nervous system activation occurs and how this impacts the symptoms that child clients are displaying is necessary. Exploring the mirror neuron system, what it means for the therapist to become the external regulator, and how coregulation supports the integration of the child's activation are also foundational elements that bridge SPT and EMDR and thus are also discussed.

When we perceive a challenge in life, our bodies are naturally designed to attempt handling the difficulty. There are two branches that exist in the autonomic nervous system to help support the ability to manage these perceived challenges. The sympathetic branch revs us up, and the parasympathetic branch slows us down. If in the moment of the perceived challenge, we have the thought or feeling, "I can do something about the challenge," the body becomes activated into a flight or fight state of sympathetic arousal. If, on the other hand, we perceive that, "The challenge is too much! I can't do anything," then the body will respond through dorsal parasympathetic activation supporting the slowing of the body to shut down, withdraw, and collapse. There is another activation of the parasympathetic branch called the ventral vagal response, which is explored later as regulation is discussed. Exhibit 4.1 lays out the various symptoms of nervous system activation.

It is important to note that the body also has a freeze response associated with sympathetic activation of the nervous system. It was Steven Porges who postulated that this freeze response can be dangerous for people and all mammals (Porges, 2011). It is important to understand that the physiology of *freeze* is not the same as *surrender* or *collapse*. The latter is a collapsed physical response related to the instinctual reaction to appearing dead to survive the predator's attack (Scaer, 2005). *Freeze*, on the other hand, is an active somatic state of fight or flight that has been *held in* because the person perceives it dangerous to act. When this energy is not able to be discharged, it is stored in the mind and body. This held-in energy leads to many symptoms, including those of posttraumatic stress disorder (PTSD).

For example, we can consider what can happen when trauma gets stored in the body. If a person is sexually abused and not able to fight or flight in self-defense, the system will store the sensory data as they were experienced, the body will remember the muscle patterns of the impact, and the fear is coded in the mind and the body (Scaer, 2005; Shapiro, 2001; Siegel, 1999; Van der Kolk, 2014). Shapiro taught that this was all stored in state-dependent form, maladaptively stored in networks in the brain, and without access to adaptively stored

Exhibit 4.1 Nervous System Symptoms of Regulation and Dysregulation

All symptoms of dys-regulation arise out of perceptions of the events in our lives. When we change our perceptions, we change the symptoms in our nervous system. It is wise to master the art of how to change our perceptions and how to manage the symptoms that arise in our bodies to help return us to a more regulated/ventral state.

Freeze, Flight, Fight Hypoarousal Symptoms	Parasympathetic/Ventral Vagal Response-Regulated Symptoms (Mindful/Attached to Self)	Parasympathetic/Dorsal Vagal Response—Collapse/Hypoarousal Symptoms
Hyperalert Hypervigilant Increased heart rate "Pounding" sensation in the head Anxious Excessive motoric activity Overwhelmed Disorganized Highly irritable, uncontrollable bouts of rage, dissociative	Think logically Think clearly Able to make conscious choices Able to make eye contact Display a wide range of emotional expression Feel "grounded" Able to notice breath Sleep cycles stable Poised Internal awareness of both mind and body "In the body" Able to communicate verbally in a clear manner	Helplessness Appear lifeless Nonexpressive Numbing Lack of motivation Lethargic/tired Dulled capacity to feel significant events Emotional constriction Isolation/depression/dissociation

Source: From Dion, L. (2018). *Aggression in play therapy: A neurobiological approach for integrating intensity.* New York, NY: W. W. Norton

memory. All of these data are stored both explicitly and implicitly. Explicit memory refers to an actual recollection of the details of the event, and implicit memory refers to the way the body has stored the patterns of activation. When this individual later encounters data in their environment that offer a reminder of the original event, the individual's system will likely respond in a defensive, protective way. Assuming the threat is over, it is possible that over time the person is able to discharge the held patterns from the body, neutralize the disturbance, and achieve new learning, which is adaptive resolution (Shapiro, 2002). If, however, the disturbance is not resolved, and/or the threat continues to occur on an ongoing basis, say, for instance, in a pattern of on-going sexual abuse, the person is likely to develop conditioned associations with the cues, and the memory networks become larger with misperceptions and interpretations of the perceived threat. This individual now walks through the world highly activated by both external and internal cues (Scaer, 2005). The brain in a sense is now hijacked, and the individual is easily and often triggered. Robert Scaer refers to *neurosensitization* or *kindling* to describe this process of spontaneous activation of the autonomic nervous system (Scaer, 2005). In a research study using rats, Goddard, McIntyre, and Leetch (1969) found the amygdala to be the easiest brain center to develop this kindling process. This concept supports our clinical understanding of the symptom in PTSD when the amygdala sends signals to the body that the person is not safe even when they are safe. Scaer believes kindling may even explain the worsening of body symptoms over time. He further describes the brain and body as being on autopilot, continuing to respond to old cues from unresolved, mostly unconsciously stored material. This process explains the repetition we often see in our clients with their emotions, sensations, and behaviors associated with trauma. An example of this would be the reenactment of the sexual behavior learned from a perpetrator by a victim of sexual abuse, or the selection of a partner much like the former perpetrator of abuse. The brilliance of this process is the individual's attempt to come in contact once again with the nonintegrated data to offer a new opportunity for integration, but tragically, the social care system misunderstands this and blames the victim for what are natural responses to trauma unresolved. This also explains how the reflexes, fascia, and muscles can hold defensive postures, often for years. The fascia becomes like shrink-wrap, restricting our muscles and distorting our reflexes. We commonly observe physical patterns with our clients, which are also memories stored from unresolved events (Ogden, Minton, & Pain, 2006).

In the face of ongoing trauma, the body experiences high levels of cortisol, and the child begins to adapt to these heightened cortisol levels. Over time, the child becomes less able to adaptively respond to stress and develops a new normal with regard to their active state of arousal. The body is constantly scanning for cues of danger, and these cues expand over time. In other words, the child is subconsciously activating the fear response even in the absence of a real external threat. This pattern of growing associations to the original trauma memory is called *neurosensitization* and is another way to describe *kindling* (Scaer, 2012). When this pattern is combined with incoming messages from others that it is not okay to express their dysregulation, the child begins to grow a bank of procedural memories connected with past events. Stored memory from these events is activated by reminders (triggers) internally and externally. Cortisol is released, and the action needed (fight or flight) is initiated. When this is thwarted, the result is the development of a repetitious pattern of autonomic dysregulation of overactivation, and, ultimately, the child will move into a collapse or dorsal parasympathetic response as the system learns to shut down. In this process, the child becomes susceptible to dissociation as the mind will do whatever is needed to protect a person from being physical and psychologically overwhelmed. Dissociation can begin at a very young age and can result from single incident trauma or continuous trauma. When trauma is ongoing and unremitting, dissociation is developed as a way to cope with attempted but failed protection (Scaer, 2012).

To review, when people are challenged by experiences that overwhelm their ability to cope or navigate successfully, these experiences, unresolved, are automatically stored in the brain and body. They are elicited by cues in the body and the environment and responded to as if the past were the present. When the person is successfully able to handle or resolve the event, they return to homeostasis. All systems in the body are involved in maintaining homeostasis, and it is the disruption of homeostasis and the return to homeostasis that create resiliency, or the ability to adapt to threat. Homeostasis is actually a connection to the self in a state referred to as relaxed and ready. When this return to homeostasis does not occur, research in the neurobiology of trauma shows us that the patterns of collapse, learned helplessness, and dissociation are adaptively learned. Conditions for these patterns include the vulnerability of the child and an external environment unresponsive in protection or aid in making sense of the child's experiences.

SYNERGETIC PLAY THERAPY AND EMDR

Sarah, aged 7, started play therapy with a synergetic play therapist for issues concerning school anxiety. She would often display signs of high-level sympathetic arousal in class. She would look around nervously, fidget with her hands, bite her lip, and have a hard time sitting still. When she was 3 years old, she witnessed multiple episodes of highly emotionally charged fighting between her parents. Her parents no longer live together, but the emotional conflict still continues between them. During her sessions, she would create play filled with anxiety and safety concerns, often placing a small puppy in the position to watch two dragons fighting.

Working with children in therapy to successfully address stored components of memory and their activation requires the therapist to assess the child's memory networks and the stored cognitive, affective, and sensory material in order to help integrate their thoughts, feelings, and bodily sensations (Shapiro, 2001, 2018). In both SPT and EMDR, the therapist aims to address all of the dominant activations that are arising moment to moment during the play and the EMDR processing.

As children play, visualize, and talk about their challenges, they are simultaneously accessing their associated memory networks. As this occurs, the child will begin to experience the corresponding nervous system activation in their own system. In other words, the child's dysregulated state will begin to emerge through the play itself and through the child's behaviors and language. When we translate this into the world of play therapy, we can see that much of what we are working on in play therapy is also supporting the repatterning of the child's dysregulated states and memory networks as they work toward integrating their challenges (Dion, 2018).

In Sarah's play, it can be speculated that she held a cognitive belief that the puppy was not safe or protected. The play itself contained feelings of fear as the puppy was set up to observe the dragons fighting. As she created this play, her body naturally became activated in a sympathetic response as she simultaneously was experiencing the fear that she was playing out. This was evident as the therapist noticed that Sarah was holding her breath to manage the anxiety that she was experiencing. All aspects of memory storage were being activated in the moment in the play. It is important to note that activation of the AIP occurs in every moment of play and is not dependent on the play therapy approach that is being used. The theoretical differences really depend on the way the therapist supports the integration of the activation.

In SPT, the play therapist meets the child where they are in time and space from the very beginning of therapy, attuning to both the self and the child in each moment of the therapy process for the purpose of coregulation. The overarching goal is the shift in the child's perception of the challenging events that have occurred in the child's life with a repatterning of the child's nervous system states, allowing the child to reconnect to themselves. EMDR would describe this process through the lens of the AIP. From an EMDR perspective, stored memory is moved into the adaptive memory networks of difficult experiences mastered and are able to link up with other adaptive memories. The result is a discharge, or letting out the stuck components of memory through desensitization. In both modalities, the resolution (EMDR) or empowerment (SPT) is a process of transformation. The child is becoming themselves, restored *and* updated.

When a child's unresolved memory is activated, a result of sympathetic and/or dorsal parasympathetic activation occurs. These states fluctuate within the child as they move through the world triggered by their nonintegrated experiences. As the child's nervous system becomes activated, the child will make whatever effort they can to regulate with the means and skills that are at their disposal. In SPT, the child's symptoms are understood as dysregulation in the nervous system (Dion, 2018). In EMDR, the symptoms are understood as the outgrowth of unprocessed memories. Both are true. When triggered to those memories, there is dysregulation in the nervous system. When this child appears in the therapy office or playroom, the therapist begins by observing the activation in the nervous system and then works directly with the activation being displayed. In other words, therapists meet children where they are as they begin the work.

Because much of the training in EMDR therapy has focused on the readiness to verbalize disturbing events, it is often difficult for the therapist to know how to support the child when the child is unable to verbalize the disturbance or is highly sympathetically or dorsal parasympathetically activated. Adler-Tapia, Gomez, Lovett, and many others (Adler-Tapia & Settle, 2016; Gomez, 2012; Lovett, 2014) have developed creative ways to adapt EMDR protocols to age and developmental levels of functioning that have begun to shed light on how to use EMDR with the younger population. Although historically there has been more emphasis in the EMDR field on cognitive and verbal work, we are beginning to see a shift toward working directly with implicit memory. Play therapists may become stuck in their attempts to help children "develop the resources" to talk about incidents, without realizing that the play itself is the child's way of talking about it and, as we saw with Sarah, also revealing the targets in present time.

In EMDR, preparation work precedes the work of processing the disturbing material. For children who are verbal and have a narrative of what has happened to them, many can be helped with the standard EMDR protocol. For children who are not verbal, who refuse to talk about what has happened to them, or who are highly traumatized, the addressing of the disturbance is not so straightforward. For this population, play therapy is the perfect way to help these children, and when the components of EMDR are woven into the play therapy experience, even deeper opportunities for integration can occur. One of the benefits of an SPT approach is that the implicit memory is worked with directly in the play. Some children are verbal about the disturbances they have experienced and, much like in verbally guided EMDR, the synergetic play therapist avoids interpretation and trusts the process. What this really means is that the therapist is open to perceiving all that the child does and "goes with" the unfolding of the process in the child, trusting that children have everything inside of themselves needed to heal.

INTEGRATION REQUIRES REGULATION

As this chapter is teaching, a primary goal for both SPT and EMDR is the integration of the challenging experiences that have been maladaptively stored and unresolved in the child's internal system. In order for integration to occur during activation, regulation is required. There is a false belief that often exists in the understanding of regulation that can impact a therapist's ability to support their client's integration of the challenging thoughts, feelings, and sensations that arise in sessions. This false belief is that regulation means calm. Regulated actually means *connected*. From an SPT perspective, the definition is extended to include *mindfulness* and *awareness of the self* (Dion, 2018). For example, in moments of regulation, individuals can think clearly, can make conscious choices, can notice their breath, are able to feel grounded, and have an experience of being in the body. We could say that these individuals are connected to themselves. For this to occur, these individuals has accessed their ventral vagal parasympathetic response, which puts a break on the flight, flight, or collapse response of the autonomic nervous system. If we review Exhibit 4.1 outlining the symptoms of the various nervous system states, we find the symptoms corresponding with the ventral vagal response, the second state of activation of the parasympathetic branch.

Stephen Porges in his polyvagal theory reveals that the vagus nerve in the parasympathetic nervous system aids in slowing the body down, but for different reasons. The dorsal parasympathetic branch of the vagus nerve responds when there is a perception of threat. The ventral vagal branch, on the other hand, responds when the person has what Porges describes as a "neuroception of safety" (Porges, 2011).

When clients are processing their traumatic experiences with EMDR or through play, therapists are working toward helping them regulate through the intensity and this requires *connection*, which is different from calm. As they mindfully track their experience, they are activating their ventral vagal response in the midst of their sympathetic or dorsal parasympathetic activation. This means that the child will be regulated and dysregulated at the same time. They will feel the dysregulation in their bodies while simultaneously knowing they are safe and not in danger. This is the concept of dual awareness, which is explored in greater detail later on and is a key understanding for EMDR and SPT. The work is for therapists to teach their clients how to mindfully be with themselves in their play and stories as they recall the challenging thoughts, feelings, and bodily sensations. This allows the client to continue to move toward the intensity without emotionally flooding or becoming overwhelmed.

The purpose of regulation is to go toward the dysregulation, go into it, and even feel it more. Integration requires moving toward, not moving away from. This is an essential understanding of modulating the intensity that can arise in the playroom and coregulation, which is why SPT emphasizes and focuses a large part of its training on the development of the therapist. The therapist must be able to hold and modulate the intensity. To sum this up, *in order to regulate, a person must move toward the intensity, not try to get away from it.*

THE THERAPIST AS AN INSTRUMENT OF THE REGULATION OF THE CHILD'S AUTONOMIC NERVOUS SYSTEM

Children need an *external regulator* to help integrate the dysregulated state in their nervous systems. In SPT, the most important role of the therapist is that of the external regulator. When babies are born, they need the support of an attuned caregiver to learn how to regulate effectively because their capacity to self-soothe is still immature in their development. The nervous system works in a hierarchical fashion and is wired toward making sure that any potential threat in the external or internal environment receives the greatest amount of attention. When something does not feel okay, a baby knows how to cry, scream, become agitated, withdraw, and even collapse, if needed. A baby also needs external support to help put the brakes on the activation, so that the baby can learn how to engage their ventral state more effectively. Allan Schore stated that "the mother is literally a regulator of the crescendos and de-crescendos of the baby's developing autonomic nervous system" (Bullard, 2015, Trauma and Development section, para. 1). We might even say that babies borrow the regulatory capacity of the caregiver as their own regulator capacity develops (Dion, 2018).

When working with children, therapists sometimes forget that their child clients are often babies disguised in big bodies and expect them to be able to regulate in ways that they cannot and in some cases never learned how to do well. When therapists are supporting children through a traumatic experience in their lives using play and EMDR, they need to keep in mind that as children recall the events in their lives, their bodies simultaneously become activated in the corresponding dysregulation and they need support to regulate through the intensity. The reason they are in therapy is because the original experience was perceived as "too much" and "too scary" so as we offer them an opportunity to approach the thoughts, feelings, and sensations, they need the support of an external regulator. Another way to understand this concept is that therapists need to help "rock the baby" to help repattern their nervous system.

BECOMING THE EXTERNAL REGULATOR

Understanding what an external regulator is and how to become one is one of the most critical elements of working with children using play or EMDR in our opinion. In order to become external regulators, therapists must be willing to:

1. Feel what is happening inside of their own bodies.
2. Move toward the uncomfortable thoughts, feelings, and bodily sensations that arise in the playroom during the play and the EMDR without wanting to avoid or become consumed by the emotional experience.

3. Regulate themselves so that they can support the child's regulation.
4. Work through their own biases and blocks that keep them from being able to attune to the client.

Going back to the example of Sarah and her play, Sarah focused her play on the components of memory and their associated thoughts, feelings, and bodily sensations that are still unresolved and maladaptively stored in her system. In Sarah's case, the focus was on the fear and anxiety that she felt while witnessing her parents fight. If the activation in her system had been too much for her, she would naturally begin to move away from her emotional states and painful memories in an attempt to avoid the intensity. This act of moving away would indicate that she was approaching the edge of her window of tolerance (Siegel, 2010). The window of tolerance is described as the optimal zone of arousal that allows a person to integrate sensory data (Ogden et al., 2006; Siegel, 1999). As she moves away from these experiences, she reinforces the message that there is a threat or challenge. This reinforcement keeps her nervous system in a state of dysregulation. This is why active coregulation is so necessary for integration and, unfortunately, is often missed as part of a play therapy or EMDR process. This same process of avoidance also can happen inside of her therapist. The therapist will also move away from her own internal states if she is not willing to feel her own bodily, emotional, and cognitive states while working toward modulating them (Schore, 1994), which could potentially leave Sarah feeling unsafe and unseen (Siegel, 2010).

When therapists are not willing or able to feel the shifts that are occurring inside of themselves during the EMDR or play, they will most likely begin to move away from those particular body sensations and emotions, denying they exist, shutting them down in some way, or emotionally flooding. Becoming the external regulator requires therapists to feel what is happening in their bodies while simultaneously regulating through it. This is also the same process therapists are teaching their clients to do with EMDR, but therapists need to lead the way. Feeling what is happening inside of the body during a play therapy or an EMDR session can be uncomfortable, and yet it is a requirement to accurately attune and hold the client's experience. From our perspective, continuing to develop a relationship with our bodies and continuing to widen our capacity to feel while staying connected to ourselves is one of the most important skills we need to develop as therapists.

While children play and share their stories, their memory network of nonintegrated thoughts, feelings, and bodily sensations will naturally arise. In these moments, they need the therapist's window of tolerance to be larger than theirs. Looking back to the metaphor of rocking the baby, the caregiver's window of tolerance must be greater than the baby's in order for the baby to borrow the caregiver's regulatory capacity. The same is true in the playroom; children need to be held in the therapist's ventral embrace, allowing them to go deeper into their feelings and move toward their challenges (Badenoch, 2017; Kestly, 2016). Bonnie Badenoch in her book *The Heart of Trauma* (2017) offers us a beautiful depiction of this describing a client's window of tolerance meeting the therapist's window of tolerance to create a joined window of tolerance. Visually, it is as if the therapist is energetically wrapping their arms around the child. It is within this window that coregulation occurs, and the child can explore sympathetic arousal and dorsal collapse while being regulated by the therapist.

DUAL AWARENESS

Matthew, aged 6, in his play picks up a very aggressive-looking tiger and moves it toward a small kitten that is sitting alone. Matthew then begins to make growling noises for the tiger as the tiger is looking toward the kitten. As the therapist observes, she notices sympathetic activation begin to arise as anxiety and fear begin to enter the play. Matthew then takes the tiger and suddenly moves the tiger toward the therapist to bite her. In this play scenario, the attuned therapist's own nervous system will begin to activate as the play is observed and experienced. The intensity will then rise in the therapist as the tiger comes toward her in an attempt to bite. It is at this moment that the therapist must practice dual awareness. The therapist becomes present with the dysregulation while simultaneously accessing her own ventral state allowing for a neuroception of safety to emerge. The therapist is then able to hold both the felt sense of the client's world and the knowledge that it is play.

In SPT, therapists learn that as we experience the activation of our own nervous system states, we have to be in the dysregulation and not in it, simultaneously. Teresa Kestly (2014) described it as the ability to track the felt sense (right hemisphere) and hold conscious awareness (left hemisphere) simultaneously. The ability to hold both or to be regulated and dysregulated at the same time is what allows the therapist to maintain a neuroception of safety through ventral vagal activation, which then allows the therapist to attune, regulate, and be present. When therapists do not hold this dual awareness, they increase the probability that they will merge with their clients or move too far away from them. On a practical level, this means that therapists have to allow themselves to know that it is the child's play, while feeling the realness of the dysregulation in their bodies that is naturally arising from the play and stories. One way to work with this in the playroom or during an EMDR process is for therapists to hold the mantra "one foot in and one foot out" in their awareness. Metaphorically, therapists can put one foot in the dysregulation and leave one foot out to access their regulatory capacity. In these moments, the therapist is working to embody the same process that the client is trying to learn.

The reality is that therapists will become triggered to their own unresolved material and blind to the presence of unresolved memory; however, when the therapist is able to regulate through the intensity, the ability to be present still exists. When the therapist is not regulating, it is likely that the therapist will steer the client away from their full expression of components of memory or steer them to the cognitive domain. This often manifests in a stuck point in the play therapy process. The client's play then becomes repetitive because the child is not able to borrow the therapist's regulatory capacity to move toward the challenge for integration.

Enhancing skills as external regulator:

- Learn how to listen with the entire body, not just the ears.
- Engage with the intention to be open, neutral, and curious.

- Engage in mind/body activities daily, such as meditation, mindful exercise, breath work, energy psychology exercises, yoga, tai chi, massage, and brainwave entrainment.
- Neutralize triggered states with EMDR therapy.

THERAPIST ACTIVATION

Understanding and normalizing the idea therapists do become triggered while facilitating a child's play or EMDR process is important. Returning to the example of Sarah, if Sarah's therapist had her own unresolved memories triggered while watching the fight scene, the therapist's own protective patterns likely would have entered the room. Allan Schore refers to this process as *mutual regression* (2019). Depending on how much the play activated the therapist's own memory networks would determine the degree to which these protective patterns would present themselves. The same is true with Matthew's therapist as he approached her with the tiger. If her own memory network was triggered, she too would have had a higher probability of responding with a protective pattern. In his book, *Right Brain Psychotherapy*, Schore explains that "mutual synchronized topographical regressions, operating at levels beneath conscious awareness, are ubiquitous in all relational, psychodynamic, affectively focused psychotherapies" (p. 118). In other words, to think that therapist activation can be avoided in the playroom is to fail to understand the workings of interpersonal neurobiology. This is one of the primary reasons why SPT focuses so heavily on the development of the therapist and the therapist's own understanding of their own nervous system activation. It is also why learning how to identify the signs of dysregulation and how to regulate through them is an essential component of the therapeutic process.

Allan Schore (2019) also discusses how these moments of mutual regression can also be one of the most therapeutic parts of the process if the therapist becomes aware that their defense patterns are surfacing. In these moments, as the therapist is able to maintain ventral activation in the dysregulated state (one foot in, one foot out), the therapist can maintain an "empathic resonance and an interpersonal right brain synchronization with the patient's dysregulation" (p. 80). Schore sums this process up like this:

> When a therapist's wounds are hit, can she regulate her own bodily based emotions and shame dynamics well enough to be able to stay connected to her patient? Can the therapist tolerate what is happening in her own body when it mirrors her patient's terror, rage and physiological hyperarousal . . . Herein lies the art of psychotherapy. (Sieff, 2015, p. 132)

THE MIRROR NEURON SYSTEM

The mirror neuron system was first discovered in the 1980s when scientists in Italy discovered the same neurons were firing in a monkey's brain when the monkey observed an individual picking up an object as when the monkey was actually grasping the object. The monkey's neurons fired as if it were performing the task even though it was an observer (Rizzolatti, Fogassi, & Gallese, 2001). The mirror neuron system helps the mind make a simulated mental model of what is being observed and then imitate what has been seen (Heyes, 2009). This mirror neuron system enables children to learn through observation (Iacoboni, 2007; Rizzolati, Fogassi, & Gallese, 2001). In another experiment demonstrating the mirror neuron system, Tanya Chartrand and John Barge, social psychologists, created an experiment where subjects were instructed to choose photos from a group of photographs. The subjects were told that they needed to find pictures that they perceived to be stimulating in some way. In the same room, another person was placed pretending to also be a subject. While the real subjects were looking through the pictures, the pretend subject was told to engage in a very deliberate action, such as rubbing his face or shaking his foot. Chartrand and Bargh found that the real subjects unconsciously began to copy the deliberate action of the test subject (Iacoboni, 2008)!

Not only does the mirror neuron system allow for the replication of actions that have been observed over and over, but this system also makes it possible to understand the actions of others (Bandura, 1977). It does not stop there as this understanding goes right into the world of emotions.

As Marco Iacoboni writes in his book *Mirroring People*,

> Our mirror neurons fire when we see others expressing their emotions, as if we were making those facial expressions ourselves. By means of this firing, the neurons also send signals to emotional brain centers in the limbic system to make us feel what other people feel. (p. 119)

It turns out that the brain is designed to help people feel what other people feel. It is as if for a moment a person imagines being the person being observed in order to create a shared experience with that individual. Whether a therapist is facilitating a child's processing with the EMDR protocol, observing the play, or engaging with the child in dramatic play, she is picking up on the child's verbal and nonverbal cues. More specifically, as therapists pick up on the various states of activation of their autonomic nervous systems, they will also begin to experience somatic shifts inside of themselves as their own autonomic nervous system is activated just as in the case examples discussed earlier. This activation happens automatically, whether the therapist wants it to or not. The saying, "monkey see, monkey do," is familiar to many people. With a deeper understanding of the mirror neuron system, this saying can now be seen as the "I feel what you feel" emotional empathy system.

THERAPIST AUTHENTICITY

As the mirror neuron system makes it possible for children to learn through observation, the old neural programming can be interrupted when children repeatedly see the therapist being authentic and present in the midst of the dysregulation that arises. As children observe, their mirror neuron system becomes engaged as they watch how the therapist relates to the intensity. When a therapist authentically moves toward the uncomfortable internal states, it creates an opening for a new experience inside of the child allowing the child to also move toward challenging internal states. As children move toward their challenging internal states, new neural connections can be created and eventually initiate new neural organization (Dion & Gray, 2014; Edelman, 1987; Tyson, 2002). Research shows that neural systems can change with dedicated amounts of repetition; however, according to Bruce Perry (2006), most therapeutic interventions do not achieve that goal.

As children observe the therapist, they will also observe what the therapist's own inner activation is, making therapist authenticity paramount. Anyone with misattunement or attachment disruptions, child or adult, is very perceptive of mismatch between word and action in their relations with others. They will spot inauthenticity "on a dime."

In Carl Roger's book *A Way of Being*, he shares the importance of being authentic and congruent in the therapeutic relationship this way:

> The more the therapist is himself or herself in the relationship, putting up no professional front or personal facade, the greater the likelihood that the client will change and grow in a constructive manner. The means that the therapist is openly being the feelings and attitudes that are flowing within at the moment. The term *transparent* catches the flavor of this condition: the therapist makes himself or herself transparent to the client; the client can see right through what the therapist is in the relationship; the client experiences no holding back on the part of the therapist. (p. 115)

When therapists are feeling emotions such as fear, anxiety, sadness, or anger and attempt to hide their experience, children are able to pick up on the nonverbal and verbal cues of the therapists (Dion, 2018). In these moments, the cues that the children are picking up are letting them know that the therapist is being inauthentic. This lack of authenticity can potentially trigger a safety threat in the brain as the child struggles to make sense of the incongruence (Dion, 2018). In addition to the potential threat to the brain, the therapist is also modeling to the children what to do in those moments when those feelings arise. As examples, if therapists change the subject, smile every time they are scared, pretend that they feel fine, and disconnect from their bodies, the children learn to do the same. As therapists work toward helping children mindfully move toward their emotions with dual awareness, it is crucial that the therapist models this movement.

Another important consideration is that when the therapist is inauthentic, it is most often a validation of what the child has already learned to be true for them in their environment. This validation then reinforces patterns already learned and can result in discouragement of the child's hopefulness of finding true connection or expression of who they really are.

It is also important to understand that attunement is not possible without authenticity, and without attunement, the therapist is not able to serve as the external regulator (Schore, 1994). In other words, authenticity plays a critical role in teaching children how to regulate their nervous systems and change their brain activity (Dion & Gray, 2014). As Badenoch (2008) and Siegel (1999) explained, when the child's mirror neuron system is activated, the therapist's mindfulness and authentic expression can trigger new brain activity that can become associated with the feelings in the neural nets of memories ultimately helping rewire the child's neural network.

In SPT, authenticity is carried into the play itself. The synergetic play therapist responds authentically to the child's own initiated play and stories. This response is different from acting or pretending to be a role. As the therapist observed Sarah's play, the therapist responded with observational statements such as, "The puppy is sitting there watching the dragons fight" and "The dragons are hitting each other." The therapist also allowed genuine responses to the play, saying, "I feel nervous watching them fight, and I am worried that the puppy may not feel safe." Therapists' ability to reflect within to make sense of their own inner experience and share it with the child is incredibly powerful as it is often these types of statements that help the child feel *felt* and *known*. As a reminder, the mirror neuron system is designed to help people feel what other people feel. Children want their therapist to feel their world, and they will do everything they can with their play, their stories, and their behaviors to help their therapist "get it," including putting the therapist in the position to experience similar thoughts, feelings, and bodily sensations that they are holding.

Again in his book *A Way of Being* (1980), Carl Rogers helps therapists understand the importance of these genuine reflections:

> Sometimes a feeling "rises up in me". . . . I have learned to accept and trust this feeling in my awareness and try to communicate it to my client. . . . I have learned that if I can be real in the relationship with him and express this feeling that has occurred in me, it is very likely to strike some deep note in him and to advance our relationship. (p. 15)

As a quick review, when children play or tell a story, their bodies become activated in either sympathetic or dorsal parasympathetic (assuming they are processing something challenging) activation. Therapists will begin to experience somatic shifts in their own bodies as they observe, listen, and interact with the child. This is the critical juncture for integration. If the therapist pulls away or denies their internal experience in some way, the child will potentially experience the therapist's incongruency and also back away from their experience. If, however, the therapist is able to hold dual attention and regulate through the dysregulation, the child's mirror neuron system will observe the therapist's authenticity and congruence while simultaneously watching how the therapist handles the intensity. In this way, the therapist's regulatory capacity disrupts the child's neural network bringing about the potential for change (Badenoch, 2017; Schore, 1994).

THE SYNERGY BETWEEN SPT AND EMDR IN THE PLAYROOM

This section begins to weave together EMDR and SPT in the playroom. Case examples are used to illustrate the phases of EMDR during synergetic play using both directive and nondirective application of EMDR during play therapy sessions.

Though children can present with a single upsetting event, often it is a pileup of events, many of which are hidden from view by their protective patterns, rules prohibiting the expression or talk of them, and painful incidents of efforts at expression met with hurt and fear. Recall in the example of Sarah that she came in primarily for anxiety that was arising at school, yet her history revealed incidents of witnessing parental fights, which emerged in her play as her primary disturbance.

It is helpful in examining the phases of EMDR along with the parts of SPT to think of EMDR Phases 1 through 3 as the beginning of treatment, and the Phases 4 through 8 as the working phases. In both EMDR and SPT, the establishment of the therapeutic relationship is central to the beginning of treatment. SPT emphasizes the development of the therapist's ability to attune and coregulate as a way to heal the neural disorganization in the brainstem and repattern the nervous system. EMDR training also addresses attunement; however, it does not teach it. It is as if the training in EMDR assumes therapists do this as a part of becoming a psychotherapist; however, not all therapists receive comprehensive training in attunement. This skill of attunement may well be one of the major factors in the making of an effective EMDR therapist over an ineffective one. Both SPT and EMDR therapies utilize the therapist's attunement to themselves and the child to help facilitate change.

With AIP in mind, the EMDR/SPT therapist addresses case conceptualization with the following parameters: the current situation, symptoms, triggers, past incidents unresolved, and future goal states. In Sarah's case, anxiety was her predominant symptom, triggered when her parents had contact with each other, and likely in many other circumstances, the connections unknown. For example, she may have been triggered at school in class and at play with peers when family topics were talked about or she perceived conflict between two people. Although the identified goals were the reduction of the anxiety symptoms she displayed at school, her parents fighting became the target as it emerged in her play. While conceptually it is true that a focus on the earliest event that precipitated disturbance in beliefs, thoughts, emotions, and body sensations is the most direct route to resolution, sometimes clients are not able to address their disturbance in this way and can only access stored memory through current triggers. The beauty of using play is that through the play itself, children can explore their triggers as they work toward being able to access the roots of the disturbance. In Sarah's case, she may or may not have consciously known the connection between her anxiety and witnessing her parent's fighting, but the play allowed the earlier memories to begin to emerge.

In EMDR, the work of history taking and preparation phases is taught primarily in directive ways, with the therapist guiding, teaching, and leading. In both EMDR and SPT, the directness of relating and the education on coping skills will occur based on the developmental age of the child and the complexity of the child's symptoms. It is useful to find many ways to explain the EMDR process to children, and often it is most effective to explain it in terms of something that is most meaningful to them. For example, working with 7-year-old Tommy who loves cars, the therapist promoted the analogy of a car that will not start and needing jumper cables to get the car started; or for Carla, aged 10, who loves to travel and fly, the therapist might use the analogy of observing her thoughts and sensations as if she were looking out a plane window at the clouds and cities below (dual attention). The therapist also works toward strengthening and/or developing an internal felt sense of safety and adaptive coping skills, including those of nervous system regulation and containment. In preparation-phase work, the child is developing mindfulness about themselves and their emotions and increasing supportive connections to resources outside themselves. This can be accomplished through play, artwork, and mindfulness or body-awareness exercises. Therapists can also teach the child how the brain works as a way to support the child with internal coping skills they can use to navigate their current environment. The ultimate goal of this preparation phase, or resource development, is the building of adaptive memory networks. As the child strengthens their networks, the child learns how to cope with life in ways they may have never learned. We believe that it is important to include resource development in every session, not just at the beginning of treatment, but as part of ongoing preparation (Korn & Leeds, 2002). In this phase, it is important to reconnect a child to adaptive memories, build new memories of positive experiences, and create mastery skills and connections to outside resources that are helping, nurturing, and protective. Using the case of Matthew discussed earlier, at the beginning of a particular session, Matthew's mom reported that he was having trouble at school with a classmate who Matthew felt was being mean to him. In response, Matthew was at times isolating himself at recess. The therapist, focusing on resource development, discovered that Matthew enjoyed drawing cartoons and asked him about his favorite characters. Matthew told the therapist that he had created three of them, and he was happy to draw them for her. In the session, he described their characteristics, and the therapist strengthened his sense of these characters as a protective circle with bilateral stimulation (BLS) and suggested he could take them with him to school. His parents and teachers noted an immediate improvement in his ability to feel more confident and that he was seeking out other classmates to play with at recess. This particular session with Matthew included the following phases of EMDR, in the order as they occurred: Phase 8, because the clinician is using reevaluation to decide how to focus the session, then Phase 2 resourcing, and then Phase 7 closure of the session.

Activating components of memory with questions requires the child be verbal and to have developed mindsight or the ability to observe their inner experience while staying within their window of tolerance (Siegel, 2010). This is a top-down activation of the memory network. It is a direct approach, yet guided in a way to be inclusive of all components of memory held in the mind and body. If the child is developmentally unable to do this, the story can be supplied by the caregivers or the therapist. The child can also express their inner experience with art and play. All of these procedures activate the components of memory and directly precede desensitization. It is the indirect expressions of stored memory that newly trained clinicians often have trouble navigating. In the playroom, the expression of stored memory can occur within minutes of the first session as the child begins to play or tell a story.

The reevaluation phase is where adaptive integration is determined directly through target-specific assessment, along with other information gathered from the caregivers about recent events and changes in symptoms and behaviors. From the perspective of working with the child *as they are that day*, the reevaluation phase is really a guide to understand where to begin the work for that session. Looking at the next session with Matthew, we began with reevaluation, where the accomplishments of Matthew of using his protective circle on his own and playing more easily with others at recess were reported by his parents. Matthew also shared that he felt a lot better at school. Next, the therapist strengthened the positive experiences, which is preparation-phase work. The therapist asked Matthew what it was like for him to take his protection circle with him when he went to school, choosing this first because it was a resource Matthew developed himself. As he described what he liked about having these three characters with him, the therapist asked him to notice where he was feeling this in his body and to let the feelings get as strong as they wanted to be while giving himself the butterfly hug, their already-established pattern for BLS.

> Therapist: *What was it like playing with the kids at recess?*
>
> Matthew: *Fun!*
>
> Therapist: *Notice where that feeling is in your body, and let it get as strong as you want it to be* (BLS).

As the therapist was listening to Matthew describe his new experience with his peers, the therapist became curious about the level of confidence he was feeling with his peers. The therapist then asked Matthew if he knew what it means to be confident, and if he did have that sense of himself at school. As he was not sure, the therapist described confidence and asked him if he would just notice if he did have that feeling sometimes. When he shared that he feels it only sometimes, the therapist noticed that his body began to move from side to side indicating that he was activated as he recalled the experiences with his peers. From there, the therapist shifted to play as Matthew needed a way to continue to process the disturbance that he was experiencing. Matthew found the small kitten that was once alone and scared by the tiger and took it over to the sand tray. There he began to bury gold coins in the sand while telling the therapist to close her eyes. After the coins were buried, the therapist was asked to find them, but before she started, Matthew said, "Kitty is going to help you. Kitty knows how to find them if they are down at the bottom of the sand." As the therapist and the small kitten worked together to find the gold coins, feelings of excitement, teamwork, and accomplishment began to enter the play. Quickly, after all of the coins were found, the tiger appeared, threatening to take them away and it was simultaneously almost time to end the session. Next came Closure, where the therapist asked Matthew if he would like to "lock up all the yuck," as Matthew's play indicated that he had not yet fully integrated the activation that he was working through in that particular session. To initiate the containment, the therapist borrowed the work "yuck," which had been spontaneously expressed by Matthew during his play. The therapist showed Matthew her padlocked dump station for hazardous waste material and asked him if he would like to scoop up all the yuck and dump it in. Matthew used a scoop and dumped in an assortment of rubber objects. He especially liked unlocking and then locking up the dump station and hanging up the keys. After this was done, they listened to one of his favorite songs for soothing; then, she talked with him about what cartoon books he was currently reading as they were walking out to the lobby (present orientation). We feel that it is important to wrap every session with resource development, or preparation-phase work if possible.

Another task in reevaluation is making sure the therapeutic goals have been achieved (targets have been integrated). The desired outcomes of the reprocessing are empowerment, a neutralization of disturbance, and the strengthening of positive affect and belief, and these need to be maintained over time for treatment to be complete. The "proof" of resolution is in the absence of symptoms and demonstrated functional behavior of the child in both the playroom and outside of sessions.

In addition to what has been mentioned, the SPT therapist is also assessing whether or not the child's emotional age corresponds to the chronological age as this indicates the child has integrated the disturbance in their memory network to the present (adaptive resolution). For example, 6-year-old Matthew's play often focused on the safety of the kitten, with the kitten being put in situations where it was not safe and could not trust. This play alone is not necessarily an indicator of an earlier emotional age; however, the themes of trust/mistrust and safety (corresponding to Erikson's developmental stages) along with Matthew's regression in body language and verbal expression (often speaking in a very young voice and using body movements indicative of earlier regression) allowed the therapist to understand that although Matthew was working on a present-day issue, the roots were historical in his development. By the end of his therapy, the kitty in Matthew's play was safe and confident and his body and verbal language were in line with the development of a 6-year-old. As Matthew integrated his disturbances, the therapist emphasized his empowerment or positive, future-oriented insights with statements such as "The kitty is safe" and "The kitty knew exactly where to find the hidden treasure."

In a way, the process of SPT operates as if EMDR Phases 3 to 6 were implemented seamlessly. This is achieved by way of the therapist becoming the external regulator (an intervention that desensitizes disturbance), using the child's mirror neuron system to model regulation, and coregulating the child through the activation of the disturbance. The coregulation also acts as ongoing preparation throughout the entire process as the child learns how to modulate the intensity that is being experienced internally. The activation itself in the moment becomes the target of EMDR. The child does not need to discuss it or identify it with the therapist. The work begins with the activated components of memory in real-time. We can liken this to the targeting of a presently held triggered state. It is at this point that the therapist must decide whether to use a directive or nondirective approach. With SPT, we are taking the child as they present, allowing the activation to be expressed from whatever component(s) of memory is brought forth in the spontaneous expressions of the child. From a neuropsychological perspective, we are beginning our work from the activated state in the mind and body. In EMDR, this would be like noticing whatever components of memory the person is reporting to us (Assessment) and using that to begin the desensitization with what is being triggered (Target). Working in this way allows us to access memory that cannot be addressed verbally, yet held in implicit memory.

In the case of Sarah, if the therapist wanted to choose a more directive play intervention, the therapist could ask Sarah if she would like to help the puppy feel less scared as the puppy watched the dragons fight (if she wanted to stay in the metaphor of the play), or the therapist could have directly asked Sarah if she wanted help to feel less anxious and scared. At that point, the therapist could have introduced BLS by either stopping the play and following the verbal steps of EMDR desensitization or using BLS as Sarah played, perhaps by tapping on her shoulders or knees. Verbal communication is not necessarily a goal here. Addressing the type of activation and expression with BLS is a choice point at every step of the process. When the therapist decides to be more directive, it would be in response to the expression of the child, and based on the therapist's clinical judgment of the next best step, much like the goal of a cognitive interweave.

From a nondirective approach, we can refer back to the mirror neurons. Consider what could happen if the therapist merely offered BLS in the child's visual field as the child played. In many ways, this is not very different than asking a client to track the therapist's fingers back and forth. The client is not receiving the input directly into their body, but rather through their visual field! As Sarah set up the play with the puppy and the activation began, the therapist (without interrupting the play) could gently rock side to side knowing that Sarah's mirror neuron system would pick up the bilateral movements. The same could be done with the therapist tapping on her own knees or the floor. There are so many ways to incorporate the BLS creatively. As the therapist offers the bilateral input, the therapist also gets the benefit of the BLS, which supports the therapist to stay in their own window of tolerance. We are going to keep bringing this back to the metaphor of rocking the baby. One of the most beautiful parts of the design of the human species is that in order to rock a baby, the caregiver must also rock themselves simultaneously. When considering the movements that a caregiver makes to soothe a baby and repattern the baby's nervous system state, it can be noticed that the majority of the movements are bilateral.

Another way to understand this is that during an SPT session, the child moves through their inner experiences in synergetic work with the therapist, whether it be with play or verbal communication, while the components of memory are being expressed and the child is following channels of association. The BLS is applied either directly from therapist to child or indirectly with the child applying BLS to themselves with the therapist doing the same, or with the therapist applying BLS themselves with the child observing this in their line of vision. As this process is occurring, the child goes in and out of their window of tolerance, expressing hypo- and hyperarousal as the therapist maintains attunement, authenticity, and regulation. The activation, which is largely somatic, is enveloped within the safety of the therapist's ventral embrace, allowing for spontaneous expression of the held memory in mind and body.

In EMDR language, stored memory components within a memory network are being processed, with the target incident possibly being largely unknown to the therapist. The results of this process are the neutralization of the disturbance, a strengthening of positive belief, followed by shifts in future behavior. The child's play will also reflect the integration and resolution. There are observable signs of physical shifts in body expression, movement, and posture as the child's system demonstrates a higher regulatory capacity. In Sarah's play, as therapy progressed, other animals joined the puppy so that the puppy was not alone anymore, and together they built fences between the dragons so that the dragons stopped fighting. The puppy and the other animals were then able to play without the anxiety or safety concerns. Sarah's body also changed from sympathetic activation to a relaxing of the shoulders; she exhibited laughter as the puppy and the other animals played, and she had the ability to take deeper breaths. All of these manifestations were indicators that there was no longer a disturbance felt in her body, providing evidence that EMDR Phases 4 to 6 have been completed.

The therapist's ability to engage their own ventral state and rest in dual awareness is what allows the coregulation to occur, just like the caregiver rocking the baby. When we think about how caregivers regulate babies, they use sound, breath, movement, and naming their experience out loud. The therapist can do these same things in the playroom to help access their own ventral state, deepen their attunement, and support the child in developing a greater capacity for their own dual awareness allowing for a more integrative experience (which also constitutes good Phase 2 preparation work). When the therapist said, "I feel nervous watching them fight, and I am worried that the puppy may not feel safe" while watching Sarah's play, the therapist then followed it up by taking a deep breath. As this occurred, Sarah observed the therapist move toward the activation and then regulate through it. More specifically, her mirror neuron system watched and tracked the pattern priming her to be able to copy the pattern. As Sarah's therapist made observational and reflective statements of her own experience, Sarah also started to become aware of her own sensations and feelings. An interesting phenomenon occurs when a person says to someone something like, "My lower back hurts." The listener automatically puts their attention on their lower back to see if they are having the same experience. The same phenomenon happens in the playroom. When the therapist makes a reflective statement about their own experience, children automatically check in to see if they are having the same experience, thereby strengthening their own dual awareness.

As mentioned earlier, EMDR training also addresses the importance of attunement to both the self and the client; however, it does not directly teach it. Because this skill is central to a successful outcome, it is important for therapists to obtain training and/or therapy to further this development of ability to attune. The inability of the caregiver to attune to the baby can prolong the baby's dysregulated state, and the same occurs in the playroom. Both SPT and EMDR therapies utilize the therapist's attunement and dual awareness to help the child facilitate change. Over time, Sarah started to take deep breaths in the midst of her own activation. This shift represents the power of synergetics. The addition of SPT coupled with EMDR allows the therapist to address the activation at the level of the survival activation of the lower brainstem and works directly with the dysregulation of the nervous system and body patterns, enabling us to get to the stored, unresolved experiences when the client is hyper- or hypoaroused, dissociated, or holding the trauma in implicit memory.

In summary, the usual EMDR treatment plan is issue-specific; it includes the present events that trigger disturbance, past experiences feeding the current disturbance, the clinical theme represented in the beliefs a person carries about themselves, and the skills and internal resources that need to be developed for adaptation in the future (Shapiro, 2002). In SPT, the therapist works with the target that is arising in the moment, recognizing that the activation, beliefs, and past-associated disturbances are all linked to the present moment. In both therapies, the therapeutic process completes when all aspects of memory held in the mind and the body are desensitized; sensory input is no longer perceived as a trigger to the adverse experience but is rather viewed *as is*. For example, the color blue would become just a color that may represent peace or healing, and not the color associated with the uniform of the police in the stored memory of trauma. The individual is not just restored to a previous level of functioning but is instead updated in their level of functioning to include adaptive learning from the experience. In SPT, this is referred to as *empowerment* where the child has the ability to stay connected to themselves and modulate their internal experiences. For SPT or EMDR to provide lasting change, both therapies must address all disturbance in the body and mind. Both therapies must also transmute to the positive in belief and action thereby creating a new future template.

ASSESSMENT: IS THE CHILD READY?

Assessing for EMDR readiness occurs in many ways and throughout the process, not just at one point in treatment. From an SPT perspective, readiness is really about recognizing whether or not the child is within their window of tolerance in any given moment and having the resources available to the child to support emotional flooding.

Because SPT works directly with the child's somatic experiences and dysregulated states of the nervous system, clients are not as readily labeled as unsuitable, or "not ready" for processing as the regulation of the dysregulated states is the focal point of intervention. The precursor for readiness is the child's ability to maintain dual awareness during the activation. Just like the therapist needs to be able to have "one foot in and one foot out," so does the child, to a certain degree. Not being able to have dual awareness leads the child toward higher levels of emotional flooding and dissociative tendencies. Emotional flooding occurs when there is an excessive amount of data coming in through the senses. In these moments, the client is not able to access a "neuroception of safety" and, therefore, is not ready for BLS. We must first help the child back into their window of tolerance and secure a sense of safety when emotional flooding and dissociation arise. An example of this is demonstrated in the subsequent section on working with parents.

As children work through the activation of stored memory, they will naturally be in and out of their window of tolerance. Therefore, the therapist must learn how to titrate the child's experience supporting their ability to stay within their window of tolerance. The word *titrate* means to continually adjust the balance. During play therapy sessions, children's windows of tolerance are changing moment to moment as they respond to their inner and outer environments. The therapist's capacity to hold the experience is adjusting as well. As we have already discussed, it is the therapist's job to maintain a window of tolerance larger than the child's in order to allow the child's activation to fluctuate between sympathetic and dorsal parasympathetic activation.

In order to effectively assess for readiness in any given moment, the therapist does need to know what to do if and when the child emotionally floods. This means that the therapist must understand the signs of emotional flooding, or else it will be more challenging to accurately attune to the child and assess their readiness to keep moving toward the challenge. Therapists must also recognize the signs of emotional flooding within themselves. As we explore the concept of emotional flooding, it is important to realize that *emotional flooding happens in every play therapy model because emotional flooding is part of a relationship*. No one is immune to the experience of emotional flooding. The attuned therapist will experience flooding in the therapy process, as will the child. In all play therapy approaches, both direct and nondirective, as well as in EMDR therapy, emotional flooding will occur.

There are two ways that the body responds to emotional flooding. One way is through excessive sympathetic activation (*escalation*), and the other way is through excessive dorsal parasympathetic activation (*shutdown* or *collapse*). Once a child has emotionally flooded, there is only one task at hand: to create a neuroception of safety and help the child return into their window of tolerance (Dion, 2018). When a brain becomes emotionally flooded, the parts of the brain that can think rationally are temporarily out of service, and their ability to govern themselves quickly diminishes. Attempting to engage children in a discussion about what is happening inside of them or about their behavior will most likely escalate the situation, yet this process is exactly what many children experience. Refer to Exhibit 4.2 for a list of ways to help children regulate their nervous system.

Exhibit 4.2 *Nervous System Regulation Activities From Synergetic Play Therapy*

Synergetic Play Therapy™—Regulation Activities

The following *are some examples of activities that can be used to help regulate a dys-regulated nervous system. It is wise to do these activities pro-actively, as well as in moments of dysregulation. It is also important to follow the body's innate wisdom back to a regulated/ventral state. These activities are important to be done alone AND with someone.*

- Run, jump, spin, dance with pauses to take deep breaths
- Make a game and have the child jump high to touch something high on a wall or in a door frame
- Run, jump, etc., and crash into something soft (i.e., jump on a bed and crash repeatedly)
- Bounce on a yoga ball
- Roll across the floor back and forth
- Sit in a chair and push up with your arms (as if trying to get out of the chair); keep some resistance
- Massages
- Deep pressure on arms and legs (you can slowly apply pressure down arms and legs in a long, stroking motion)
- Eat (particularly something crunchy)
- Drink through a straw

(continued)

Exhibit 4.2 *Nervous System Regulation Activities From Synergetic Play Therapy (continued)*

- Take a bath or shower
- Wrap up in a blanket and snuggle (a little tightly for some pressure); of course, do this safely
- March or sing during transitions
- Play Mozart music in the background during challenging times of the day if in hyperarousal
- Play Hard Rock/Fast/Bass music if in hypoarousal
- Carry heavy things or push heavy things around
- Do isometrics—wall pushups or push hands together (looks like you are praying)
- Walk quickly
- Run up and down steps
- Shake head quickly
- Hang upside down off of a bed or couch
- Play sports
- "Doodle" on paper (this one can be a bit more distracting, but sometimes works)
- Hold or fidget a Koosh ball, rubber band, straw, clay
- Rub gently or vigorously on your skin or clothing
- Put a cold or hot wash cloth on face
- Dim the lights if in hyperarousal
- Turn on the lights if in hypoarousal
- Read a book
- Swing
- Learn about "Brain Gym"—tons of ideas
- Yoga
- Snuggle
- Dance
- Move, move, move—any way that it feels good to your body
- Describe what is happening in your body out loud—"My tummy is going in circles"; "My legs feel heavy"; etc.
- Breathe, breathe, breathe—make sure that your inhalation is the same length as your exhalation

Source: From Dion, L. (2018). *Aggression in play therapy: A neurobiological approach for integrating intensity.* New York, NY: W. W. Norton.

In the counseling profession, therapists are easily drawn into the focus on solutions, with pressure from caregivers, teachers, and insurance companies to fix problems with their clients. Therapists want their clients to experience relief and success, so they are easily lured into helping their clients to calm down and have short-term solutions. Especially when there is pressure from the child's environment, sometimes therapists exchange comfort for the opportunity for growth. Growth occurs when a person is comfortably uncomfortable, not when a person is completely comfortable. From a neuroscience perspective, the child must stay on the edge of their window of tolerance for maximum integration. Also, it is important to know that research shows an attuned caregiver is actually only attuned 30% of the time (Tronick, 2007). This means that even in the best-case scenario, the majority of the time relationship is actually a dance of navigating misattunement! When therapists are overly attached to the idea that they must be attuned for the majority of the time and things like emotional flooding should never happen, they actually miss one of the most important building blocks for creating safety in the therapeutic relationship. It is the act of having an interactive repair that strengthens emotional connection (Bullard, 2015). In fact, it is the dance between the therapist and the child as they repair the ruptures and misattunement that strengthens their relationship and develops trust. Rupture and repair are actually necessary to create attachment!

In the discussion of emotional flooding, it is important to also discuss boundaries. Boundaries are an incredibly important part of the process as they support containment and emotional regulation. From an SPT perspective, the primary reason for setting boundaries during a session that is focused on trauma resolution is to help the therapists stay within their windows of tolerance. When therapists are facilitating the repatterning and the release of stored patterns in the body, it is important that therapists not stop the expression and instead *redirect it*. What this means is that the moment the therapist is no longer able to hold the dysregulation, it is important that a boundary is set to help the therapist continue to access their ventral state and be able to modulate the intensity. Having said this, if there is ever a safety issue, it is important that the therapist does whatever is needed to maintain the safety in the room. When setting a boundary, the first step is to acknowledge the child and the second step is to redirect their expression. In the story of Matthew, there was a moment when he took the tiger and threatened to bite his therapist. If the therapist had felt that this was too activating for her nervous system, the therapist could have set the boundary the following way: "Matthew, you really want me to know how this feels. Show me another way." Notice in this example that Matthew was not told, "No," and his expression was not shut down. Instead, the therapist acknowledged the wisdom in his attempt and then simply told him (not ask) to show her another way so that she could stay present with him in his play. "Show me another way" is considered to be one of two golden phrases in boundary setting in SPT. The other is "I don't have to hurt to understand."

As the therapist sets boundaries, the following are important:

- Taking a deep breath to be grounded.
- Being present so that the child can energetically feel the therapist.
- The therapist uses a nonthreatening yet serious voice.
- Making eye contact when possible, but not forced.
- Acknowledge the child's need before redirecting.
- Keep the therapist's feelings out of it!

As readiness continues to be assessed in the sessions with the child, the other things to look for are the child's current stability not just in the session but also in the child's life. The child's moods and behavior patterns, ability to problem-solve, ability to regulate through emotions, and patterns of sleep, nourishment, and relationships with peers and caregivers are all considered as all of these influence the child's window of tolerance.

There are many reasons that a child may need the support of play therapy and EMDR. Sometimes, it is single-incident events such as auto accidents, fires, personal injuries, experiencing or witnessing a disturbing event that bring a child in for treatment. In other instances, children come to therapy because their symptoms and behaviors are causing disruption to the child, family unit, school, or other social situations. Whatever the reason that brings the children to the therapy, there is one thing they all have in common: Children are struggling with regulating through their dysregulation and integrating whatever aspect of their experience that they perceived or currently are perceiving as challenging. When assessing for the child's readiness, it is equally important to assess the adults' readiness to support the child in their healing. It is often that parents do not fully understand the impact of the events that their child has experienced and so they often dismiss the impact; this too needs to be a part of treatment.

THE PARENT–CHILD DYAD IN THE PLAYROOM

Henry, aged 7, was taken to therapy specifically for EMDR. His mother had experienced EMDR in her own therapy and felt the therapeutic benefit from it and thought that EMDR could help her son through some of his challenges. Henry was adopted from Russia at age 1 and since then has struggled with anger outbursts, often hitting and screaming at his parents. This behavior became so intense that getting him to school in the mornings was often challenging as he would often become violent.

When Henry and his parents sat down on the couch, the therapist could immediately tell that all of them were overwhelmed and emotionally flooded. Henry was not able to make eye contact, his body appeared agitated, and it was clear that he was highly sympathetically aroused. As his parents sat next to him, the therapist could see their own anxiety and fear as Henry's agitation increased. The therapist also sensed that his agitation was not about being in the session; rather this was his ongoing state of activation. His body was in a perpetual fight or flight response, and he was not able to regulate or settle.

In order to begin to regulate Henry to a place where EMDR was even a possibility, she was going to have to regulate his parents first. It is important to share that this therapist was already familiar to Henry, as she often saw him in the waiting room with his father as they waited for his mother to finish her own therapy with another therapist. On a few occasions, they smiled at each other and had a few playful verbal exchanges, a beginning sense of safety.

When parents enter the therapeutic space, it is so important that they are involved. Too often parents are simply witnesses to the play or EMDR. The danger in a parent just being an observer is that the parent is feeling all of the emotions that are arising in the session, even while observing the child doing EMDR, which leads to potential emotional flooding and even retraumatization if the parent was somehow involved in what the child is processing. When a parent is in the room, the therapist is in charge of three nervous systems: the child's, the parent's, and their own. For this reason, it is important to have the parent actively engaged in the process and not be just an observer. It is equally important to prepare parents for the session by helping them understand what to expect and setting them up for success through a separate session with the parents to explain, role play, and prepare.

As the therapist noticed Henry's parents trying to manage his behaviors, she gently explained that in order for them to support Henry, they needed to regulate themselves first to help create a sense of safety and containment for him. She asked them to each take a few deep breaths and notice what they were experiencing inside. His parents were both able to share that they felt nervous and worried about Henry. She invited them to keep breathing and keep noticing. As she worked on helping his parents to let go of attempting to manage Henry's agitation and instead mindfully place their attention on their own experience, Henry immediately began to shift his state. From a neurobiological perspective, as his parents started to regulate themselves in the midst of their own dysregulation, Henry was able to begin to borrow their nervous system regulatory capacity. In SPT, the therapist regulates the parent so that the parent can regulate the child.

Once his parents were grounded in their dysregulation, the next step was to support Henry through his emotional flooding to help him access his own regulatory capacity. As discussed, children must first be within their window of tolerance before applying BLS to decrease the chances of more emotional flooding and dissociation. While the therapist observed Henry, she noticed that his body kept trying to touch everything around him; he would push into pillows, push up against his parents, move around on the couch, and so forth, seeking proprioceptive input in an attempt to ground himself. Proprioception is sometimes referred to as our sixth sense and is the sense of self-movement and body position. While the therapist asked his parents to gently push back toward him to provide a little resistance, she watched Henry very carefully to see his response. When we work with a child in the playroom and especially when the child is right at the edge of their window of tolerance, it is so important to attune moment to moment to watch for signs of emotional flooding or indicators that it is too much. When it is too much, the therapist needs to stop, contain, and create a neuroception of safety. Unless therapists are attuned to themselves and are able to feel what is happening in their own bodies, it will be challenging to attune to the child and to the child's parents. This process is the ongoing personal work as therapists.

Henry responded back with a push and a slight smile. As he pushed, his parents pushed back. Imagine a game of peek-a-boo, except with the body. "Are you there?" his body asked. "We are here," his parents responded. Back and forth and back and forth. It is interesting to point out that he was moving his body from left to right, as he pushed one way into one parent and then the other way into the other parent. He was already seeking out bilateral input organically!

As Henry's affect and body began to indicate that he was starting to internalize the regulation and was back into his window of tolerance, the therapist invited his parents to slowly begin to share what they noticed about the difficulties Henry often experienced in the mornings. As they shared, she invited his father to begin to rub Henry's back with both hands—focusing on pressure in the left hand and then the right hand. Directive EMDR processing had begun. Whenever a parent is invited to touch their child in a session, it is also necessary to tell the child that at any point they get to say, "Stop." They also get to ask for more or less or for the touch to happen in a particular way. It is so important that the child has a voice in how they are touched. This is similar to asking an adult client whether or not they need the BLS to be eye movement, tactile, or sound, to be faster or slower, or louder or quieter. Clients know the level of input they need. As Henry listened to the narrative of his mornings, his father provided the BLS needed to support integration. Also, as his mother shared, the therapist invited her to gently rock back and forth. From this description, it can be recognized that she was including everyone in the process and making sure that everyone was receiving BLS because everyone was affected by the mornings with Henry. As this occurred, the therapist supported the process through her own tracking and breathing. Everyone was coregulating everyone! What happened as a result was quite magical.

Henry's body started to process the story being shared by his parents, moving from a dysregulated affect to a more regulated affect. His face softened. His shoulders dropped. His legs relaxed. His body started to slow down. His eyes closed. Once they finished processing the events of the morning times, he was curled up in a fetal position on his mother's lap. At this point, they moved right into installing the positive cognition using "I am safe." His mother repeated softly, "You are safe," while his dad alternated between tapping and rubbing his back. Henry quietly took deep breaths as he let the message enter his body that lived in a daily state of not feeling safe.

Here is another example of how to work with the parent–child dyad when the parent is in the room and the child engages in play. Six-year-old Laura and her mother walked into the playroom. As her mother sat on the couch, Laura grabbed the handcuffs and handcuffed her. Her mother, stunned, did not know what to do. Feeling the shock, the therapist immediately oriented to the mother to support her. Her mother had been a part of their play therapy sessions before and therefore knew to have an authentic and genuine reaction to the play, but before she could say anything Laura had grabbed a scary puppet and was moving quickly toward her mother. "I feel scared. I am trapped and I am not safe," her mother was finally able to say. The therapist supported her by breathing with her through the intensity. Laura's face indicated that she knew her mother understood what she was trying to say. She then walked over to the sand tray and began sifting the sand back and forth in her hands. Her mother and the therapist proceeded to sit next to her as she explored the sand. As she sifted the sand, the therapist quietly said the words "left," "right," "left," "right" as she moved the sand bilaterally back and forth. Ten minutes later, Laura announced that she saw something scary. She begins to share that she had a friend over at her house last week. Laura had left the room to use the restroom and when she returned to the living room, her friend had turned the television on and had the screen held on pause waiting to show her a trailer to a movie that had just come out. The trailer included a violent scene where people were being attacked by sharks, and it terrified her so much that she had regressed at night and was now having trouble sleeping.

It is worth pausing for a minute to understand the play that she initiated with her mother when they first walked into the room. In less than a minute, Laura created an experience with the handcuffs and the puppet to help her mother feel the shock, the fear, and the sense of being trapped that she felt the moment the trailer played. Her mother allowed herself to feel it, she regulated through it, and she named it. This experience is what allowed Laura to feel *felt* by her mother, which allowed the play to then shift toward regulation in the sand and eventually allowed her to be able to safely talk about what happened.

Once the therapist heard the story about what happened, the therapist made a decision. She could have continued with imaginative play, adding in BLS when necessary, but this time asked Laura if she would like to do something to help her not feel so scared. Laura said she would. The therapist then explained the EMDR process to her, and they spent the rest of the session using the standard EMDR protocol to help clear both the fear and shock that were still stuck in her body. Incorporating parents into the play process can be incredibly impactful, but there are a few considerations that need to be made when figuring out whether or not to have the parent be a part of the play or the EMDR process. Here are a few things to consider:

- Does the therapist know the parent's trauma history?
- Does the parent want to be in the session? (Sometimes, a resistant parent in the room can create a barrier, so the therapist needs to be willing to work with the resistance.)
- How wide is the parent's window of tolerance for what the child is trying to integrate?
- How developed is the parent's regulatory capacity?
- How emotionally available is the parent?

Knowing the answers to these questions can guide the therapist to know how much preparation work may be needed to do with a parent and whether or not having the parent in the room will be a supportive experience for the child as the child works toward integration. Regardless of whether or not the parent is a part of the sessions, it is important to have their involvement as much as possible.

DEVELOPING EMOTIONAL RESOURCES

As mentioned earlier, we see resource work as important to include in every session. Developing emotional resources is just one area of resource development; however, it is at the core of the loss experienced with a child's chronic misattunement with caregivers. In the case examples we have given thus far, we have shown that the resolution of upsetting events results in the repatterning of the nervous system. The process of working through the activation of unresolved memory does enable children to develop emotional expression and capacities for handling life experiences. Case examples presented have also illustrated the use of the reevaluation and closure phases of EMDR for resource development. In the preparation phase of EMDR, therapists assess the child's ability to access inner resources, and resources for connection in their environment. Preparation phase is focused on the building of adaptive memory networks, which are made up of both positive experiences and difficult experiences mastered. This phase is not one a client goes through once to get ready to face their work, but it is used continuously throughout the treatment process. Preparation-phase work in EMDR will take place at any time a child needs a strengthening or building of adaptive networks. The AIP system is always operating on our behalf, except when it has become stuck with whatever we have experienced that has overwhelmed our system. Likewise, our emotional signals are also operating continuously on our behalf unless they have become stuck because the expression is met with shaming or intimidation from the external environment. These important signals are then deemed as a threat to survival and are subsequently distorted or shut off. The suppression of emotion stops the flow of energy in our system. Chronic suppression leads to the numbing of the signals and can also be the catalyst for the development of anxiety, depression, and pain patterns in the body. It is true there can be a wide variation of the amount of resource development each child needs. All of these factors affect the level of expression of the child in therapy.

The emotional resources needed to navigate life include being able to feel emotions in the body, the ability to settle ourselves down when upset, to have patterns of healthy self-care, and to reflect on our experiences. Children are in the developmental stages of discovery and highly reliant on adult caregivers to teach them how to navigate these stages. Lucky is the child who has a caregiver who experienced the successful navigation of all these tasks!

What parents did not learn, they cannot pass on. Teaching skills to children with the parent or caregiver present is an opportune time to teach to the caregiver a skill they may not have ever learned. It can be done in a way that honors the caregiver as a mentor, and when asked to do it with the child, allows them to learn it themselves. There are many creative ways to help children learn about emotions, and healthful expression of them. Many parents need this education as well. Learning and practicing state change repeatedly in therapy are usually necessary before a child can use it independently. Music, metaphor, and story are ways to reach beyond the conscious mind. State change skills combined with mental rehearsal for upcoming difficult experiences are resources needed to manage life in between therapy sessions. Neuroplastic treatments have been developed to treat a host of neurological and physical problems and impairments. Examples include biofeedback, neurofeedback, meridian, and sensorimotor therapies. It is important for therapists to understand the need for physical health treatment modalities, which also bring change to the neurology of the brain.

REPROCESSING TRAUMA WITH SPT/EMDR

In the following case study, the therapist was able to flow back and forth between directive and nondirective EMDR application while engaging the child in SPT.

Scarlet first began play therapy to support her through her parent's divorce. Scarlet often found herself in the middle of her parent's tension and anger during hand-offs, and, as a result, Scarlet would often act out before and after. Scarlet had a successful SPT experience as the therapist worked with both her and her parents to resolve many of the challenges and create a new experience for Scarlet during the transitions. One day, the therapist received a phone call informing her that there had been an incident between Scarlet and a neighborhood boy. Scarlet was 8 years old, and the neighborhood boy was 11 years old. The mother shared that Scarlet had gone over to his house and according to Scarlet, the boy asked her to go into a back bedroom and then had coerced her into having intercourse with him.

When Scarlet came in to the next session, the therapist first allowed her to just begin to play. Through Scarlet's play, she began to bring to life the thoughts, feelings, and sensations that she experienced during the event. Scarlet engaged the therapist in dramatic play telling her that she was going to go on an adventure to a castle. The therapist embodied the role, authentically expressing her excitement about the adventure. Once the therapist arrived at the castle, Scarlet became a scary monster making noises trying to scare the therapist. At this point, the therapist activated her ventral state by taking deep breaths, becoming the external regulator and beginning to regulate through the intensity to support Scarlet's ability to stay within her window of tolerance, activate dual awareness, and keep her moving toward the activation that was occurring inside of her. The therapist continued to respond authentically, knowing that Scarlet was offering her an opportunity through the play to experience the fear that she had experienced; then, the therapist modeled how to regulate through it. The therapist did not force Scarlet to talk about what happened.

In the second play therapy session, the therapist decided to share with Scarlet that she knew about what had happened as an invitation to discuss it directly. The therapist simply said, "I just want you to know that I know what happened." That was all that was said. This type of statement gives the child permission to choose whether or not they want to verbally talk without feeling pressure from the therapist to talk about it. We understand that play is the child's primary form of communication and will say everything they need to without the use of words. Scarlet did choose to share. After she shared what had happened, the therapist decided to talk to her about using EMDR as a way to help integrate her experience. Scarlet was open to this idea.

When EMDR was first introduced to Scarlet, it was with the demonstration of BLS. When the therapist placed the buzzers, a common nickname for a tactile BLS device, in her hands and turned them on, Scarlet immediately flooded. This was not a result of the intensity or speed of the vibration, but rather that there was a vibration. What became clear immediately was that part of what Scarlet was attempting to integrate was the felt sense of the experience in and on her body. Her body was hypersensitive and defensive to touch, so the vibration was too much. The therapist recognized the flooding and quickly began to create a neuroception of safety for her. They stood up and coregulated by breathing deeply and moving to release the activation from her body. Keep in mind that the flooding occurred before Safe Place or containment were established, so the therapist adjusted quickly to help Scarlet. Once Scarlet was able to return to her window of tolerance, the therapist invited her to think about a Safe Place. Scarlet chose a scene of an ocean that was hanging on the wall in the play therapy room. Scarlet chose to imagine herself there as she stood in front of the picture and was instructed to gently rock back and forth while looking at it to help lock it into her adaptive memory network.

Once the resourcing was complete, the therapist chose to allow her to process through play the rest of the session. Scarlet continued with themes of fear and lack of safety. The therapist continued using observational and reflective statements, modeling regulation and creatively incorporating BLS when possible.

At the third session, the therapist decided to try again with directive EMDR application. Recognizing that any form of input directly into the body would be too much for Scarlet, the therapist knew that tapping on her or even the audio beep would most likely be outside of her window of tolerance. This part of the story is highlighted because it is so important that we continuously work toward making sure that the client is near the edge of their window of tolerance but not over it. In order for this to occur, therapists must be willing to feel the activation in their own bodies or else they will miss the cues that allow for attunement. Scarlet and her therapist eventually decided to use art for the desensitization phase; for further containment, they created a folder in which she could keep the art. At the end of every session, Scarlet would place the art in the folder and she and the therapist would put it away for safekeeping. Due to the intensity of the work, the therapist worked carefully to titrate the experience, constantly watching for signs of flooding. Most of the sessions were a combination of directive EMDR and play, with nondirective EMDR woven in to enhance the continued integration in the play.

To prepare for the art, the therapist asked Scarlet to think about what bothered her most about the incident. As Scarlet was thinking about it, she said, "I didn't feel safe," which was already the offering of the negative cognition. The therapist asked her how she would like to feel as she thought about it. Scarlet's answer was quite interesting. She said, "Do you know what I really want to be able to do?" She then shared that she wanted to be able to see the boy in the neighborhood and not feel scared. Notice that Scarlet was already identifying for herself what empowerment and integration would look like. She was also identifying "I am safe" as her positive cognition. Together they decided to set this as a treatment goal. Scarlet was then asked to notice where in her body she felt the activation when she recalled the incident. The final question before drawing was asking Scarlet to show her with her hands how disturbing the incident felt. Scarlet stretched her arms out wide to her sides and said, "this much." Scarlet was then asked to draw *whatever came to mind* as she thought about the incident.

Scarlet's first drawing was of a spider with red eyes. Once she completed the drawing, the therapist asked her to track the therapist's fingers back and forth to apply the BLS for 45 seconds. The therapist then asked Scarlet to draw *what came to mind next*. Her second drawing was a page of many spiders, and then BLS was applied for 45 seconds. Her final drawing was a stick figure person lying down looking up while spiders came down toward her from up above. A few of the spiders had reached her body (BLS again).

Recall what happened to Scarlet. Now, imagine that was you. Read it again, if needed.

Notice the activation inside of you. Are you feeling anxious? What feelings are you noticing?

What is happening in your body? How is your breathing?

(continued)

(continued)

> Whatever you are experiencing is quite possibly a glimpse of what you would also be experiencing if you were watching her create the drawings in front of you. Your mirror neurons and nervous system activation are helping you get a felt sense of her experience during the trauma.
>
> Now, practice being the external regulator right now!
>
> Activate your ventral state as you feel the dysregulation. Take a deep breath. Name your internal experience to yourself. Move your body. Whatever feels right for you right now in this moment.
>
> The risk of not doing this is that the activation will get stored in your system, and you will set yourself up over time for compassion fatigue and vicarious trauma.

Once the third drawing was complete, the attuned therapist sensed it would be helpful to move back to play to give Scarlet a break from the intensity of the anxiety that was arising through her drawings. This time Scarlet engaged the therapist in a scene where an intruder came into the home to attack the therapist. And as the dysregulation and intensity arose in the play, the therapist continued to be the external regulator modulating the intensity with external regulation and BLS.

The next three sessions progressed in a similar way. Sometimes, they would play first and then make art, and sometimes they would make art first and then play. Her art progressed as follows: The spiders turned into a figure of a boy with red eyes. Then, the stick figure who now looked like a girl was lying down yelling "Help!" From there a scene emerged where the girl was being laughed at by the boy. And finally, the trauma itself emerged in a scene with the boy lying on top of the girl, who now had a face. All of her drawings were black and white, with the exception of the red eyes. During each session, her play paralleled the feelings that she was recreating in the art. Although she never literally played out the scene, what did emerge was the implicit memory and stored activation. The feelings of intrusion, anxiety, paralysis, being trapped and overwhelmed, as well as a loss of control all emerged. During her play, BLS continued to be applied wherever possible. Sometimes, the therapist would sway side to side or engage in other bilateral movement in her visual field. On one occasion, Scarlet picked up a set of simulated play swords (foam pool noodles cut in half) and banged them on the wall, one in each hand. This came at a point in the play where a monster was about to attack and no one could move. Scarlet grabbed the swords in self-defense (empowerment), stood up, and hit the wall. Her body was repatterning and releasing the implicitly stored trauma. The therapist quickly jumped up and grabbed another set of swords and stood next to her and invited her for a minute to just alternate hitting the swords back and forth on the wall. The therapist did it with her for support. On another occasion, the therapist was set up to be trapped; as Scarlet watched her, the therapist squeezed her own arm and then her other arm, alternating the squeezes. As Scarlet watched, her mirror neuron system activated a similar experience inside of her body. As this case illustrates, there are so many ways to weave BLS into play, making this work creative, spontaneous, organic, and attuned to the child's needs. Whether Scarlet was processing her trauma through EMDR or play, it was the therapist acting as the external regulator and modulating the intensity that allowed the child to process quickly and fluidly. Scarlet's desensitization process was four sessions in total. On the fourth session, Scarlet drew two final drawings. The first was an image of the girl yelling at the boy, "No! Stop! I am going to tell!" and the boy appearing scared. In this drawing, for the first time, the girl was much larger in size than the boy. In Scarlet's final drawing, she drew a sun. Under the sun stood the girl and the boy. The girl was smiling and looking at the boy and out of her mouth were the words, "Hi!" In her final drawing, the goal Scarlet identified was achieved. Her drawing was in full color. In her play, there were no intruders or monsters. She finally felt safe.

CONCLUSION

Whether you are an EMDR therapist learning play therapy, or a play therapist learning EMDR, common elements in both therapies (when emphasized and combined) allow the therapist and child to flow together in seamlessly blending modalities, creating new opportunities for integration. The phases of this combined therapy process are able to be both directive and nondirective in application, determined by the interchange between child and therapist, the task at hand, and the expressed communications from the child. The therapist, becoming the external regulator, creates a neuroception of safety so the child is able to rock within the embrace of their ventral states leading to faster and deeper transformation. It is the synergy of the therapist's authenticity, attunement, congruence, and nervous system regulation that supports the child to continue to safely move toward the maladaptively stored memories and ultimately process these memories to adaptive resolution and empowerment.

REFERENCES

Adler-Tapia, R., & Settle, C. (2016). *EMDR and the art of psychotherapy with children, infants to adolescents.* New York, NY: Springer Publishing Company.
Badenoch, B. (2008). *Being a brain-wise therapist: A practical guide to interpersonal neurobiology.* New York, NY: W. W. Norton.
Badenoch, B. (2017). *The heart of trauma.* New York, NY: W. W. Norton.
Bandura, A. (1977). *Social learning theory.* Upper Saddle River, NJ: Prentice Hall.
Bullard, D. (2015). *Allan Schore on the science of the art of psychotherapy.* Retrieved from www.psychotherapy.net/interview/allan-schore-neuroscience-psychotherapy
Dion, L. (2018). *Aggression in play therapy: A neurobiological approach for integrating intensity.* New York, NY: W. W. Norton.

Dion, L., & Gray, K. (2014). Impact of therapist authentic expression on emotional tolerance in synergetic play therapy. *International Journal of Play Therapy, 23,* 55–67. doi:10.1037/a0035495

Edelman, G. M. (1987). *Neural Darwinism.* New York, NY: Basic Books.

Fuller, R. B., & Applewhite, E. J. (1975). *Synergetics: Explorations in the geometry of thinking.* New York, NY: Macmillan.

Goddard, G. V., McIntyre, D. C., & Leetch, C. K. (1969). A permanent change in brain function resulting from daily electrical stimulation. *Experimental Neurology, 25*(3), 295–330. doi:10.1016/0014-4886(69)90128-9

Gomez, A. (2012). *EMDR therapy and adjunct approaches with children.* New York, NY: Springer Publishing Company.

Heyes, C. (2009). Evolution, development and intentional control of imitation. *Philosophical Transactions of the Royal Society B, 364,* 2293–2298. doi:10.1098/rstb.2009.0049

Iacoboni, M. (2007). Face to face: The neural basis for social mirroring and empathy. *Psychiatric Annals, 37*(4), 236–241. doi:10.3928/00485713-20070401-05

Iacoboni, M. (2008). *Mirroring people: The new science of how we connect with others.* New York, NY: Farrar, Straus and Giroux.

Kestly, T. (2014). *The interpersonal neurobiology of play: Brain-building interventions for emotional well-being.* New York, NY: W. W. Norton.

Kestly, T. (2016). Presence and play: Why mindfulness matters. *International Journal of Play Therapy, 1,* 14–23. doi:10.1037/pla0000019

Korn, D., & Leeds, A. (2002). Preliminary evidence of efficacy for EMDR resource development and installation in the stabilization phase of treatment of complex posttraumatic stress disorder. *Journal of Clinical Psychology, 58*(12), 1465–1487. doi:10.1002/jclp.10099

Lovett, J. (2014). *The trauma attachment tangle: Modifying EMDR to help children resolve trauma and develop loving relationships.* New York, NY: Taylor & Francis.

Ogden, P., Minton, K., & Pain, C. (2006). *Trauma and the body: A sensorimotor approach to psychotherapy.* New York, NY: W. W. Norton.

Perry, B. D. (2006). Applying principles of neurodevelopment to clinical work with maltreated and traumatized children: The neurosequential model of therapeutics. In N. B. Webb (Ed.), *Working with traumatized youth in child welfare.* New York, NY: Guilford Press.

Porges, S. (2011). *The polyvagal theory: Neurophysiological foundations of emotions, attachment, communication, and self-regulation.* New York, NY: W. W. Norton.

Rizzolatti, G., Fogassi, L., & Gallese, V. (2001). Neurophysiological mechanisms underlying the understanding and imitation of action. *Nature Review Neuroscience, 2,* 660–670. doi:10.1038/35090060

Rogers, C. (1980). *A way of being.* New York, NY: Houghton Mifflin.

Scaer, R. (2005). *The trauma spectrum: Hidden wounds and human resiliency.* New York, NY: W. W. Norton.

Scaer, R. (2012). *8 keys to brain-body balance.* New York, NY: W. W. Norton.

Schore, A. N. (1994). *Affect regulation and the origin of the self: The neurobiology of emotional development.* New York, NY: Erlbaum.

Schore, A. N. (2019). *Right brain psychotherapy.* New York, NY: W. W. Norton.

Shapiro, F. (2001). *Eye movement desensitization and reprocessing (EMDR) therapy: Basic principles, protocols, and procedures* (2nd ed.). New York, NY: Guilford Press.

Shapiro, F. (Ed.). (2002). *EMDR as an integrative psychotherapy approach.* Washington, DC: American Psychological Association.

Shapiro, F. (2018). *Eye movement desensitization and reprocessing (EMDR) therapy: Basic principles, protocols, and procedures* (3rd ed.). New York, NY: Guilford Press.

Sieff, D. F. (Ed.). (2015). *Understanding and healing emotional trauma: Conversations with pioneering clinicians and researchers.* London, UK: Routledge.

Siegel, D. J. (1999). *The developing mind: How relationships and the brain interact to shape who we are.* New York, NY: Guilford Press.

Siegel, D. J. (2010). *The mindful therapist: A clinician's guide to mindsight and neural integration.* New York, NY: W. W. Norton.

Tronick, E. (2007). *The neurobehavioral and social-emotional development of infants and children.* New York, NY: W. W. Norton.

Tyson, P. (2002). The challenges of psychoanalytic developmental theory. *Journal of the American Psychoanalytic Association, 50*(1), 19–52. doi:10.1177/00030651020500011301

Van der Kolk, B. (2014). *The body keeps the score.* New York, NY: Penguin Random House.

5

Treating Trauma in Young Children: Integrating EMDR, Child-Centered Play Therapy, and Developmental Play Therapy

ROXANNE GROBBEL

"He dropped into my lap and allowed me to gently rock him from side to side. I could feel him starting to relax as I hummed a song that I used to sing to my own children while I tapped his left and right knees interchangeably."
—Excerpt from the case of Peter, a 5-year-old boy

INTRODUCTION

In this chapter, we review how clinicians can combine play therapy skills with eye movement desensitization and reprocessing (EMDR) therapy to treat young children who have experienced trauma. We present a descriptive approach to integrating play therapy skills with the EMDR protocol for therapists already using play to facilitate trauma. Young children's trauma often arises from early neglect and abuse, resulting in emotional dysregulation and inappropriate behaviors. This type of interpersonal trauma impacts all areas of their development, especially attachment. Child-centered play therapy (CCPT), developmental play therapy (DPT), and EMDR are interventions that address these issues and are also effective relational therapies that can be even more powerful when combined. These therapies complement each other to allow successful treatment of complex trauma in our youngest clients. Through examples and a case study, therapists will appreciate how play therapy and EMDR work well together and how clinicians' play therapy skills can be easily incorporated into all phases of the EMDR protocol.

A CASE STUDY FOR INTEGRATING CCPT, DPT, AND EMDR: INTRODUCING PETER

Peter was a 5-year-old boy who had recently been adopted by his mother's maternal aunt, Suzie (all names and identifiable information have been changed in this case study to protect the client's and his family's privacy). Peter had arrived at my office with a history that included numerous diagnoses: attention deficit hyperactivity disorder (ADHD), oppositional defiant disorder, and bipolar disorder. He was on several medications when Aunt Suzie had gained custody, but she had been weaning him off of the medications because she did not think that any of them worked. Peter's mother had reportedly used and sold drugs, and it was believed that she had not had stable housing while Peter was with her. Peter's father had not been a part of his life. Peter had come into state custody after the police responded to a call about a toddler wandering the street at 10 p.m. At that point, the police had found 3-1/2-year-old Peter, unkempt, wearing a diaper that had not been changed in days, malnourished, and with bruises on his body. He had been removed from his mother's custody and placed in numerous foster care homes as well as with several different members of his mother's family. Family and foster families would not care for Peter very long because his behavior was aggressive and "out of control." At one point, he slept at a different place every night for a full month.

TRAUMA AND ADAPTIVE INFORMATION PROCESSING

Sadly, Peter's case is far from rare. Young children (under 6 years of age) are a vulnerable population as they have the highest rate of neglect, representing almost 50% of child maltreatment victims in the United States (U.S. Department of Health and Human Services, 2018). The majority of children coming into therapy have a history of some form of trauma or neglect. Young children are often referred for services due to behaviors such as refusal to follow directions, hitting, kicking, biting, crying, temper tantrums, and an inability to get along with peers. Frequently, parents or caregivers report that they have tried everything, that their child acts out for "no reason," and that they are angry and frustrated. Many of those children may even be facing expulsion from school (or preschool). These children are often given negative labels such as bad, defiant, or manipulative or even given inaccurate mental health diagnoses such as ADHD, ODD, or bipolar disorder because their behaviors are not recognized as symptoms of trauma and/or neglect. However, in reality these children are doing the best they can do to get their needs met in the face of trauma (Perry & Dobson, 2009; van der Kolk, 2005, 2014). In the case of Peter, this line of thinking had led him to be heavily medicated rather than being given trauma-informed therapy services. As such, there is a need for continued education of both trauma theory and interventions among providers.

In order to understand how trauma affects the brain, knowledge of EMDR's Adaptive Information Processing (AIP) model is helpful. This model suggests that the client's symptoms result from these events being maladaptively recorded in memory and/or incompletely processed (Shapiro, 2017), consequently becoming traumatic. Such traumatic events are stored in fragments in implicit memory, where they cannot be recalled, but where they continue to run in the background and easily become triggered (van der Kolk, 2014), thus producing symptoms. For example, children who were physically abused by a caregiver record those memories maladaptively in implicit memory. This means that the memory is stored in fragmented pieces in the subconscious mind. Negative learned beliefs ("I'm not good enough," "Adults are dangerous and can't be trusted") and corresponding emotional responses (panic, terror, guilt) and behavioral reactions (run, fight, shut down) develop as the child attempts to make sense of their world. These negative memories continue to run in the background of their minds so that any similar event triggers an immediate reaction, as if the traumatic event was actually happening again. This explanation helps in understanding why abused children, like Peter, will often continue to mistrust adults, and when an adult raises his voice, Peter may react aggressively or try to run away, even if this is an adult who has never actually hurt Peter. In this case, the message that Peter learned was that adults cannot be trusted and that he must always fight to keep himself safe. He would frequently be triggered by things that reminded him of his abuse from his mother (although he was not able to identify those triggers as the memory was stored in his subconscious mind). These trauma-reactive behaviors continue to happen even when children are in a safe home with safe adults, because they are often triggered by similar events and respond to the old, unprocessed trauma. Children cannot access those events stored in implicit memory in order to change their behavior or emotions, and unfortunately, they develop self-beliefs that they are not good enough or that they are not deserving of love. These beliefs and isolated memories become activated when triggered by similar reminders and cause them to respond with aggressive behaviors and high emotions to keep themselves safe from the perceived threat.

Not only do children with a history of trauma often respond to trauma triggers, they are also more likely to perceive future events as dangerous and be more vulnerable to future trauma (van der Kolk, 2014), thus compounding the problem. Those children are triggered by perceived threats (which others often see as nonthreatening) and respond for survival. In Peter's case, he would often perceive many actions as threatening, such as another child touching/bumping him and/or an adult telling him it was time to leave. Similarly, traumatized children adopted into safe homes often continue to lie, be defiant (refuse to follow directions), and act impulsively (stealing, hoarding) in response to the trauma that they have experienced. Unfortunately, these are trauma survival behaviors that are often mislabeled as deliberate, bad, and punishable.

TRAUMA'S LONG-TERM EFFECT ON SOCIAL, EMOTIONAL, AND BEHAVIORAL DEVELOPMENT

The negative effect of neglect and abuse on social, emotional, and behavioral development has been well documented. Children who have suffered through abuse, neglect, chronic stress, and interventions such as removal from home, foster care, or legal system frequently will have increased emotional and behavioral issues as opposed to children who have been living in nurturing and supportive environments (Stirling & Amaya-Jackson, 2015). And yet, these traumatized children are often expected to immediately change their behaviors when taken from an abusive situation. Being removed from parents, even neglectful, abusive ones, can be traumatizing in itself. Chronic stress, abuse, and neglect cause the brain to wire for the environment, and it takes time and intervention for the brain to reorganize (Keyser & Ahn, 2017; Painter & Scannapieco, 2013; Perry, 2009). Adverse childhood events occur more frequently and across economic and social statuses than most people, even therapists, believe. The extent and magnitude of their impact extends well into adulthood (Felitti et al., 1998), with a correlation between the number and types of childhood trauma and the complexity of symptoms in adulthood, including family/peer/work relationships, physical health, problems with the legal system, and educational and career achievement (Cloitre et al., 2009; Felitti et al., 1998). And yet, there are people who still believe that because an event happens at 3 years of age, it will not have a lasting effect. I remember a child welfare worker trying to reassure me about a little boy who had been badly neglected and abused: "Don't worry. He is only 3, and he'll never remember it." Hopefully, in time providers across the board will be adequately educated.

TRAUMA AND ATTACHMENT

In additional to complex trauma, Peter had also experienced severe neglect during the formative years when his attachment system was developing (ages 0–3). Attachment is the reciprocal, enduring, emotional, and physical connection between a child and a caregiver (Bowlby, 1969). Those early attachment relationships between the infant and caregiver determine lifelong relationships and physical, emotional, and brain development. When children have a stable, attentive caregiver, who responds in a consistent manner the majority of times, children are able to explore their world, gain a sense of safety and trust, learn cognitive skills, and develop social skills and relationships (Bowlby, 1988; Schore & Schore, 2014). Attentive caregivers provide a sense of direction, a scaffolding of how to act and what to do in the world. From these responses, children develop positive self-beliefs, the ability to trust, the capacity to regulate, and the capability to form and maintain relationships from secure attachments (Bowlby, 1969). Children also learn to regulate and self-soothe through this attachment relationship. When an infant is distressed, it is through closeness to their caregiver that stress is reduced (Bowlby, 1988). In order words, the caregivers coregulate the sense for the distressed infant (and later toddler/child), who over time will internalize this regulation independently. As such, the attachment relationship allows brain rhythms to be in tune and, ultimately, for infants to manage stress. Children's ability to emotionally and physically regulate is learned through attachment behaviors such as when the child cries and the caregiver responds by picking up the child and rocking them. That sense of being soothed is encoded in implicit memory and becomes the mental model of attachment (Siegel, 1999), which fosters what Bowlby termed the internal working model (Bowlby, 1969, 1988; Schore, 2009). By being understood and cared for by the caregiver, children learn to regulate, develop positive beliefs about themselves, and trust themselves. This dance of accurately perceiving and responding to children's signals increases the children's positive emotional states and helps to modulate their negative states. It allows children to understand themselves in relation to others and interact in appropriate ways (Siegel, 2012).

No one had been there to provide such responses and coregulating activities for Peter during the early years of this life. He had not learned to regulate his emotional or physical state. As is often the case in neglect or abuse and where attuned attachment responses are lacking, he had also become fearful to initiate actions, had difficulty concentrating/following directions, and had poor social skills and relationships. This also caused him to struggle with anxiety/fear; lack of trust; speech and motor skill delays; hyperarousal; and compromised emotional, physical, and mental development (Perry & Dobson, 2009). As we will see later, Peter struggled with negative beliefs about himself (I'm not good enough, I'm bad, I'm not lovable) due to his trauma and lack of attachment. Eventually, he had been labeled as bad and defiant and blamed when he could not "settle down" or "control himself."

In summary, young children with ruptured/insecure attachment and complex trauma often present with such extensive developmental delays and mental health problems, including dissociative disorders, affect dysregulation, loss of impulse control, concentration difficulties, self-perception difficulties, and somatization and personality disorders (Cloitre et al., 2009; van der Kolk et al., 2005), that clinicians and researchers have proposed a distinct diagnosis of developmental trauma disorder (D'Andrea, Ford, Stolbach, Spinazzola, & van der Kolk, 2012; Spinazzola, van der Kolk, & Ford, 2018; van der Kolk, 2005). Complex trauma causes extensive damage and has far-reaching impact psychologically, biologically, and interpersonally on young children. In order to treat children and prevent the long-term effects, therapists must understand how complex trauma impacts children's developmental stages, brain development, and attachment, resulting in inappropriate behaviors and defenses (Cloitre et al., 2009; Kinniburgh, Blaustein, Spinazzola, & van der Kolk, 2005). Without an attachment relationship, there is no opportunity for the child to develop appropriately neurologically, socially, emotionally, or behaviorally. Therapists can utilize interventions such as CCPT, DPT, and EMDR in order to repair this lack of attachment and foster social, emotional, and behavioral growth.

TREATING CHILDREN WHO HAVE SUFFERED TRAUMA AND NEGLECT: WHY PLAY THERAPY?

Play therapy has long been used by therapists to allow children to process trauma within a safe attuned relationship (Axline, 1947; Gil, 2016; Goodyear-Brown, 2010; Landreth, 2012). The Association for Play Therapy defines play therapy as "the systematic use of a theoretical model to establish an interpersonal process wherein trained play therapists use the therapeutic powers of play to help clients prevent or resolve psychosocial difficulties and achieve optimal growth and development" (Association for Play Therapy, 2019b). The processing often takes the form of repetitively playing out those aspects of the event that are painful and allowing the trauma story (actual or in metaphor) to find an adaptive ending (Gil, 2016; Goodyear-Brown, 2010; Landreth, 2012). Through play, social and emotional skills are learned in a relationship context that can positively impact attachment. Most importantly, play therapy is a relational therapy (Axline, 1947, 1969; Brody, 1997; Gil, 2016; Landreth, 2012).

Play allows for a sensory expression of the trauma event and healing, a mind–body integration that is key to trauma resolution (van der Kolk, 2014). It has a "bottom-up approach" versus a "top-down approach," such as with cognitive behavioral therapy, in that it starts with the brainstem and action versus the cortex and thinking (Perry, 2009). Play and expressive art can enhance children's ability to communicate, retrieve memories, and link implicit and explicit memories (Malchiodi, 2014). These interventions also help children physically regulate in response to emotion or test new ways to regulate, resulting in a sense of relief in being able to master their bodies' responses to trauma (Levine, 2002; Malchiodi, 2014). Research has verified that play and relationship can therapeutically alter the brain structure (Siegel, 2012). It has been found that just the experience of play can be regulating (Hong & Mason, 2016; Panksepp & Biven, 2012) and rhythmic, and that repetitive play helps to organize/reorganize the brain (Perry, 2009). Since play therapy establishes a warm, caring relationship, it is consistent with brain research findings that feeling understood and connected to an adult is necessary for calming a child's limbic system and regulating a child's developing brain (Hong & Mason, 2016; Panksepp & Biven, 2012; Perry, 2009; Schore, 2001; Siegel, 2012; Sroufe, Coffino, & Carlson, 2010).

Today there are numerous play therapy models under the play therapy umbrella in addition to CCPT and DPT: sandtray/sandplay, family play therapy, filial play therapy, group play therapy, gestalt play therapy, Theraplay, and FirstPlay® therapy. While this chapter focuses on CCPT and DPT, therapists should have a number of play modalities with which they are familiar. Young children often require the use of varied models to meet their diverse and shifting needs.

CHILD-CENTERED PLAY THERAPY

CCPT has become a highly researched intervention and has been found to be effective with diverse populations of children and issues (Bratton, Ray, Rhine, & Jones, 2005), and as a result, it has gained acceptance in the clinical community. CCPT is "a way of being" with a child rather than a set of prescribed activities. Virginia Axline (1947) developed CCPT from Carl Rogers's (1980) person-centered theory. Axline applied the person-centered principles of congruence, acceptance, empathy, and unconditional positive regard to her work with children, ultimately naming it nondirective play therapy (Axline, 1947). An extensive body of research, including four meta analyses, supports the effectiveness of CCPT as intervention for children with a wide range of mental health issues with positive outcomes for externalizing and internalizing behaviors, caregiver–child relationship stress, self-efficacy, social/emotional adjustment, and academics (Bratton, Ray, Rhine, & Jones, 2005; Lin & Bratton, 2015; Ray, Armstrong, Balkin, & Jayne, 2015).

CCPT is based on the tenet that children communicate naturally through play as it is their first language and toys become their words. In CCPT, children are allowed to freely express themselves through play so they may act out what they are unable to verbalize; as such, it is the most effective means through which adults can understand and guide children (Axline, 1969; Kottman, 1995; Landreth, 2012). This is especially important when working with younger children who are at a great disadvantage communicating verbally or when working with children like Peter who are unable to verbalize traumatic experiences at first. Through play children express feelings and thoughts; develop physical, cognitive, and social skills; foster relationships; and learn about their world (Axline, 1969; Landreth, 2012).

The principal healing feature of CCPT is the therapeutic relationship (Axline, 1969; Landreth, 2012). This relationship is essential so that children feel safe enough to express themselves and process the trauma. Within that relationship, children can use toys and play to express their feelings and demonstrate how they have been affected by what they have experienced, while the therapist allows them to be "heard" and provides a corrective emotional response. For example, when Peter would play out being hurt, as a play therapist I needed to respond with empathy and nurturance, which may be different from what he had previously experienced, such as being ignored or yelled at. In this way, he could begin to process the trauma or neglect he had experienced, and I could help him to better understand the experience while fostering attachment (Perry & Dobson, 2009).

Because of its focus on relationship, CCPT can help facilitate engagement with children with complex trauma who lack trust (Struik, Ensink, & Lindauer, 2017) and help them to regulate emotions and process trauma by creating a safe, accepting, nonjudgmental relationship (Axline, 1969; Brody, 1997; Landreth, 2012). Therapy proceeds at the child's pace, creating time for trust to develop and for the therapist to make a more thorough assessment regarding the children's fears, responses, trauma history, triggers, and negative beliefs. Parents or caregivers can participate in the play process through filial therapy (Guerney, 1964), in which parents learn the therapeutic skills of CCPT. In my work with Peter, I also included Aunt Suzie in many sessions so she was able to respond to Peter in a therapeutic manner at home. Parental involvement can increase the effectiveness of EMDR and play therapy (Gomez, 2013; Wesselmann, Armstrong, Schweitzer, Davidson, & Potter, 2018), as was the case with Peter.

I consider CCPT as my foundation intervention with children. Although I am a CCPT therapist, I recognize its limitations and that there are times that I need to be more directive and offer choices that are more appropriate for what the child is experiencing. Being attuned and responsive to the child requires flexibility on the part of the therapist. If Peter came to the session dysregulated and operating from his brainstem, I would limit his options for play to those involving rhythm and movement in order to help him regulate, such as the sit and spin, rocking, or swaying like an elephant. There are times that I may offer or attempt exercises from DPT in order to connect with the child on a more basic preverbal level. DPT can help the child experience co-regulation and relationship, which can also foster regulation.

DEVELOPMENTAL PLAY THERAPY

DPT was founded by Viola Brody in the early 1960s. Brody (1997) believed that appropriate nurturing touch in DPT can help healthy developmental growth and allow healing of earlier trauma and neglect. DPT was influenced by the work of many clinicians and theorists, including Bowlby (1969) and Brazelton and Cramer (1990), as a relationship-focused approach that incorporates pleasurable playful activities to engage and stimulate young children (Brody, 1997; Courtney, Velasquez, & Bakai Toth, 2017).

DPT focuses on the importance of touch as a means of healing, since touch is the first form of communication for an infant beginning in utero and powerful form of emotional communication that is inherently reciprocal (Brody, 1997; Courtney & Gray, 2014; Field, 2014). This loving nurturing touch is integral in developing healthy attachment and an internal working model for attachment (Bowlby, 1988). However, not all children experience nurturing caring touch during early childhood. Children, such as Peter, who have experienced negative hurtful touch, will need to learn to experience caring touch in order to heal (Brody, 1997).

Unlike other play therapy models, toys are not the center of the play; the relationship is the focus of the therapeutic work. A typical DPT session may include a rug, a rocker, a table, chairs, paper, crayons, and body lotion. The rug may define the space; a rocker promotes contact and rhythmic relaxation; the table, chairs, paper, and crayons encourage expression; and the lotion may be used for soothing touch (Brody, 1997; Courtney & Gray, 2014; Courtney & Siu, 2018). DPT utilizes a presymbolic form of play in which children's play is consistent with the child's and object's conventional roles, such as stirring a pot with a spoon, hugging a baby doll, or rolling a ball. The therapist initiates caring, playful touch, which may be defined loosely and can include playful singing, humming, tone of words, or games like peekaboo. The therapist identifies and respects the child's concerns or preferences in regard to touch and must be attuned and responsive to the child's cues (Courtney & Gray, 2014). Activities may include peekaboo or singing while appropriately touching/moving body parts, for example, "I see a hand. There is your other hand. Where is your nose? Oh, there it is." The therapist is mindful of the child's shifting needs, and with each playful interaction the child builds trust in the relationship and develops a sense of self. These interactions are reciprocal communications between the therapist and the child, allowing the child to feel heard, noticed, and understood (Brody, 1997; Courtney & Gray, 2014; Courtney & Siu, 2018). For example, in a game of patty cake, the therapist must read the child's level of enjoyment and may need to adjust the touch based upon the child's cues or stop if the child isuncomfortable. Children can experience a corrective experience of touch when they have not had it before and begin to see themselves as lovable, important, and deserving, as mirrored by the therapist. When touch becomes a positive comfortable experience that children enjoy, they may initiate more appropriate interactions (Courtney & Gray, 2014; Courtney & Siu, 2018).

These DPT activities are also healing because they allow children to go back to an earlier stage of life to retrieve the developmental attachment experiences that they were denied and still need, such as the need for being held and touched, rocked, and fed. Children usually realize what they need emotionally and play it out in the present for their growth and development (Brody, 1997). These are not regressive behaviors that should not be indulged, but rather they are examples of children instinctively seeking what they need for survival, attachment, and a sense of safety. An example would be cradling, where the therapist or caregiver initiates a gentle holding by noticing the needs of the child and physically adjusting to make it possible (Courtney & Gray, 2014; Courtney & Siu, 2018). The therapist may offer the rocker or sit on the floor to allow the child to initiate being held or rocked. Unlike holding, it is done without force to foster a sense of safety, relaxation, and calmness, which is how infants learn to regulate. The child may suck their thumb or request a baby bottle or blanket, and the rhythmic motion produces a calming effect (Perry, 2009). The warmth and security can be felt emanating from the therapist, who is acknowledging the child's needs, allowing for co-regulations (Badennoch, 2008). It is a developmental attachment behavior that fails to occur for neglected traumatized children, like Peter. This becomes a wonderful exercise for resourcing by using bilateral stimulation (BLS) to tap in this calming nurturing experience, as described later in our case of Peter.

Discussion of DPT and touch within the clinical setting often raises ethical concerns due to the inherent power differences, boundary issues, or fear of it leading to inappropriate touch, misunderstandings, and potential legal consequences (Association for Play Therapy, 2019a; Courtney & Gray, 2014; McNeil-Harber, 2004). Touch can occur in all forms of play therapy. As a play therapist working with young children, it is impossible to imagine a session in which touch does not occur. For children, touch is a normal part of play, and they often initiate it, freely taking the therapist's hand to lead them, touching the therapist while putting her down for a pretend nap, sitting on her lap to hear a story, or grabbing her arm to get her attention (Association for Play Therapy, 2019a; Courtney & Siu, 2018; Grobbel, Cooke, & Bonet, 2017). Touch within the DPT model refers to the use of appropriate gentle touch. It is through the modeling and experiencing of appropriate touch that children who have only experienced touch as negative/painful can begin to heal through this corrective emotional response. This touch can begin to build new memory networks of adaptive information that can be useful when using EMDR.

EMDR THERAPY

EMDR has become widely accepted to be an effective evidence-based treatment for posttraumatic stress disorder (PTSD) and is recommended for children and adolescents with PTSD (American Psychiatric Association [APA], 2004; Substance Abuse and Mental Health Services Administration [SAMHSA], 2012; U.S. Department of Veterans Affairs [VA], 2019; World Health Organization [WHO], 2013). Research has shown its effectiveness (Chen et al., 2014; Shapiro, 2014). EMDR was initially found effective for PTSD; however, research has found it effective for a wide range of trauma-related issues, including childhood abuse, neglect, reactive attachment, and repairing ruptured attachment (Shapiro, 2017).

EMDR is a therapeutic approach developed by Francine Shapiro (2017) to reprocess traumatic events by using BLS. It is an eight-phase protocol that addresses reprocessing traumatic memories to an adaptive form so they may be integrated into working memory. EMDR is a client-centered approach that incorporates elements from many different treatment models, including psychodynamic, cognitive, cognitive behavior, experiential, and somatic body therapies, as well as a focus on a client's past, present, and future (Shapiro, 2017). Modifications have been made to the approach as new information was discovered, and this process continues (Shapiro, 2017).

EMDR is based on the AIP model which allows the client to activate the maladaptively recorded memories and to connect with the client's rational adaptive information so the memories can be functionally integrated. In this way the client is able to make sense out of the negative event. For example, after being physically abused by his mother, Peter may act aggressively and mistrust his aunt, even though she is not his mom and has never abused him and there is no danger.

When Aunt Suzie tries to set a limit with Peter, his memory of his mom hurting him may be triggered, and he may respond with the same emotion, belief, and reaction as if the event is occurring. His knowledge that this is not someone who will hurt him is not connecting with the "stuck" trauma memory. EMDR activates the processing system so the trauma memory can connect with the adaptive knowledge and no longer trigger the emotional reaction.

EMDR AND CHILDREN

EMDR has become recognized as an effective treatment for children who have been traumatized (International Society for Traumatic Stress Studies, 2018; WHO, 2013). The EMDR protocol has been successfully adapted for use with children, and there are several reviews of studies and meta analyses indicating the efficacy of its use with children (Beer, 2018; Chen et al., 2018; Moreno-Alcázar et al., 2017; Verardo & Ciccolanti, 2017). However, there are only a few studies on the effectiveness of EMDR with young children, including three single-case studies with a child as young as 17 months (Swimm, 2018), a 2-1/2-year-old child (Robbins, 2000), and a 5-year-old child (Rathore, 2018), and two with preschoolers (Greenwald, 1994; Hensel, 2009).

EMDR has been successfully combined with play therapy techniques, including CCPT, sandtray therapy, art therapy, and narrative therapy (Adler-Tapia & Settle, 2009; Gomez, 2013; Lovett, 1999, 2015; Parnell, 2013), when working with traumatized children. EMDR therapy has been integrated with play, art, sensorimotor support, storytelling, metaphors, family therapy, and parent support (e.g., Adler-Tapia & Settle, 2017; Gomez, 2013; Greenwald, 2005; Lovett, 1999, 2015; Shapiro, 2017; Struik et al., 2017). Young children especially will not be able to reprocess memories as adults do, visualizing the memory while sitting on a chair and following the therapist's fingers with their eyes. Playful adaptations can help the therapist overcome many possible obstacles regarding gaining cooperation, regulation, safety, and trust with complex, highly dysregulated children.

Play therapists are already accustomed to helping children process trauma as well as exploring attachment issues through play (Gil, 2016; Goodyear-Brown, 2010, Landreth, 2012). They are accustomed to using language that is developmentally appropriate and have experience in working with resistant or uncooperative young clients, as many young children begin as mandated clients (it is rare that a 5-year-old child requests to see a therapist!). Play therapists have an advantage over therapists not trained in play therapy, in that they recognize the various ways that trauma processes in play and have skills to facilitate it with empathy, support, and acknowledgment. Children process the traumatic events of their lives through play since they do not have the verbal skills to express themselves the way an adult would. Trauma also impacts their ability to verbally report the event. Children use toys and creative arts to connect with these memories and process them, often playing out the event repetitively and trying different endings to their stories, all in an attempt to adaptively process or make sense out of what has happened (Axline, 1969; Gil, 2015; Landreth, 2012).

Play therapists who are also EMDR therapists can creatively combine the two approaches by considering and incorporating the theories of each intervention.

The AIP model of EMDR posits that traumatic memories must be activated and desensitized with BLS so they can be integrated into memory (Shapiro, 2017), and play in play therapy already serves as the means by which children activate and process memories. Play therapists can easily use the familiar forms of play that they are currently using to process traumatic memories (DPT, CCPT, sandtray, etc.) to accomplish the processing portion of desensitization in Phase 4. Additionally, forms of play or playful exercises can be utilized to learn about the child's history for Phase 1 and to prepare the child for processing during Phase 2.

PLAY THERAPY AND EMDR HISTORY/CASE CONCEPTUALIZATION

Phase 1 of EMDR requires a thorough trauma history in order to identify the adverse events that caused the child's symptoms and can then be targeted for reprocessing. A complete clinical history is also necessary in order to identify strengths, deficits, targets, possible challenges, and inappropriate cognitions; only then can case conceptualization be completed. However, obtaining this history can be difficult when working with children. Defining trauma for clients or parents can be challenging because they are unsure what constitutes a "trauma." Some parents assume that trauma is only physical or sexual abuse and may not consider negative events involving shame, guilt, or neglect.

The word *trauma* may be off-putting and is not necessary. It can be described to parents as subjective negative experiences that have a lasting effect on the way children think about themselves and emotionally and physically respond to future events. Events become traumatic when they overwhelm a child's nervous system, subsequently altering the way memories are processed and recalled (van der Kolk, 2014). Sometimes having the caregiver think of a negative event from their own life that still has an impact on how they feel today can help them better understand. For instance, Peter's Aunt Suzie remembered being shamed in front of her second-grade class for not knowing an answer and freezing. She noticed how she still could feel that shame when triggered and sometimes would think about herself even today: "I'm stupid." This helped her to better understand how Peter's experiences (which were far worse) can have a lasting impact and what may constitute a trauma experience for him.

Clinicians often need to ask about history in a more conversational manner to discover what has happened to the child by asking open-ended questions about the child's life. Some questions I asked Aunt Suzie were as follows: *Does Peter like his preschool? Tell me about when Peter was born. Do you know about Peter's mother's pregnancy? What was happening then? Who is Peter closest to in the family? Whom does he go to when he is hurt? Are you able to soothe him? Tell me about things that calm Peter. What are his strengths? What makes you proud of Peter? Where were Peter and his mother living when he was born? Who lived in the house with them?* Clinicians also need answers to all of the typical history and symptom questions, including the parents' trauma history. Questions regarding the parents' or caregivers' attachment history can be extremely helpful, not only to better understand the relationship between them and the child, but to help parents make connections between how they were raised and what is happening in their relationship with their own child. Remember, the mother's attachment is an important predictor of the child's attachment.

A history must by obtained directly from the child as well, no matter their age, because parents are often unaware of events that children have experienced. Obtaining the trauma or neglect history from young children can be challenging because it is difficult for children to convey their story due to their developmental level as well as trauma affecting their ability to access the words to describe the experience (van der Kolk, 2014). Thankfully, play therapists have natural ways for children to "tell" their history or trauma story, through their language of play. Children experience and play out their negative experiences in the playroom if they are given a safe space to do so. Clinicians must watch and listen carefully for children's experiences, fears, self-beliefs, strengths, and emotions to be expressed in the playroom. Reflections that expand the meaning can help clarify and expand on what is communicated by the child. When the negative events are identified, those memories can be targets for reprocessing. During this initial "getting to know each other" time, therapists will develop trust, identify trauma events, and recognize strengths, fears, and negative self-beliefs, which are all necessary for the history, preparation, and case conceptualization.

In Peter's case, as mentioned earlier, he had been removed from his mother and bounced around in foster placements for over a year before being placed with his maternal aunt, her husband, and their 21-year-old son. Neither Child Protective Services nor the relatives were sure what had happened to him in those early years. However, through CCPT I learned a great deal as he played out many of his experiences in the playroom. For instance, Peter would repetitively gather all of the food and hide it. I reflected that he was hungry and worried, and he nodded and was able to add angrily that he was mad. He said he could get Mom's foods sometimes too, and he showed me with the play food. In play he teased or taunted me with the food, pretending to give it to me and taking it away as I reached for it. In one session, he also said his mom was mean. In fact, Peter said that not just was his mom mean, but the monsters were too. He then showed me how to hide behind the chair covered with pillows and be quiet so the monsters could not get us. I followed his lead, and we played hiding from the monsters for several sessions. I added to his history and trauma timeline: not being fed as well as possible physical abuse by his mom and others. I learned that he was angry and upset with his mother, whom he identified as mean, yet he was resourceful and knew enough to hide to protect himself as well as to hide food so he could eat. Using play therapy, I was able to obtain his history from Peter while developing a relationship and identify strengths and targets for EMDR.

Case conceptualization should not be skipped just because the client is a toddler or preschooler: A plan is necessary. The clinician must piece together information from parents' reports and what children share through their play to determine a trauma history. From that information, the clinician can decide what resourcing is necessary, the type of trauma experienced, targets for reprocessing, and where to start. Keeping in mind that EMDR is a client-centered therapy, clinicians should start where the child is, proceed at their pace, and remember that therapists are not in session to parent the child or to teach behaviors, rather to support and build trust in order to heal the child. An awareness of the inherent power differential and any countertransference is essential to help the therapist to refrain from coercion and threats that recreate and trigger prior traumatic experiences during which the child may have been coerced, threatened, and harmed.

PLAY THERAPY AND RESOURCE DEVELOPMENT AND INSTALLATION IN EMDR

Resource development and installation (RDI) is used for stabilization in EMDR, and as such it is an important part of phase-oriented treatment for trauma. Most trauma models include a broad stabilization phase to prepare the children for treatment (Shapiro, 2017; van der Hart, Brown, & van der Kolk, 1989). Since children with complex trauma face many obstacles to successful treatment, RDI in the early stages of EMDR is necessary because it helps the child feel safe, develop adaptive coping skills, regulate emotionally and physically, and foster self-capacities before targeting the traumatic memories (Kinniburgh et al., 2005; Leeds, 2009; Parnell, 2013; Shapiro, 2017; Wesselmann et al., 2018). RDI can be used to increase the child's abilities to change emotional and behavioral states to more positive or adaptive forms by increasing their access to functional memory networks or creating new ones. These positive memory networks are strengthened without disturbing traumatic memory networks (Korn & Leeds, 2002; Leeds, 2009; Shapiro, 2017). Focusing on the positive states in the early stages of therapy can be very valuable for developing trust, determining pace of treatment, and engagement with children. Fewer, slower sets of BLS are used to access and strengthen these positive networks while generating relaxation and comfortable feelings (Amano & Toichi, 2016). The resources strengthen through EMDR because the BLS appears to increase the emotional intensity of the stimulated memory network and vibrant associations to other positive memory networks (Korn & Leeds, 2002).

The safe place exercise for regulation is a standard part of the EMDR preparation phase (Leeds, 2009; Shapiro, 2017) and can be developed through the use of play, including in the sand tray, through expressive arts, or while running around outside. After these activities, the feelings, emotions, and sensations can be tapped in with BLS. While an adult client can perform a "safe place exercise" without external props, young children need the assistance of play therapy. Similarly, a container exercise to hold scary memories and overwhelming feelings can be developed by using a real box, drawing, painting, or just being imagined. Both of these can be created early in therapy to help children regulate through Phase 1.

Resourcing can also support children to overcome deficits by strengthening existing skills (e.g., the ability to ask for help), developing new skills (e.g., telling another child not to take your toy instead of hitting him), or developing self-capacity (e.g., confidence, caring, importance, trust). CCPT's play objectives of developing mastery of skills, forming positive self-beliefs, building relationships, and experiencing control (Landreth, 2012) match with those of RDI. Through play and interaction with an attuned therapist, CCPT and DPT provide opportunities for young children to understand and learn ways to emotionally and physically regulate as well as learn new responses to stimuli. DPT allows for the resourcing of missing attachment experiences so that they come to learn that touch can be positive. Clinicians increase these positive effects by adding BLS to intensify and strengthen the positive networks that are created through these play activities. For example, if a child has fun safely playing with goop, squishing between their hands and the therapist's hands, this feeling of joy and safety can be tapped in as a resource. This newfound ability to regulate and accomplish tasks gives the children a sense of pride, encouragement, and control.

Play can provide the vehicle for building self-capacities and skills that young children are lacking by installing positive experiences/skills that occur naturally in the playroom, whether they are spontaneous or directed exercises. Traumatized children often lack self-capacities, and play can help identify the child's deficits and then strengthen/resource them (Kinniburgh et al., 2005). Play therapists already utilize exercises to increase children's positive beliefs about self and self-capacities (reading books, telling stories, acting out scenes with a puppet, processing in a sand tray, etc.). This effect can be strengthened further by adding BLS. There are numerous opportunities for what I refer to as spontaneous resourcing in the playroom. BLS can be used to install any skill or capacity acted out (being caring, patient, or proud), positive/mastery experiences that the child shares (being able to ask for help/being able to focus and work to put the dress on the doll), transitional objects that are found and used for a variety of strengths (a picture of a pet for feeling calm), real or imaginary attachment figures (adoptive mom, strong lion character), or a protector or superhero for strength such as Superman (Parnell, 2013; Shapiro, 2017). Some children may benefit from creating and installing a resource team (superhero to represent strength, a favorite teacher for wisdom, adoptive mom for love, pretend pet for calmness, etc.). Noting a child's genuine emotion during play and installing it with BLS can develop emotional literacy, and by having them also note the sensation in their body, we can foster body awareness, which is often lacking (Adler-Tapia & Settle, 2009; Gomez, 2013; Lovett, 2015).

The therapist can use RDI for a child to strengthen their experience of using of a coping skill at school or home. Once when Peter came into a session excited and proud that he had been able to remain calm by using his happy place when the teacher said it was time to go back into the class, I immediately had him notice how good he felt, the emotions, physical feeling and the belief that he can stay calm, and had him tap it in with BLS.

Many playful activities can be used as resources. By having a child do some breathing exercises and noticing the peaceful calm feeling in the moment and installing with BLS, children can learn mindfulness. Many other approaches can be used, which include attachment, relational (both discussed later), and ego state. An example of ego state resourcing would be to have the child draw the different positive parts of themselves—the strong self, funny self, loving self—and then have them recognize the emotions and sensations as they thinks of that part and install it with BLS (Leeds, 2009; Parnell, 2013).

RESOURCING THROUGH ATTACHMENT PLAY

Resourcing can also be accomplished by fostering attachment. Utilizing attachment activities involving therapists or caregivers/parents as part of the resourcing has been developed and found successful in treating relational trauma by numerous EMDR therapists (Gomez, 2013; Greenwald, 2005; Lovett, 1999, 2015; Parnell, 2013; Wesselmann, Schweitzer, & Armstrong, 2014; Wesselmann et al., 2018). Using EMDR with the caregiver and child allows the caregiver to develop the skills for attachment and promote feelings of love, connectedness, and acceptance for the child, while also healing the child (Wesselmann et al., 2012, 2014, 2018). This bond and attunement between the child and caregiver can be strengthened using planned activities or spontaneous moments of connection.

The qualities required of the EMDR therapist in attachment work fit naturally with those of a play therapist, since attunement and a safe, congruent therapeutic relationship is central to the healing process in both (Axline, 1969; Brody, 1997; Landreth, 2012; Shapiro, 2017). For the necessary attachment work, therapists must be able to respond to the child's needs, recognize nonverbal cues, and connect right brain to right brain (Schore & Schore, 2014). By listening to internal cues and being present, flexible, authentic, and stable for the client, the therapist may allow emotional resonance; be able to feel love, acceptance, and compassion for the client, and communicate it in a safe, appropriate way (Parnell, 2013; Shore & Shore, 2014). In this way, the therapist provides co-regulation and an emotionally corrective response for a child who has not experienced acceptance, love, and empathy. The safety of the relationship allows the child to engage their positive social engagement system and disengage their defense systems that are chronically engaged by perceived threats (Porges, 2011). This attachment attunement in EMDR exercises mirrors the tenets of CCPT and DPT. Therapists must be skilled in reading and discerning children's verbal and nonverbal communication and responding empathetically.

There are many opportunities for attachment work in the playroom, which may include the sense of being nurtured and regulated by having a parent feed a child or helping a child complete a frustrating puzzle (Adler-Tapia & Settle, 2017; Lovett, 2015; Parnell, 2013). Positive body sensations can be noticed, strengthened, and installed with BLS by resourcing developmentally appropriate nurturing activities in order to replace the fear and dysregulation caused by early trauma (Adler-Tapia & Settle, 2017). Caregivers or therapists can create a sense of safety, of being cared for and connected by feeding a child (actually or pretend), rocking them, or putting them to sleep. Exercises in which the caregiver lists all of the things they love about the child, speaks about how they felt when they first saw the child, or lists the child's attributes, followed by installation with BLS can foster attachment (Adler-Tapia & Settle, 2017; Lovett, 2015; Parnell, 2013). By seeing themselves in a new positive way through nurturing, loving interactions with their caregivers, children's negative beliefs about themselves learned from neglectful abusive caregivers can be altered. Positive beliefs and emotions can be strengthened with BLS.

A note of caution when involving others in resourcing or attachment work: The children's comfort level with the adult must be considered. The therapist should consider if the children are ready for touch or closeness, if they have fears or concerns regarding the adult, and if the adult is linked to the traumatic events in a way that must be considered. Children should not be coerced into uncomfortable situations with the attachment figure. Their concerns and reluctance should be identified and respected (Lovett, 2015; Parnell, 2013). Therapists must also determine if caregivers are comfortable with the resource or EMDR exercises and able to interact or respond appropriately. If not, the exercises should not be conducted, and more preparation work should be done with the caregiver or child. More importantly, therapists must consider whether or not caregivers have their own trauma history for which they should be referred for their own work (Wesselmann et al., 2014).

The resourcing process is important to the success and effectiveness of EMDR and can improve the outcomes of therapy (Adler-Tapia & Settle, 2017). Once these skills are developed and rehearsed through play, they can easily be strengthened with the application of BLS. In addition to healing or alleviating any deficits or capacities, resourcing allows the clinician to ascertain if the client can maintain dual attention, refrain from dissociation, be present in their body, focus on positive memories, and demonstrate an ability for affect tolerance and regulation (Korn & Leeds, 2002; Leeds, 2009; Shapiro, 2017). These resources can be used to help children be successful in the eight phases of EMDR as well as used in the children's daily lives (Leeds, 2009; Parnell, 2013; Shapiro, 2017).

A CASE STUDY FOR INTEGRATING CCPT, DPT, AND EMDR: PETER'S THERAPY

As mentioned earlier, Peter had been removed from his mother's care at age 3-1/2 years. At the time I met him, he had been living with his maternal aunt, Suzie, her husband, and their 21-year-old son for 6 months. CCPT and DPT were used throughout treatment, and Peter's aunt learned some CCPT techniques so she could use the same skills at home. Sessions were flexible; often EMDR was conducted during half of the session, and half was play therapy. For EMDR he was introduced to both tapping and the tappers. When using tapping, the therapist taps bilaterally on the child's shoulders, arms, or knees (an appropriate body location in which the child can still engage in their processing activities). For example, I tapped bilaterally on Peter's shoulders as he processed in a sand tray. The tappers are electric devices with two small paddles that buzz alternately for the BLS. Children can hold these paddles, or they can be placed in socks, pockets, or waist bands. During RDI, Peter usually used tapping, and during EMDR desensitization, Peter preferred the tappers.

There were times that Peter did not want to do EMDR at all. He just wanted to play. Resistance and avoidance are parts of trauma symptomology and are often based on earlier experiences and beliefs. However, he would usually engage in EMDR with the use of reflection and choice, for example, "It's hard not to think about scary things. It's time to tap the scary stuff away, and then we can play your song on the phone and dance." While there were successful play and EMDR sessions, there were many sessions in which Peter was dysregulated or triggered, resulting in him being defiant, resistant, and/or uncooperative. During those sessions, resources, CCPT, movement, breathing, and therapeutic limit setting (Landreth, 2002) were used to help him regulate and recognize the lack of threat. There were many other memories that were targeted for EMDR processing besides those used in this case study, and not all were completed in a single session as in this case presentation.

History and Preparation: Caregiver

I initially met with Peter's Aunt Suzie alone so she could freely give me a history of Peter's life without him present. She had read some material about trauma and acknowledged that she didn't know how to handle Peter's behavior and help him overcome all the horrible things that he had experienced. She reported Peter's symptoms as temper tantrums, rages, difficulty transitioning, refusal to follow directions, defiance to anyone in authority, and inability to focus. She also stated that he would hit her or other people and appear to have no remorse or empathy afterward, as well as having difficulties with sleep, overeating, and possible sensory integration issues. I explained to her that the neglect and abuse Peter endured may have caused dysregulation in Peter's brainstem, the part of the brain that regulates our bodies' functioning (Perry, 2009; Siegel, 2012; van der Kolk, 2014).

Suzie was dismayed that everyone involved in his case ignored all of the trauma Peter had experienced and only wanted to medicate him. She gave me what little information she had from Child Services and what other details she had been able to piece together from Peter. She was shocked when she realized how badly he had been treated and how he had been let down by everyone who was supposed to protect him, including his parents, their family, and the state.

Discussion of Peter's behaviors with Suzie provided an opportunity to explain in depth how trauma affects children so she could better understand Peter and the work we needed to do. I illustrated the three parts of the brain using my fist as a model: the brainstem as the area near my wrist, limbic system as my thumb in the center, surrounded by my closed fingers as the cortex and how they control executive thinking, emotions, and survival, respectively (Siegel, 2012; van der Kolk, 2014). Since Peter perceived many actions as more threatening due to his early trauma, his brainstem was often activated, and he would want to fight or flee. This was compounded by his lack of attachment and underdeveloped limbic system. His defiance and acting out resulted from his learned belief that he cannot trust others to care for him, that he is not lovable or good enough, and that he is not safe. Subsequently, he believed that he will be rejected and left alone again. Suzie came to understand that his controlling and avoidant behaviors were defensive responses to his feelings of helplessness or powerlessness developed from the trauma experience (Perry & Dobson, 2009; Shapiro, 2017; van der Kolk, 2005).

Discussions regarding discipline can help caregivers who are feeling overwhelmed. Suzie said that Peter's anger was the worst when he was told "no" and with any transition of activities, both of which signal the fear of being out of control and being taken from something familiar to something unknown and frightening. I suggested that a possible consequence for his behaviors might be "time-in" instead of time-out. A time-out might confirm his belief that he is not loved and will be rejected whereas a time-in gives him support to learn to regulate.

Traumatized children like Peter often become distressed, and since they have not had caregivers to restore a sense of safety and control, they often become helpless and overwhelmed. As a result, they may become hypo-aroused and dissociate or hyper-aroused and act out. Peter often became hyper-aroused when transitioning or being told no: yelling, hitting, physically resisting, and crying. His behavior was an attempt to modulate these overwhelming feelings. Peter was only trying to gain a sense of control, but his behavior was viewed and labeled as bad, defiant, and oppositional. Disciplining him for this behavior was not working because he was operating from the limbic and brainstem areas of the brain rather than the prefrontal cortex (Siegel, 2012; van der Kolk, 2014). In this state, he was unable to process or integrate what was happening (van der Kolk, 2014), so he could not learn from what was happening. Peter was often triggered by his old memories of neglect and abuse. When this happened, the emotional part of his brain, the limbic system, took over, and he was flooded with emotions (fear, anger, terror). These emotions alert the brainstem of danger, so he reacted with a fight, flight, or freeze response. It was as if the limbic system or brainstem hijacked the brain, and the prefrontal cortex, which controls executive thought (decision-making and understanding consequences), went offline. He simply could not process these events or learn from them (Siegel, 2012; van der Kolk, 2014).

Aunt Suzie began to think about which area of Peter's brain was "in control" when she was trying to direct him, because if it is the brainstem or limbic system, reasoning will not work. She learned that if he was operating from his brainstem, she could help him feel safe by giving them space to move and regulate: breathing, rhythmic, somatosensory experiences such as drumming, swaying, jumping, rocking, or dancing. If he was operating from his limbic system and emotionally dysregulated, she would allow him a means to express emotions or try DPT-directed activities to engage him in a safe emotional response from an adult.

We also met alone to consider possible interventions for Peter's treatment plan, which would include EMDR, CCPT, and DPT. It was agreed that we would meet twice a week in order to allow Peter to learn skills, process memories, and heal more quickly. Peter's relational trauma and disrupted attachment needed to be addressed as well as the abuse and neglect he had suffered. I explained that these interventions could help develop attachment, since he never received consistent nurturing; no one had held him, rocked him, or fed him when he needed it, and as a result, he never learned to regulate emotionally or physically, leading to an insecure attachment.

Suzie and I further prepared by going over the CCPT and DPT modalities, and Suzie received handouts and resources for each. We role-played some CCPT reflective responses and ACT limit setting that involves Acknowledging the feeling, Communicating the limit, and Targeting acceptable alternatives (Landreth, 2002). I also described DPT and demonstrated a couple of exercises we would be using in session so she would be able to respond appropriately. Finally, I explained EMDR, the different forms of BLS, and how EMDR would be used along with play therapy as resource development and to reprocess those earlier memories and shift his negative beliefs about himself and his emotional and behavioral responses to reminders of his trauma. Suzie shared that she was looking forward to Peter no longer believing he was bad or that he could not trust anyone, especially her. I sent Suzie home to practice reflective responses and limit setting as homework.

Preparation: Child

Preparation is a necessary part of EMDR, and due to the severity of the trauma in Peter's case, it took numerous sessions. Single incident trauma is processed quickly and often does not require as much preparation as complex trauma. Therapists must be attentive to children's strengths and deficits as well as note how each may impact desensitization. Children's readiness and comfort levels must determine the pace of therapy. Peter's play allowed me the means to engage, develop rapport, ascertain history, determine possible targets for case conceptualization, recognize negative beliefs, discover deficits, and resource strengths.

When I first met Peter, he appeared alert and curious, yet he was initially reluctant to come to the playroom and held onto his aunt. I knew I would have to work to earn his trust. No one had saved him from the abuse, and his lack of trust regarding the reliability and predictability of others resulted in his anxiety, anger, and helplessness, making it difficult to rely on others for help. Using CCPT skills I was able to engage with him. I got down to his eye level and reflected that he was unsure about coming to the playroom. I didn't pressure him but rather enticed him and matched his pace by allowing him to lead and decide whether and when to go. I reflected that it was okay, that new places can be scary, and that Aunt Suzie could come too. He slowly made his way to the playroom. Once there, I told Peter, "This is your special time to do most anything you would like. I'll let you know if there is something you may not do," and I continued to use CCPT skills. In each session of CCPT, Peter would play out and reveal a new aspect of his history: another time someone hurt him, a time that he was angry, another loss. I also learned about his strengths and progress through his play; he was bright, a problem-solver, and curious.

In early sessions, the themes of his play included safety, sleeping, and eating. He played hiding from the monsters, making the baby dolls go to sleep by screaming at them, and bringing the play food to Suzie and me and then telling us we couldn't have any. He also hit the baby doll and said it was bad. Through play, Peter was able to share some of his traumatic experiences and the feelings around them. I was able to reflect many of the feelings for Peter to begin to allow him to be heard and understood. Much of this trauma play was repetitive play, in which he was able to express these painful events and attempt to understand what had happened or to discover a different ending to his story (Campbell & Knoetze, 2010; Gil, 2016; Landreth, 2012). Peter's play revealed several targets for reprocessing (being hurt by his mother, being removed from his mother, moving from foster home and family constantly), triggers (being told "no", transitioning, being touched), and negative cognitions (I'm not good enough, I am bad, I'm not worthy or lovable). He often got angry when a limit was set (e.g., "You're angry. Hard toys are not for throwing. You can throw the soft ball.") as well as during any transition in session.

One of the toys Peter focused on was the policeman figure. In one CCPT session, he had the policeman take the baby and placed them together on the table. I watched mindfully while tracking his action and reflecting possible feelings.

Therapist: *Oh, he's taking the baby over there.*

Peter: *He's making him safe.* (Then he took the baby doll and threw it on the ground.)

Peter: *He's bad.* (He looked up to ensure that I was watching.)

Therapist: *You wanted me to see you do that. You want me to know the baby is bad.*

Peter: *Uh-huh. The baby can't stay here.*

Therapist: *The baby feels sad that he can't stay anywhere.*

Peter: *Very…and mad.*

This play with the baby occurred repeatedly over our first couple of sessions, and often the policeman figure was used too. My interpretation of this was that

Peter was letting me know he believed that he was bad; that he wanted to be good and safe. While the adults were supposed to keep him safe, this had not always happened.

When Peter first came into treatment, he lacked an emotional vocabulary or any means of expressing emotions appropriately. Traumatized children often have difficulty expressing emotions, which can result in intense emotional states and difficulty calming down. As a part of preparation and through the use of reflection, I wanted to help Peter appropriately develop an emotional vocabulary and express emotions so he wouldn't need his old coping skills. After a reflection, he would stop and ponder what I had said and then repeat it or reject it. We also played games with the "emotion ball" (a ball with colored squares with an emotion word in each). One game we played was a form of dodge ball, which he had taken the lead in creating. He would run back and forth, and I would throw the ball at him. If I hit him, we would look at the emotion word his thumb was on when he picked up the ball. He would then describe or enact the emotion and/or think of a time he felt that way. When it was my turn, he would throw the ball, and I would be hit. This gave me the opportunity to claim that my thumb landed on an emotion about which I knew he needed to learn and express. After playing this game a few times and with the use of reflection, he began developing an emotional vocabulary. I had also identified several negative beliefs that he held about himself, which included he was bad, could not trust others, and was not good enough. He viewed many actions as threatening and believed that any transition meant danger, to which he often would respond aggressively with fear for survival.

In our third session as part of preparation, I introduced breathing as a way to feel calm and less angry or upset by saying, "Aunt Suzie has to do this activity with us because adults have times when they are upset or angry too." Peter seemed to feel comforted by the realization that adults can have a hard time controlling their feelings too. Before working with Peter on breathing, I asked Peter what he liked to smell. "What is something that smells good?" He answered, "Chocolate chip cookies!" I asked, "Have you ever blown out a candle?" When he said "yes," I demonstrated how to breathe by breathing in and saying, "Smell the cookies," and then exhaling and saying, "Blow out the candles." He was excited to show me how much he could breathe in and out. Then it was Aunt Suzie's turn to breathe in and out. He was excited as he chanted, "Smell the cookies, blow out the candles," as she took her breaths. We all practiced breathing and worked on noticing different parts of our bodies relaxing. Last, I asked them to come up with a funny word that they would use to cue each other that one or both of them needed to take a breath to relax. Peter picked the word *mosquito* because yesterday he and Aunt Suzie had been teasing that the silly mosquitoes needed to find someone else to bite and not them. They took turns practicing as each of them said "mosquito" and they both took nice slow breaths. They each promised to stop and breathe no matter who said the word *mosquito*.

I introduced the idea of EMDR and the tappers to Peter by explaining that the tappers turned on a switch in your brain to help make scary or yucky feelings go away. He was intrigued by the tappers and experimented with them and the controls. He liked the idea of using them to make him feel better. I told him we could also "tap good things in" (Parnell, 2013) by tapping on his shoulders, arms, or legs, which I demonstrated on Suzie. Peter did not want anyone to tap on or touch him, but he was willing to tap on Aunt Suzie. Peter perceived touch as dangerous and

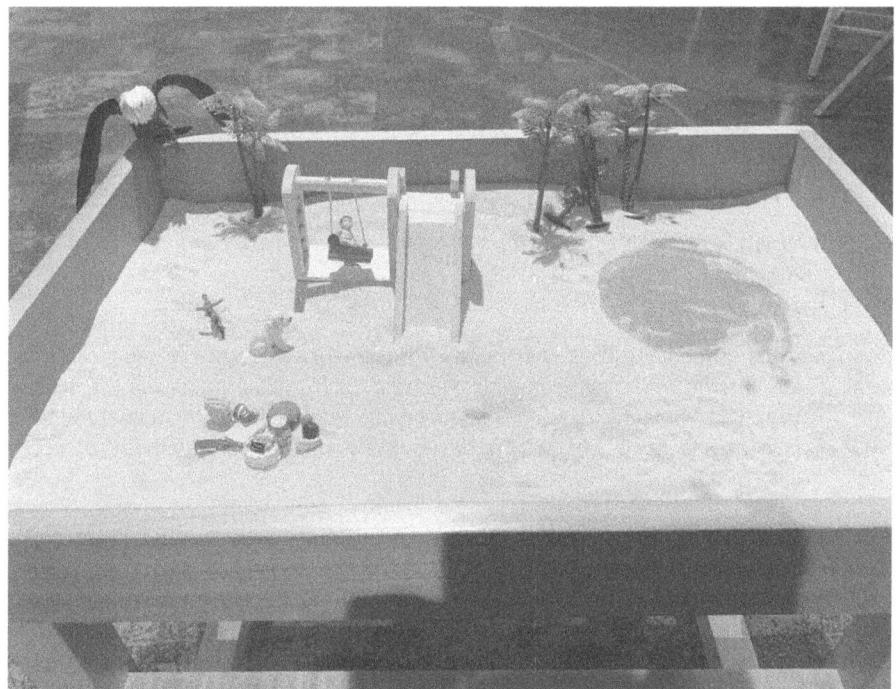

Figure 5.1 *Peter's Safe Place in the Sand Tray*

uncomfortable, as he had not experienced much touch that was good in his short lifetime. I showed Peter how he could tap in "the good stuff" himself, and he excitedly followed my lead, slapping his hands alternatingly on his legs. I used encouragement ("You were able to follow my pattern!") to reinforce the behavior. Then we practiced in earnest. Both he and Aunt Suzie did their breathing and "tapped in" the calm relaxed feeling.

On the fifth session, Peter had asked for Aunt Suzie to be in the room. Suzie reported that most of the time Peter was willing to practice breathing, and it seemed to help him regulate if she could cue him before he was too upset. Since Peter was still vigilant about touch, we practiced tapping our hands onto our legs again, following the slow pattern I set. Peter slapped his thighs more than tapped them. I again used encouragement as he did it: "Great, you can really keep the rhythm. You are following along."

Once I was sure the BLS was established, I asked Peter to create a place in the sand tray that would be calm and happy. He placed many of his favorite things into the tray: a dog, a bike, food, a lake, and trees. I prompted him to make it so it was just his special place; he put an eagle on the edge of the tray for protection, and he said it had a special shield to make it invisible (Figure 5.1).

> Therapist: *What would you be doing there to make you feel calm and happy?*
>
> Peter (smoothing all of the sand and adding a boy figure and a swing set): *I love to swing.* (swinging toy back and forth)

Therapist: *Picture yourself on the swing. Notice how your body feels as you picture swinging back and forth. Notice the air moving across your face and how high you are going. Notice any sounds or smells.*

Peter: *I hear myself laughing! I like to go high so no one can get me.*

Therapist: *Notice that thought.*

Peter: *I'm flying free!*

Therapist: *Notice that while we tap our legs. Can you make the feeling get any stronger?*

Peter: *Yes!* (more BLS)

Therapist (anchoring the experience with the word swing): *You can go back to swinging on the swing in your mind and having this great feeling whenever you want. All you have to do is take a breath, think of the word* swing, *and go there in your mind. This good feeling is inside you, and you can feel it whenever you want.*

We practiced it again toward the end of the session by having Peter close his eyes, picture his happy place, and imagine the feeling of swinging again. I asked him and Aunt Suzie to practice this every day, because it becomes easier and more helpful with practice. We did not test this resource's effectiveness in that session because I wanted him to practice and be successful. Testing by bringing up something mildly upsetting may not work without practice, and then children feel like they have failed or that these skills will not work.

We continued to further develop and practice the resource of the happy place during the next few sessions. Aunt Suzie reported that they practiced at home and confided that she found it helpful for herself and that they often used the breathing and happy place as part of the bedtime ritual. In a subsequent session we tested it by Suzie helping Peter think of something a little upsetting, like being told he had to eat dinner in order to get dessert. He stated that he felt a little upset thinking about that scenario, and then we asked him to use his safe place. He said "swing" and took a breath. He then smiled and reported that it had worked. He was imagining that he was swinging and it felt good. I began to sway my arms back and forth in front of me, and he followed with his arms. We both laughed, and the movement seemed to calm him further. We also did the breathing exercises and installed the feeling of calmness that it brought Pete and Suzie. I included Aunt Suzie in the development of resources so she understood what was developed, how he could use the resource/safe word to regulate, and so she would be able to prompt him to practice and use them at appropriate times. I try to involve caregivers who are appropriate and supportive in resourcing because young children need help in practicing these resource exercises and identifying times they should be used. Additionally, most caregivers like Suzie need resourcing too!

Aunt Suzie joined us for the sixth session, which we began in my "adult office" that does not have toys, which I felt might distract Peter for the DPT and EMDR attachment resource exercises I had planned. These DPT exercises also help children develop sensory awareness, which can increase the sense of safety and also reduce dissociative factors (Waters, 2016). I had brought a bottle of hand lotion with me, and I initiated a game with touch using the lotion on his hands.

Therapist: *Did you bring your hands with you today?*

He laughed at the silly question and showed me his hands. I counted his fingers, touching the tip of each one as I counted.

> Peter: *Did you bring yours?* (counting mine)
>
> Therapist: *Did Aunt Suzie bring her hands?* (planning to use the lotion on Suzie if Peter is not ready for a game involving touch)
>
> Peter (laughing): *Yes!*
>
> Therapist (putting a little lotion on hands and rubbing them together to warm it): *Which hand should get to feel the warm lotion first?*
>
> Peter: *Neither!* (Not surprisingly, pulling back. This was a new game, and he seemed unsure what was going to happen.)
>
> Therapist to Aunt Suzie: *Did you bring your hands with you? May I gently rub the lotion on your left hand?* (She nodded, and we started in with the lotion.)
>
> Aunt Suzie: *Feels so good. Can we put some on my right hand? It wants a turn too.*
>
> Peter (watching with interest): *I want a turn too!*
>
> Therapist (talking to Peter's hands): *Which one wants to go first?* (softly singing a song about rubbing lotion and counting fingers while lotioning)
>
> Peter: *This feels really good.*

I gave the bottle of lotion to Aunt Suzie; she put some in her hand, and then she gently reached out for Peter's hand to rub the lotion. He hesitated briefly and then put his hand in hers. I helped Suzie attune to Peter's responses and reflect what Peter was feeling, making statements like, "I wonder which finger wants some lotion?" "It looks like Peter wants to switch hands." "It feels good to have someone who loves you touch you gently." "Hands can be for caring."

After Aunt Suzie rubbed the lotion on Peter's hands and arm, we tapped in the good feeling using slow BLS. At the end, Peter wanted to be the one to rub the lotion on Aunt Suzie, and he asked her to sing a song.

Impromptu RDI

Resourcing can be a planned activity as with the hand lotion, or it may occur from a spontaneous opportunity. During session nine while using CCPT, Peter seemed agitated and upset when he dropped into my lap and allowed me to gently rock him from side to side. I could feel him starting to relax as I hummed a song that I used to sing to my own children while I tapped his left and right knees interchangeably. I took this as an opening and shifted to a DPT mode. His body felt tense and stiff; his breathing was rapid. I cradled him slightly and began rocking gently. I wasn't sure if he would accept this form of touch. Both Peter and Aunt Suzie had reported that Peter still did not like to be touched or hugged and that he would often pull away when she tried to physically comfort him. I also began humming a melody, one I used when rocking my own children to settle them down. At first, he remained stiff and seemed unsure whether he wanted to get up. I continued to rock and was surprised when I felt him begin relaxing in my arms. I continued to hum and began to sing a little song reflecting the positive changes in his body, singing words about how his body was relaxing and his breathing was getting slower and how good it felt to be calmer. I began to gently tap on his legs, left and right.

> Therapist (singing): *Notice your body relaxing, your breathing getting slower, feels so good to be rocked and held* (gentle BLS).

He then started to suck his thumb and looked into my eyes as he laid there (see Figure 5.2).

> Therapist: *Feeling calmer, feeling relaxed, feeling cared for…wonder what else you are feeling?*
>
> Peter: *Feeling happy, feeling like a baby.*
>
> Therapist: *Notice how your legs feel, so relaxed, notice how your tummy feels, notice how your heart feels* (continuing to tap).

He stayed in my arms for several minutes rocking, then smiled up at me and got up to play (see Figure 5.3).

When asked how he was feeling now, he picked up our body scanner, an old TV remote control, which we would move up and down his body and he would make beeping noises when it hit an area of disturbance. In earlier sessions, we had created the "scanner" to use for any body scans we did for EMDR. This time, we used it to scan for good feelings, and he reported he felt good all over, so we tapped in that good feeling.

We were close to the end of our session, and I let him know that we had 5 more minutes left before it was time to leave. I prepared for an emotional response; however, this time he remained calmer. He did not yell or run as he had done during previous sessions. He was upset but seemed sad rather than angry to leave.

> Therapist: *You're upset but able to leave the playroom calmly. It's hard to leave when you did hard work in here and it felt so good. Do you want to think of swinging and your safe place?*
>
> Peter: *I want to think of the rocking.*

We tapped the rocking in again as a resource, and he left the playroom peacefully.

In that session, Peter gave me the opportunity to spontaneously use developmental play as resource development in EMDR. He was able to initiate touch and then relax and notice how good it felt to be nurtured, accepted, and cared for. He was allowed to remain in control and relax his threat response. When he chose to get up from my lap, he did so freely but turned back to give me a smile. During those minutes of being held and rocking, we were in attunement. I was responding to his state of arousal and adjusted according to his facial expression, his body language, and other nonverbal communication in order to help regulate

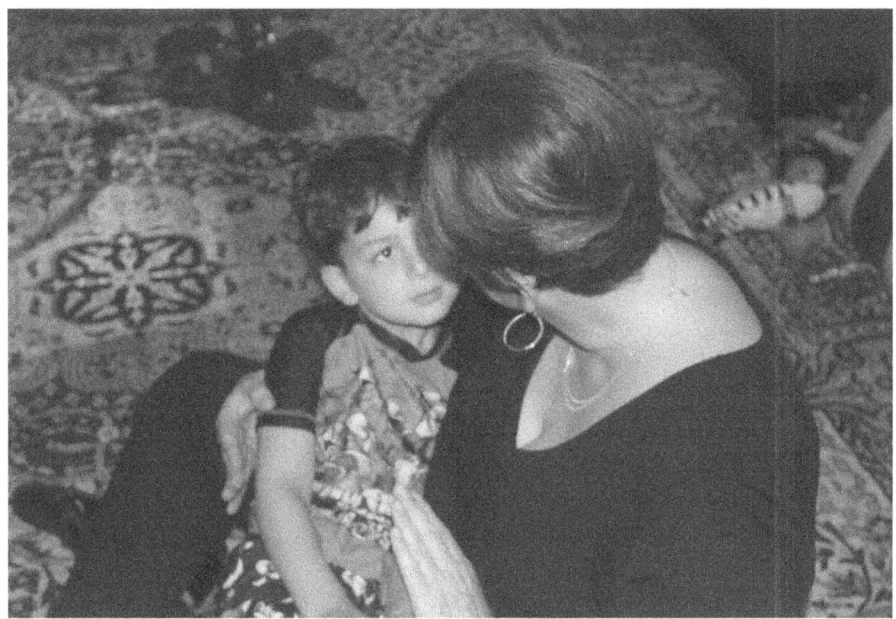

Figure 5.2 *During Rocking Play "Feeling Like a Baby"*

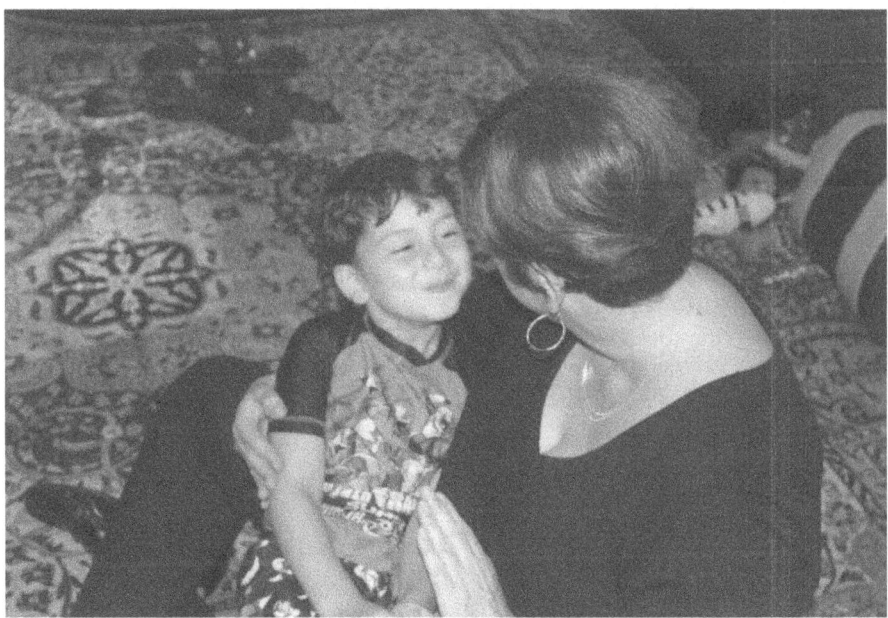

Figure 5.3 *Smiling After DPT With BLS to Install the Feeling*
BLS, bilateral stimulation; DPT, developmental play therapy.

his nervous system. This was a type of touch that he had not experienced in early childhood, nurturing caring touch, an attachment behavior.

I consider this session the perfect storm of resourcing. Peter was able to overcome his initial perception of touch as a threat from previous DPT and CCPT. The attunement provided an opportunity for Peter to be "heard" on every level. His arousal was met with warmth, acceptance, and understanding. It appeared to be the first time that Peter could sense a safe adult's emotional state and regulate by internalizing the adult's response (Siegel, 2012). This ability to self-regulate through co-regulation is developed through right brain to right brain attunement. This right brain communication is conveyed through a gentle tone of voice, expressing kindness through our eyes and facial features, openness and acceptance in our body language, and calm breathing/heart rate (Badennoch, 2008; Schore & Schore, 2014). Such an attuned response requires the therapist to have knowledge of their own mental health and have a keen awareness of their own feelings and self-regulation in order to serve in this capacity (Badennoch, 2008; Courtney & Gray, 2014). This attuned cradling is a DPT exercise used to develop the attachment relationship and trust. Rocking and cradling are the type of focused, patterned, repetitive somatosensory activities related to self-regulation, attention, arousal, and impulsivity, which help the brain organize (Gaskill & Perry, 2014). In Peter's case, EMDR and BLS were added to the DPT experience to strengthen and "tap in" the resource. Since our self-capacities are developed in the context of the attachment relationship (Briere, Hodges, & Godbout, 2010), it is advantageous to utilize attachment experiences and BLS to develop and strengthen them.

After that session Peter was excited to share with Aunt Suzie how we rocked together. Later in private, Aunt Suzie expressed her excitement and yet disbelief that Peter had sat in my lap while I rocked him and tapped in the positive feeling. She was also surprised that I had let him suck on the baby bottle and pretend to be an infant. She had been told by a previous therapist not to encourage those behaviors because they are regressive and to urge him to be a "big boy" instead. I explained to her that these behaviors are some of the developmental pieces he missed as an infant and toddler. He sought them out to repair what he missed in earlier developmental stages (Brody, 1997; Vereshack, 1993). In doing so, his brain is making new positive neuro-networks (Shapiro, 2017) and learning to regulate his body much in the way an infant would learn to do but which he had not had the opportunity to do because of an abusive, neglectful mother. He was also making the connection that touch could be pleasant and calming. These new positive emotional and physical responses were building connections in the brain, which could lead to new positive beliefs about himself.

Continuing to Build the Attachment

Before the next session, I talked with Suzie and asked her to make a list of all of the unconditional things she loved about Peter. I gave her examples, such as "I love your smile," "I love how warm your hugs are," and "I love how your eyes are so blue." I told her that she was going to do an attachment exercise with Peter, which is based on Wesselman, Schweitzer, and Armstrong's attachment resource,

Messages of Love (2014). Suzie had sent me the list of things before the session so I could review them to ensure the statements are appropriate. Conditional statements such as "I love you when you pick up your toys" and "I love how you go to bed without crying" are not appropriate for this intervention. The messages must convey unconditional love. I told her that we had communicated love through the hand touching and rocking and now, we would give him more words to associate love with himself while enjoying the physical comfort as well.

During the next session, Peter was playing and came over to me and sat in my lap so we could again rock and sing while tapping. He got up after a minute and went to Suzie to ask her to rock him. She rocked him just as I had done, that is, loosely cradling him and singing her own song about his feelings. Peter looked up at Suzie, and I suggested that she could tell him some of the things she loved about him. Before Suzie started, I asked Peter if I could "tap in the good stuff" by tapping on his legs so he could enjoy the rocking. He agreed. While Suzie completed this exercise, I gently tapped on Peter's legs. Peter appeared to enjoy both the physical "message of love" and the verbal messages from Aunt Suzie. He seemed relaxed, made eye contact with Aunt Suzie, and smiled. They appeared attuned, and Aunt Suzie was able to help Peter regulate, both physically and emotionally. After Aunt Suzie was finished with the attachment statements, I said, "It looks like Peter is really enjoying this. I wonder if he would like to have Aunt Suzie continue to rock and sing." I said this to foster Aunt Suzie's awareness of Peter's internal state and desire, much as therapists do with parents and infants (Meins et al., 2002). She recognized how he was feeling and asked Peter if he would enjoy that, and he eagerly agreed. Peter seemed able to remain relaxed for longer periods of rocking. We continued to notice how relaxed his body felt, how he could feel safe and calm, while Aunt Suzie used slow BLS to tap in the feeling as a resource. I reminded Peter that he could picture Aunt Suzie rocking him anytime he needed to comfort himself, and she could help Peter practice by bringing up these feelings when they were at home and he could go to her for hugs or to be rocked anytime.

In accordance with phase-oriented trauma work, a great deal of time was spent in Phase 2: preparing Peter for trauma work. Most importantly, Peter needed a trusting safe relationship with me to complete the trauma work as well as with his aunt for support in his daily life. This takes more time for a child with such an extensive abusive history with little reason to trust adults. I wanted to ensure that Peter developed memory networks relating to his strengths and positive feelings, emotions, and behaviors so this adaptive information would link with traumatic material when we processed with EMDR (Shapiro, 2017). Peter also needed to be able to emotionally regulate and have useful coping skills to be successful in the EMDR process, to give strength during processing, and to emotionally or physically regulate after sessions or at home and school.

EMDR Assessment and Reprocessing

Once I was confident that Peter was able to use breathing exercises, his happy place, resources, and was able to accept and seek comfort from his aunt, Peter was ready to try to process some of his traumatic memories. Aunt Suzie was included in the session because she was a safe person for Peter and he wanted her there.

He had had hours of CCPT during which he played out many of the things that had happened to him. I had been able to identify traumatic events and possible negative beliefs Peter had developed about himself. During those sessions, I had been able to offer him adaptive information through reflections such as "All babies are good"; "It is the mommy's job to love the baby and feed him, rock him, and love him"; and "Even when a child does something bad, they are still good. They are just learning." He also learned to express emotions through my use of reflection, such as "It's scary when you can't get away," "You learned to protect yourself," and "You learned that it wasn't safe to trust your mom."

I started the assessment phase by reminding Peter, "You had some scary things happen to you with Mommy before you came to Aunt Suzie's house."

He said, "I know. We drew some of them." He still had nightmares about people hurting him and would worry that they would come and get him. Many nights he would still be confused about where he would sleep, and he would ask Suzie, "Where am I? Am I staying here with you?"

We had previously tried the tappers, and Peter was now able to use them. I told Peter that I thought it was time to use the tappers to make the memories less scary. I asked him if he wanted to use the sand tray or the art supplies (crayons, markers, paper) with the tappers. He picked the sand tray/miniatures/toys.

> Therapist: *Can we work on a scary time when Mommy hurt you where you used to live?* (He had played out and spoke of numerous times of Mommy hurting him that were cluster memories, which he often referred to it as the bad things.) *Do you remember a really bad time that you felt hurt and sad at your old house with your mom?*
>
> Peter: *Yes, when I was bad and Mommy was mean and hurt me bad.*
>
> Therapist: *What was the scariest part?*
>
> Peter: *Me crying and Mommy hitting and yelling.*
>
> Therapist: *Peter, when you think about that time, what do you think about yourself? Like "I'm bad," "I'm not important," or "I'm not good enough?"* (Because he had played out the belief, "I'm bad" while he played scenarios of his mom being mean to him, I gave him some related options for his negative cognition.)
>
> Peter: *I'm bad.* (His negative cognition was straightforward, he said it in his description of the memory, and it was a belief that he played out over and over in the playroom.)
>
> Therapist: *What would you like to be able to say about yourself?*
>
> Peter: *I am a good boy.*

We skipped the Validity of Cognition (VoC) score of the positive cognition, as he was very dichotomous and often rating things as either 0 or 10, with no in-between.

> Therapist: *What emotions do you feel when you think of the scary time?*
>
> Peter: *Scared, mad, and sad.*
>
> Therapist: *How scary or upsetting is it to think of that time?*

Peter: *All the way* (indicating a 10 with his arms stretched out all the way).

Therapist: *Where do you feel it in your body?*

Peter: *My tummy* (using the scanner—an old TV remote control).

By this point, he was pretty fidgety, and the assessment phase had only taken a couple of minutes. I had given him a choice of using the tappers in his socks or waist band or me tapping on his shoulders. He chose the tappers in his socks. I told him to think of the memory of Mommy hurting him. He went to the toys and selected the gorilla family. He took a "mother" figure and a "baby" figure. He put both of them together. Then, he had the mother figure hitting the baby.

Peter: *You're bad!*

Therapist: *Babies and children aren't bad. They just try to let people know what they need.*

Peter: *Yes they are. I'm bad.* (He walked over to the shelves and got a figure of a small child and had the mother figure hit that figure too.)

Peter: *No crying. You're bad!* (screaming while hitting the figure; see Figure 5.4).

Therapist: *Remember, little children and babies can't talk, so they cry to let parents know that they are hungry or hurting. It is the mommy's job to help him so he can stop crying.* (He paused and appeared to think about it but had the gorilla hit the baby again.) *Mommies should rock their children so they feel better and stop crying. Mommies are supposed to be nice and love their babies. Sometimes mommies are sick, and they don't know how to be loving mommies, even though the baby is good.*

Peter: *Mommies should rock their babies* (getting the baby doll and starting to rock her). *My mommy was mean and hurt me because I was bad.*

Therapist: *Go with that* (BLS while he continued to play in the sand). *What is happening now?*

Peter: *The baby is scared.*

Therapist: *Okay, go with that* (Peter continued to play that the baby was scared).

Peter: *My mommy was mean.*

Therapist: *Your mommy was mean because she was sick and could not be nice, and that is why she is not allowed to take care of you anymore.*

Peter: *Because she did bad things to a good baby?* (Looking at the baby doll) *The baby's crying, but he is good?*

Therapist: *Yes, just notice that.*

Peter (getting other figures to hit the little gorilla): *Sometimes, monsters hurt children too.*

Therapist: *No one should hit babies or little children.*

Peter (pausing): *Even when they are mad?*

Therapist: *No one should hit, even when they are mad. People aren't for hitting.*

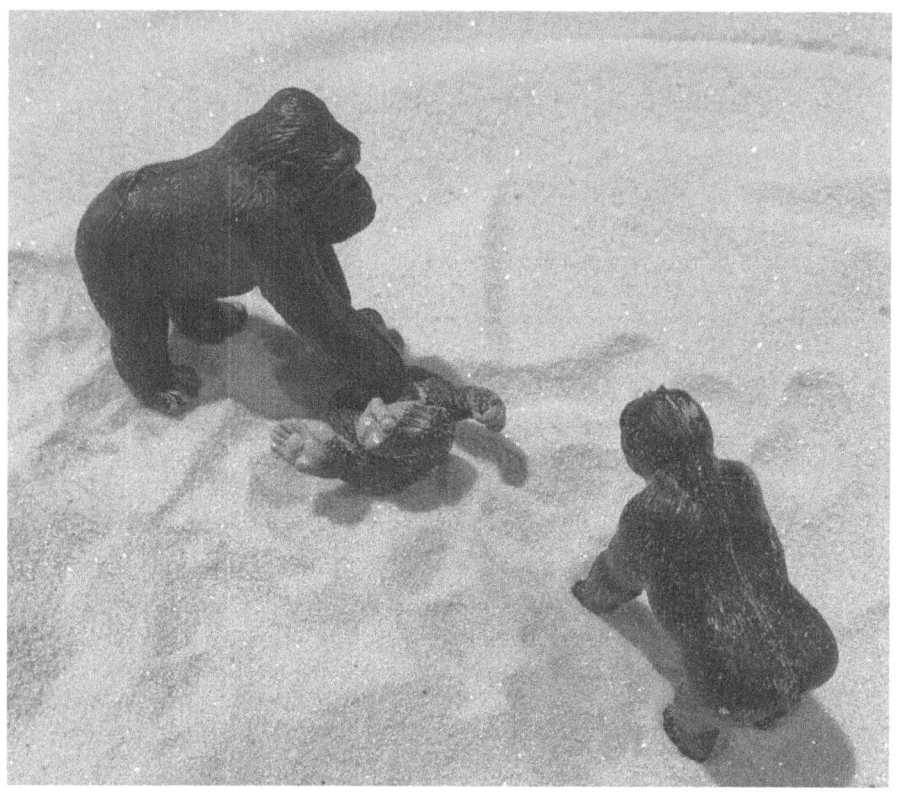

Figure 5.4 *The Gorilla Family During Processing*

Peter (getting the policeman figure to take the mother and others away): *Aunt Suzie doesn't hit me, even when I am bad.*

Aunt Suzie: *You are good even if you do something you are not supposed to.*

He walked over to the shelves and got three figures to represent his Aunt Suzie, Uncle Bob, and cousin Matthew, which he named. He put these figures in the sand tray. He took the little boy figure and said, "He lives here now." He then added play food, a bike, a bed, and a basketball player to the sand tray.

Therapist: *What else do you notice?*

Peter: *No one hurts me now.*

Therapist: *What else is happening?*

Peter (pointing to the little boy figure, then looking at Aunt Suzie): *I'm not hungry, and I don't have to hide food.*

Therapist: *What else?*

Peter: *No one hurts me. I'm okay. My mommy and the monsters can't be mean to me anymore.*

Therapist: *What else?*

Peter (taking tappers out of his socks): *I'm done.*

Therapist: *Do you believe, "I am good"?*

Peter: *Yes.*

Therapist: *How scary is it to think of the memory of Mommy hurting you?*

Peter put his hands together, indicating a 0. He then climbed into his aunt's lap on his own accord.

Therapist: *Think "I am good" while you think about the scary memory* (BLS). *Let's get the scanner and scan your body one more time for any yucky feelings.*

Peter got up and grabbed the TV remote and scanned his body with it.

Peter (after using the TV remote scanner): *I'm good.* (He crawled into his aunt's lap again, and she began gently rocking and singing to him.)

Therapist: *This is how mommies make children feel better and feel loved.* (He smiled while Aunt Suzie tapped these good feelings in.)

Peter was able to complete most of the assessment components without difficulty. Each was completed using developmentally appropriate modifications. He could not understand the VoC score. When working with young children, therapists may not be able to scale that component in assessment as children have great difficulty understanding how it is to be measured; even adults often struggle with the concept. Some EMDR writers have suggested eliminating the left brain scaling questions in order to allow the client to maintain right brain memory activation VoC (Parnell, 2013) and the scaling activities for young children can be frustrating and distracting due to their developmental level.

During desensitization I did not count each set exactly but was aware of the set length while allowing Peter's emotions, desire to share, and body language determine when to turn the tappers off. Therapists need to be flexible when working with young children. Young children may get distracted by the tappers going on and off or require additional time as they "play out their work," so the therapist should consider the temperament and needs of each young client. Peter began his processing using a metaphor, the monkey family that included a mommy monkey and baby monkey. It was easier for Peter to access the traumatic memory in a metaphor as it is a less intrusive way (Gil, 2016; Gomez, 2013). Metaphoric play allows children to project the experience onto objects so it does not trigger the trauma response and is less emotional. Since children do not have the same coping skills or understanding of the world, metaphoric play allows them to safely explore disturbing events, understand what has happened, express thoughts and feelings, and create solutions or different endings (Landreth, 2012; Gil, 2015; Gomez, 2013). It also facilitates access to healing as it is a right brain activity (Gomez, 2013). Here, Peter could safely begin the story of his trauma in metaphor and then shift as he desensitized the memory and felt safer (Gomez, 2013). The metaphor can also provide an escape route; if the experience is too overwhelming, the child can pretend that it was just a story. Peter was able to process and play out the trauma that occurred for him. Toward the end of the desensitization, he was able to process without metaphor. His processing led him to positive memories about his current situation, which included food, safety, and love. He was able to move through the frightening memories to the present with a new understanding about himself today and his role in the past events.

Many cognitive interweaves had to be used with Peter because as a 5-year-old, he still did not have sufficient information or experience to understand that he was not bad or that it was his mother's role to love him and care for him. So, therapists must use more cognitive interweaves when working with children. Interweaves introduce information through the form of statement, question, thought, or imagery to activate information the client has or introduce new information, which can then link with the isolated traumatic memory in order for it to be recorded with a healthier perspective. Interweaves were used to allow him to shift his understanding of himself and the world ("I'm bad. Crying babies are bad") and to challenge these beliefs with rational information such as "It is the mommy's job to be nice to the child to help him stop crying"; "Mommies should rock their children so they feel better and stop crying"; and "Sometimes mommies are sick, and they don't know how to be loving mommies, even though the baby is good." Peter was able to use this information to help reprocess those early memories.

After trauma processing sessions some children need more together time, while others need some solitary time. Children may feel tired, aroused, anxious, or relaxed, but the important thing is to monitor what their needs are and attempt to meet them in the best way possible. Suzie and I had discussed this, and she had several plans for postsession activities, including the swings at the park if he was aroused, a float in the pool if he was anxious, or perhaps a frozen yogurt as a treat.

CONCLUSION

Play therapy and EMDR can be blended to allow even young children to process their trauma and eliminate negative self-beliefs and inappropriate emotional and behavioral responses so they can lead a healthy, productive life. Play therapists already use play to develop skills, foster attachment and relationship, and process trauma events. Play provides a developmentally appropriate means for conducting all phases of EMDR with young children. It allows the child to engage with the therapist, provides history, demonstrates strengths and weaknesses for resourcing, conveys attachment issues, expresses negative self-beliefs, and processes memories and their meanings. Play in the form of nondirective CCPT or directive attachment and DPT activities provides the perfect vehicle for young children to imagine positive beliefs and states for resourcing as well as to build attachment. EMDR desensitization can be completed through play and expressive arts. The play therapist needs to consider children's developmental levels and regulation in order to substitute a form of play for the adult method of processing in Phase 4 of EMDR. As demonstrated in the preceding case, CCPT can be valuable in all phases of EMDR and DPT and can be invaluable when working with the youngest clients with attachment issues stemming from trauma.

REFERENCES

Adler-Tapia, R., & Settle, C. (2009). Evidence of the efficacy of EMDR with children and adolescents in individual psychotherapy: A review of the research publish in peer-reviewed journals. *Journal of EMDR Practice and Research, 3*(4), 232–247. doi:10.1891/1933-3196.3.4.232

Adler-Tapia, R., & Settle, C. (2017). *EMDR and the art of psychotherapy with children: Infants to adolescents*. New York, NY: Springer Publishing Company.

Amano, T., & Toichi, M. (2016). The role of alternating bilateral stimulation in establishing positive cognition in EMDR therapy: A multi-channel near-infrared spectroscopy study. *PLoS One, 11*(10), e0162735. doi:10.1371/journal.pone.0162735

American Psychiatric Association. (2004). *Practice guideline for the treatment of patients with acute stress disorder and posttraumatic stress disorder*. Arlington, VA: American Psychiatric Association Practice Guidelines. Retrieved from https://www.apa.org/ptsd-guideline/ptsd.pdf

Association for Play Therapy. (2019a). *Paper on touch clinical, professional and ethical issues*. Retrieved from https://cdn.ymaws.com/www.a4pt.org/resource/resmgr/Publications/Paper_On_Touch.pdf

Association for Play Therapy. (2019b). *Why play therapy?* Retrieved from https://www.a4pt.org/general/custom.asp?page=WhyPlayTherapy

Axline, V. (1947). *Play therapy*. Cambridge, MA: Houghton Mifflin.

Axline, V. (1969). *Play therapy*. New York, NY: Ballantine.

Badennoch, B. (2008). *Being a brain-wise therapist: A practical guide to interpersonal neurobiology*. New York, NY: W. W. Norton.

Beer, R. (2018). Efficacy of EMDR therapy for children with PTSD: A review of the literature. *Journal of EMDR Practice and Research, 12*(4), 177–195. doi:10.1891/1933-3196.12.4.177

Bowlby, J. (1969). *Attachment and loss, Vol. 1: Attachment*. New York, NY: Basic Books.

Bowlby, J. (1988). *A secure base: Parent-child attachment and healthy human development*. New York, NY: Basic Books.

Bratton, S., Ray, D., Rhine, T., & Jones, L. (2005). The efficacy of play therapy with children: A meta-analytic review of treatment outcomes. *Professional Psychology: Research and Practice, 36*, 376–390. doi:10.1037/0735-7028.36.4.376

Brazelton, T. B., & Cramer, B. G. (1990). *The earliest relationship*. Reading, MA: Addison-Wesley.

Briere, J., Hodges, M., & Godbout, N. (2010). Traumatic stress, affect dysregulation, and dysfunctional avoidance: A structural equation model. *Journal of traumatic Stress, 23*, 767–774. doi:10.1002/jts.20578

Brody, V. A. (1997). *The dialogue of touch: Developmental play therapy* (2nd ed.). Northvale, NJ: Jason Aronson.

Campbell, M. M., & Knoetze, J. J. (2010). Repetitive symbolic play as a therapeutic process in child-centered play therapy. *International Journal of Play Therapy, 19*(4), 222–234. doi:10.1037/a0021030

Chen, R., Gillespie, A., Zhao, Y., Xi, Y., Ren, Y., & McLean, L. (2018). The efficacy of eye movement desensitization and reprocessing in children and adults who have experienced complex childhood trauma: A systematic review of randomized controlled trials. *Frontiers in Psychology*. doi:10.3389/fpsyg.2017.01750

Chen, Y. R., Hung, K. W., Tsai, J. C., Chu, H., Chung, M. H., Chen, S. R., . . . Chou, K. R. (2014). Efficacy of eye-movement desensitization and reprocessing for patients with posttraumatic stress disorder: A meta-analysis of randomized controlled trials. *PLoS One, 9*(8), e103676. doi:10.1371/journal.pone.0103676

Cloitre, M., Stolbach, B. C., Herman, J. L., van der Kolk, B., Pynoos, R., Wang, J., & Petkova, E. (2009). A developmental approach to complex PTSD: Childhood and adult cumulative trauma as predictors of symptom complexity. *Journal of Traumatic Stress, 22*(5), 399–408. doi:10.1002/jts.20444

Courtney, J. A., & Gray, S. W. (2014). A phenomenological inquiry into practitioner experiences of developmental play therapy: Implications for training in touch. *International Journal of Play Therapy, 23*(2), 114–129. doi:10.1037/a0036366

Courtney, J. A., & Siu, A. F. Y. (2018). Practitioner experiences of touch in working with children in play therapy. *International Journal of Play Therapy, 27*(2), 92–102. doi:10.1037/pla0000064

Courtney, J. A., Velasquez, M., & Bakai Toth, V. (2017). FirstPlay® infant massage storytelling: Facilitating corrective touch experiences with a teenage mother and her abused infant. In J. A. Courtney & R. D. Nolan (Eds.), *Touch in child counseling and play therapy: An ethical and clinical guide* (pp. 48–62). New York, NY: Routledge.

D'Andrea, W., Ford, J. D., Stolbach, B., Spinazzola, J., & van der Kolk, B. A. (2012). Understanding interpersonal trauma in children: Why we need a developmentally appropriate trauma diagnosis. *American Journal of Orthopsychiatry, 82*(2), 187–200. doi:10.1111/j.1939-0025.2012.01154.x

Felitti, V. J., Anda, R. F., Nordenberg, D., Williamson, D. F., Spitz, A. M., Edwards, V., . . . Marks, J. S. (1998). Relationship of childhood abuse and household dysfunction to many of the leading causes of death in adults: The Adverse Childhood Experiences (ACE) Study. *American Journal of Preventative Medicine, 14*(4), 245–248. doi:10.1016/S0749-3797(98)00017-8

Field, T. (2014). *Touch* (2nd ed.). Cambridge, MA: MIT Press.

Gaskill, R., & Perry, B. (2014). The neurobiological power of play: Using the Neurosequential Model of Therapeutics™ to guide play in the healing process. In C. Machoidi & D. Crenshaw (Eds.), *Creative arts & play therapy for attachment trauma*. New York, NY: Guilford Press.

Gil, E. (2016). *Posttraumatic play in children: What clinicians need to know*. New York, NY: Guilford Press.

Gomez, A. M. (2013). *EMDR therapy and adjunct approaches with children: Complex trauma, attachment, and dissociation*. New York, NY: Springer Publishing Company.

Goodyear-Brown, P. (2010). *Play therapy with traumatized children: A prescriptive approach*. Hoboken, NJ: Wiley.

Greenwald, R. (1994). Applying eye movement desensitization reprocessing (EMDR) to the treatment of traumatized children: Five case studies. *Anxiety Disorders Practice Journal, 1*, 83–97.

Greenwald, R. (2005). *Child trauma handbook: A guide for helping trauma-exposed children and adolescents*. New York, NY: Routledge Mental Health.

Grobbel, R., Cooke, K., & Bonet, N. (2017). Ethical use of touch and nurturing-restraint in play therapy with aggressive young children, as illustrated through a reflective supervision session. In J. A. Courtney & R. D. Nolan (Eds.), *Touch in child counseling and play therapy: An ethical and clinical guide*. New York, NY: Routledge.

Guerney, B., Jr. (1964). Filial therapy: Description and rationale. *Journal of Consulting Psychology, 28*, 304–310. doi:10.1037/h0041340

Hensel, T. (2009). EMDR with children and adolescents after single-incident trauma an intervention study. *Journal of EMDR Practice and Research, 3*, 2–9. doi:10.1891/1933-3196.3.1.2

Hong, R., & Mason, C. M. (2016). Becoming a neurobiologically informed play therapist. *International Journal of Play Therapy, 25*(1), 35–44. doi:10.1037/pla0000020

International Society for Traumatic Stress Studies. (2018). *Practice guidelines*. Retrieved from http://www.istss.org/treating-trauma/new-istss-prevention-and-treatment-guidelines.aspx

Keyser, D., & Ahn, H. (2017). Predictors of mental health and developmental service utilization among children age birth to 5 years in child welfare: A systematic review. *Journal of Public Child Welfare, 11*(4–5), 388–412. doi:10.1080/15548732.2017.1339656

Kinniburgh, K. J., Blaustein, M., Spinazzola, J., & van der Kolk, B. A. (2005). Attachment, self-regulation, and competency. *Psychiatric Annals, 35*(5), 424–430. doi:10.3928/00485713-20050501-08

Korn, D., & Leeds, A. M. (2002). Preliminary evidence of efficacy of EMDR resource development and installation in the stabilization phase of treatment of complex posttraumatic stress disorder. *Journal of Clinical Psychology, 58*(12), 1465–1487. doi:10.1002/jclp.10099

Kottman, T. (1995). *Partners in play an Adlerian approach to play therapy*. Alexandria, VA: American Counseling Association.

Landreth, G. L. (2002). Therapeutic limit setting in the play therapy relationship. *Professional Psychology: Research and Practice, 33*(6), 529–535. doi:10.1037/0735-7028.33.6.529

Landreth, G. L. (2012). *Play therapy: The art of the relationship* (3rd ed.). New York, NY: Routledge.

Leeds, A. M. (2009). *A guide to the standard EMDR protocols for clinicians, supervisors, and consultants*. New York, NY: Springer Publishing Company.

Levine, P. (2002). *In an unspoken voice: How the body releases trauma and restores goodness*. Berkley, CA: North Atlantic Books.

Lin, D., & Bratton, S. (2015). A meta-analytic review of child-centered play therapy approaches. *Journal of Counseling and Development, 93*, 45–58. doi:10.1002/j.1556-6676.2015.00180.x

Lovett, J. (1999). *Small wonders: Healing childhood trauma with EMDR*. New York, NY: The Free Press.

Lovett, J. (2015). *Trauma-attachment tangle: Modifying EMDR to help children resolve trauma and develop loving relationships*. New York, NY: Routledge/Taylor & Francis.

Malchiodi, C. A. (2014). Neurobiology, creative interventions, and childhood trauma. In C. A. Malchiodi (Ed.), *Creative interventions with traumatized children* (2nd ed.). New York, NY: Guilford Press.

McNeil-Harber, F. M. (2004). Ethical consideration in the use of nonerotic touch in psychotherapy with children. *Ethics & Behavior, 14*(2), 123–140.

Meins, E., Fernyhough, C., Wainwright, R., Das Gupta, M., Fradley, E., & Tuckey, M. (2002). Maternal mind-mindedness and attachment security as predictors of theory of mind understanding. *Child Development, 73*(6), 1715–1726. doi:10.1111/1467-8624.00501

Moreno-Alcázar, A., Treen, D., Valiente-Gómez, A., Sio-Eroles, A., Pérez, V., Amann, B. L., & Radua, J. (2017). Efficacy of eye movement desensitization and reprocessing in children and adolescent with post-traumatic stress disorder: A meta-analysis of randomized controlled trials. *Frontiers in Psychology, 8*, 1750. doi:10.3389/fpsyg.2017.01750

Painter, K., & Scannapieco, M. (2013). Child maltreatment: The neurobiological aspects of posttraumatic stress disorder. *Journal of Evidence-Based Social Work, 10*(4), 276–284. doi:10.1080/10911359.2011.566468

Panksepp, J., & Biven, L. (2012). *The archaeology of mind: Neuroevolutionary origins of human emotions*. New York, NY: W. W. Norton.

Parnell, L. (2013). *Attachment-focused EMDR: Healing relational trauma*. New York, NY: W. W. Norton.

Perry, B. D. (2009). Examining child maltreatment through a neurodevelopmental lens: Clinical applications of the neurosequential model of therapeutics. *Journal of Loss and Trauma, 14*, 240–255. doi:10.1080/15325020903004350

Perry, B. D., & Dobson, C. D. (2009, March). Surviving childhood trauma: The role of relationships in prevention of, and recovery from, trauma-related problems. *Counselling Children and Young People*, 28–31. doi:10.4135/9781446288894

Porges, S. (2011). *The polyvagal theory: Neurophysiological foundations of emotions, attachment, communication, and self-regulation.* New York, NY: W. W. Norton.

Rathore, H. E. (2018). Trust and attunement-focused EMDR with a child. *Journal of EMDR Practice and Research, 12*(4), 255–268. doi:10.1891/1933-3196.12.4.255

Ray, D., Armstrong, S., Balkin, R., & Jayne, K. (2015). Child centered play therapy in the schools: Review and meta-analysis. *Psychology in the Schools, 52,* 107–123. doi:10.1002/pits.21798

Robbins, J. (2000, December). Brief trauma treatment of a toddler using EMDR. *EMDRIA Newsletter, 5*(Special Edition), 25–27. Retrieved from https://emdria.omeka.net/items/show/16686

Rogers, C. R. (1980). *A way of being.* New York, NY: Houghton Mifflin.

Schore, A. N. (2001). The effects of early relational trauma on right brain development, affect regulation and infant mental health. *Infant Mental Health Journal, 22,* 201–269. doi:10.1002/1097-0355(200101/04)22:13.0.CO;2-9

Schore, A. N. (2009). Relational trauma and the developing right brain. *Annals of the New York Academy of Sciences, 1159,* 189–203. doi:10.1111/j.1749-6632.2009.04474.x

Schore, J. R., &. Schore, A. N. (2014). Regulation theory and affect regulation psychotherapy: A clinical primer. *Smith College Studies in Social Work, 84*(2–3), 178–195. doi:10.1080/00377317.2014.923719

Shapiro, F. (2014). The role of eye movement desensitization and reprocessing (EMDR) therapy in medicine: Addressing the psychological and physical symptoms stemming from adverse life experiences. *The Permanente Journal., 18,* 71–77. doi:10.7812/TPP/13-098

Shapiro, F. (2017). *Eye movement desensitization and reprocessing: Basic principles, protocols and procedures* (3rd ed.). New York, NY: Guilford Press.

Siegel, D. J. (1999). *The developing mind: How relationships and the brain interact or shape who we are.* New York, NY: Guilford Press.

Siegel, D. J. (2012). *The developing mind: How relationships and the brain interact to shape who we are* (2nd ed.). New York, NY: Guilford Press.

Spinazzola, J., van der Kolk, B., & Ford, J. D. (2018). When nowhere is safe: interpersonal trauma and attachment adversity as antecedents of posttraumatic stress disorder and developmental trauma disorder. *Journal of Traumatic Stress, 31,* 631–642. doi:10.1002/jts.22320

Sroufe, L. A., Coffino, B., & Carlson, E. A. (2010). Conceptualizing the role of early experience: Lessons from the Minnesota Longitudinal Study. *Developmental Review, 30,* 36–51. doi:10.1016/j.dr.2009.12.002

Stirling, J., & Amaya-Jackson, L. (2015). Understanding the behavioral and emotional consequences of child abuse. *American Academy of Pediatrics.* doi:10.1542/peds.2008-1885

Struik, A., Ensink, J. B. M., & Lindauer, R. J. L. (2017). I won't do EMDR! The use of the "Sleeping Dogs" method to overcome children's resistance to EMDR therapy. *Journal of EMDR Practice and Research, 11*(4), 166–180. doi:10.1891/1933-3196.11.4.166

Substance Abuse and Mental Health Services America. (2012). *Comparative effectiveness research series: Eye movement desensitization and reprocessing therapy: An information resource.* SAMHSA's National Registry of Evidence-based Programs and Practices. Retrieved from https://cdn.ymaws.com/www.emdria.org/resource/resmgr/research/treatment_guidelines/samhsa.2012.nrepp-comparativ.pdf

Swimm, L. (2018). EMDR intervention for a 17-month-old child to treat attachment trauma: Clinical case presentation. *Journal of EMDR Practice and Research, 12*(4), 269–279.

U.S. Department of Health & Human Services, Administration for Children and Families, Administration on Children, Youth and Families, Children's Bureau. (2018). *Child maltreatment 2016*. Retrieved from https://www.acf.hhs.gov/cb/research-data-techno logy/statistics-research/child-maltreatment

U.S. Department of Veterans Affairs. (2019). *PTSD treatment basics*. Retrieved from https://www.ptsd.va.gov/understand_tx/tx_basics.asp

van der Hart, O., Brown, P., & van der Kolk, B. A. (1989). Pierre Janet's treatment of post-traumatic stress. *Journal of Traumatic Stress, 2,* 379–395. doi:10.1007/978-1-4899-1034-9_12

van der Kolk, B. (2014). *The body keeps the score: Brain, mind and body in the healing of trauma*. New York, NY: Viking Penguin.

van der Kolk, B. A. (2005). Developmental trauma disorder: Toward a rational diagnosis for children with complex trauma histories. *Psychiatric Annals, 35*(5), 401–408. doi:10.3928/00485713-20050501-06

van der Kolk, B. A., & Fisler, R. (1995). Dissociation and the fragmentary nature of traumatic memories: Overview and exploratory study. *Journal of Traumatic Stress, 8*(4), 505–525. doi:10.1002/jts.2490080402

Verardo, A. R., & Cioccolanti, E. (2017). Traumatic experiences and EMDR in childhood and adolescence: A review of the scientific literature on efficacy studies. *Clinical Neuropsychiatry, 14*(5), 313–320. Retrieved from http://ezproxy.fau.edu/login?url=http://search.ebscohost.com/login.aspx?direct=true&db=a9h&AN=126203881&site=ehost-live

Vereshack, P. (1993). *The psychotherapy of the deepest self*. Toronto, ON, Canada: Life Perspectives.

Waters, F. S. (2016). *Healing the fractured child: Diagnosis and treatment of youth with dissociation*. New York, NY: Springer Publishing Company.

Wesselmann, D., Armstrong, S., Schweitzer, C., Davidson, M., & Potter, A. (2018). An integrative EMDR and family therapy model for treating attachment trauma in children: A case series. *Journal of EMDR Practice & Research, 12*(4), 196–207. doi:10.1891/1933-3196.12.4.196

Wesselmann, D., Davidson, M., Armstrong, S., Schweitzer, C., Bruckner, D., & Potter, A. E. (2012). EMDR as a treatment for improving attachment status in adults and children. *European Review of Applied Psychology/Revue Européenne de Psychologie Appliquée, 62*(4), 223–230. doi:10.1016/j.erap.2012.08.008

Wesselmann, D., Schweitzer, C., & Armstrong, S. (2014). *Integrative team treatment for attachment trauma in children: Family therapy and EMDR*. New York, NY: W. W. Norton.

World Health Organization. (2013). *Guidelines for the management of conditions specifically related to stress*. Geneva, Switzerland. Retrieved from https://apps.who.int/iris/bitstream/handle/10665/85119/9789241505406_eng.pdf;jsessionid=246B0F019F87BD6F37438497A96858C3?sequence=1

6

EMDR and Creative Arts Therapy: How Creative Arts Therapies Can Extend the Reach of EMDR With Complex Clients

ELIZABETH DAVIS

INTRODUCTION

The utilization of eye movement desensitization and reprocessing (EMDR) therapy alone, as Francine Shapiro has discussed (Shapiro, 2018, p. 328), presents challenges when working with children, particularly with complex relational trauma. Limits for the effectiveness of EMDR include the developmental immaturity of the child and missing adaptive information, the impact of trauma on skill development, and lack of trust due to the impact of relational trauma. This chapter explores how creative arts therapy holds the potential as a special form of mentalization therapy that can support and strengthen the skills required for success in EMDR in Phase 4 processing. This approach emphasizes how the expressive arts, when used strategically, can extend the reach of EMDR by utilizing the indirect dyadic process of art making within a therapeutic relationship increasing trust, building metacognitive functioning, elevating concrete thinking through experiential learning, and taking a curious, open, and playful stance that helps grow self-reflective capacity.

The advent of EMDR revolutionized the possibilities for treating the impact of trauma. Most EMDR therapists will recall how their own first experiences with EMDR changed what they thought was possible for helping their clients heal. As revolutionary as EMDR is, however, difficulties implementing the protocol remain with some clients, and particularly with adults and children who suffer with complex trauma. As a clinician who learned EMDR while working primarily with children in residential treatment, I found myself frustrated that this powerful healing approach was so often out of reach for the youth I served. Could it be that some complex cases are contraindicated for EMDR? Is it possible to use art therapy strategically for increasing the possibility that EMDR might be effective? My career path as an EMDR clinician, a formally trained artist, and art therapist has naturally led me to these questions.

THE DEVELOPMENT OF ART EXPRESSION AND EXPERIENCE

For a clear understanding of the utility of integrating EMDR and art therapy, an examination of the psychological experience of art and creative expression is foundational. Art expression is not an adjunct technique or new scripted protocol. Art appreciation and expression is intertwined with human development and behavior as well as social, political, and historical narrative. Spontaneous art making appears early as a natural behavior, reflective of the stages of maturity. Every culture and time also has its accompanying artist and art objects that narrate the culture's identity and beliefs. As expressive art experience is, therefore, a complex, multifaceted topic, an understanding of the meaning and function of it is required.

Developmentally, art creation emerges in the behavior of children beginning in the toddler years. Initially most excited by the associated sensory experience, a child begins making marks. A few months later, the scribbled form gets a corresponding name, like "Firetruck," as one 3-year-old client proclaimed of his red scribble drawing. This emerging connection of expression and form represents the *scribble stage* of artistic development (Lowenfeld & Brittain, *Stages of Artistic Development* in Anderson, 1978; see Figure 6.1).

As the child's mind matures, so too do their artistic expressions. Early representational depictions emerge more recognizable, heads growing arms and fingers, depicting a concrete representation of a growing sense of a physical self. Emerging schema of physical representations evidence the *preschematic stage*

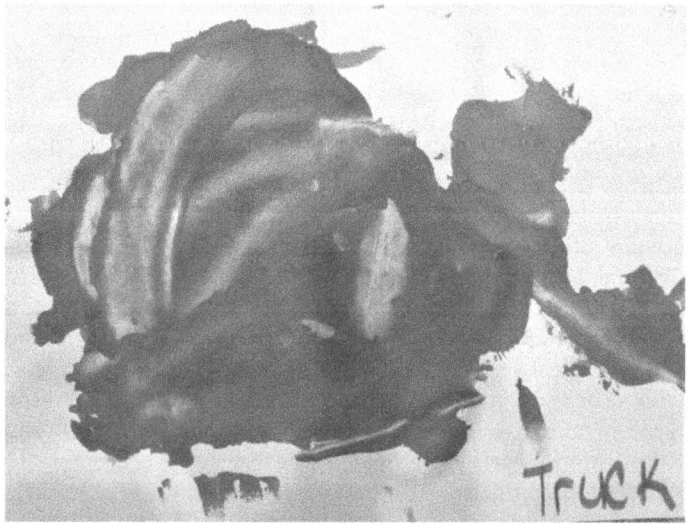

Figure 6.1 *Example of Scribble Stage: Firetruck*

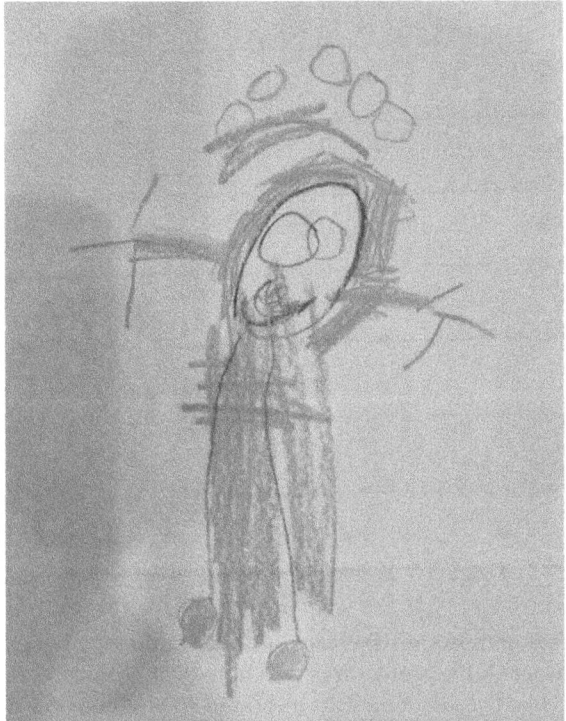

Figure 6.2 *Example of Schematic Stage: Girl and Crown*

of artistic development (Lowenfeld & Brittain, *Stages of Artistic Development* in Anderson, 1978). A 4-year-old girl creates a colorful body and head with arms with round circles on top, her "princess crown" (see Figure 6.2).

As the child grows, the sophistication of expression matches the maturing development of the complex experiences of the self. The adolescent's focus becomes typically embedded in the self in relation to their peer group denoting the *dawning of realism* or *gang age* (Lowenfeld & Brittain in Anderson, 1978). An 11-year-old creates the image of herself and peers depicting their individual styles while demonstrating unison of form with peers through body posture (see Figure 6.3).

Artistic expression follows a developing conceptualization of the connection of self to others and to the world. The creative art process becomes, like words, a potential creative tool for developing meaning. But ultimately what function does art expression serve, even as it emerges spontaneously through development?

The 20th century philosopher John Dewey (1934/1980) spoke of art as "bound to experience" in his famous Harvard Lectures, *Art as Experience*. He states, "The actual work of art is what the product does with and in experience" (p. 2). Dewey argues that art is significant in its meaning for and in experience and creates an awareness in the present moment. To Dewey, the artist and art spectator engage in a reflective behavior bringing together both inner and outer dimensions of experience to create a new awareness in the present moment.

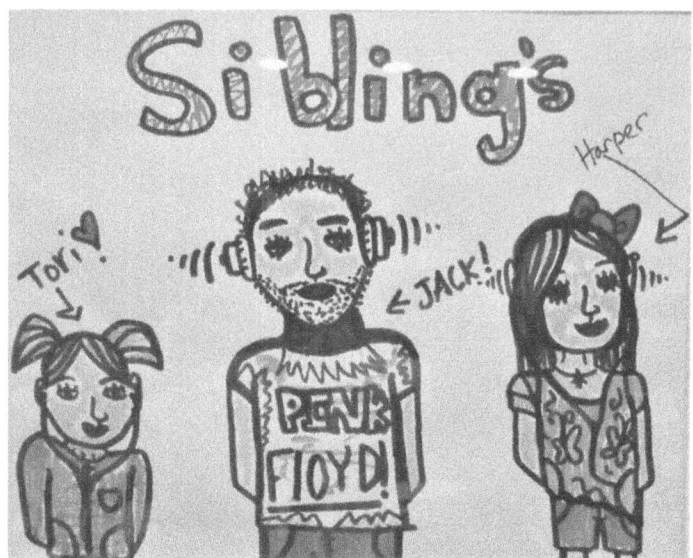

Figure 6.3 *Example of Gang Age: Peer Group*

Contemporary authors on the topic of art experience have shared similar views. Ellen Winner (2019), professor of psychology at Boston College and director of the *Arts and Mind Lab*, discusses art as bound to emotion and the attitude and experience of the individual in time. She proposes replacing "What is art?" with the question "When is art?" (p. 15).

The great 20th century psychoanalyst D. H. Winnicott (1971/2005) wrote of art and creativity in this way as well. Winnicott (1971/2005) writes "[Creativity] belongs to the approach of the individual to the external world" (p. 91). He emphasized further in this quote the important function of art psychologically:

> It is assumed here that the task of reality acceptance is never completed, that no human being is free from the strain of relating inner and outer reality, and that relief from this strain is provided by an intermediate area of experience which is not challenged (art, religion, etc.). This intermediate area is in direct continuity with the play area of the small child lost in play. (p. 18)

Here, Winnicott seems to suggest that the stance of the artist, or creator of art, is one of relieving the tension between inner and outer experience, as a means for managing psychic reality. Therefore, art expression appears to function, at least in part, as a modality of holding experiences that remain uncertain, ambiguous, and unresolved in a concrete form that can contain the tension and allow for a kind of management or framing of the experience.

But what of art's role beyond synthesizing ambiguous or uncertain experience in an external form? Why do humans seem to make art instinctually? The neurobiologist Bruce Perry describes that expressive arts are not only embedded in every culture and time but also naturally arrived at means for healing and transformation. Perry (2015) suggests that arts across expressive modalities provide a holistic neurobiological experience that culture after culture has converged on to address the healing needed in the brain and nervous system. He writes, "These practices emerged because they worked. People felt better and functioned better, and the core elements of the healing process were reinforced and passed on" (p. xxi). In this view, expressive experiences are understood as a type of culturally arrived at system of digesting stress.

Nobel Laureate, psychiatrist, and neuroscientist, Eric Kandel, one of the pioneers of the relatively new field of *neuroesthetics*, which seeks to understand the importance of art for human development, takes this view one step further. Eric Kandel's work looks at how art is an evolutionary adaptation, an instinctual response that aids in survival. He and his contemporary at University College of London, Semir Zeki, have set out to understand the neuroscience behind aesthetic experience and why it matters to humans. Kandel (2012) writes of his research, "The arts... encode information, stories, and perspectives that allow us to appraise courses of action and the feelings and motives of others in a palatable, low-risk way" (p. 501). This adaptive response, Kandel asserts, allows for an assimilation of information both emotional and factual in a way that increases adaptation and ultimately survival. In this way, expressive arts is both healing and protective as a means to increase resilience.

EVIDENCE FOR USING A CREATIVE ARTS APPROACH FOR HEALING

In spite of centuries of philosophical and experiential validation, as well as emerging neuroscientific understandings, creative arts therapy as a field of psychotherapy has struggled to define itself in the age of evidence-based practice. One practical reason is the complex nature of researching a field full of diverse methods embedded into different psychological paradigms and consisting of therapists from diverse training backgrounds. Though case studies exist, few are quantitative and methodologically sound. The last systematic review on art therapy and trauma (Schouten, de Niet, Knipscheer, Kleber, & Hutschemaekers, 2015) concluded that although there are a handful of studies that do show promise, the number is few (only six passed the methodological parameters of this review). Schouten and colleagues, who conducted this systematic analysis for the *Journal of Trauma, Violence, and Abuse*, further point out that the field of art therapy generally lacks an established research tradition. Artists are not known for their love of doing research. Another systematic review from 2018, studying art therapy for anxiety, came to a very similar conclusion. Abbing and colleagues (2018) concluded, "To get high quality evidence of effectiveness of AT [art therapy] on anxiety (disorders), more robust studies are needed" (p. 10). Both reviews were focused on the adult population. Even less research exists for how art therapy works treating traumatized children. Perhaps Bessel van der Kolk (2015), in his book reviewing the state of trauma treatments, *The Body Keeps the Score: Brain, Mind and Body in the Healing of Trauma*, captures the overall problem best when he writes:

> There are thousands of art, music, and dance therapists who do beautiful work with abused children, soldiers suffering from PTSD, incest victims, refugees, and torture survivors, and numerous accounts

attest to the effectiveness of expressive therapists. However, at this point we know very little about how they work or about the specific aspects of traumatic stress they address, and it would present an enormous logistical and financial challenge to do the research necessary to establish their value scientifically. (p. 244)

A growing number of researchers in the field of art therapy are beginning to follow a different strategy to identify how the expressive therapies function for healing. As with Kandel's investigation on the neuroscientific basis of art and art making, researchers are now looking for the underlying common experiences, or elements, inherent in expressive therapies that offer the most promise for mental health healing.

Noah Hass-Cohen and Joanna Clyde Findlay (2015), in their book, *Art Therapy and the Neuroscience of Relationships, Creativity, and Resiliency: Skills and Practices*, have proposed an approach to art therapy following the tenets of interpersonal neurobiology. They aptly call their approach Art Therapy Relational Neuroscience. They assert that expressive therapy modalities work in the relational sphere. Their approach focuses on how creative experiences activate the brain hemispheres both horizontally and vertically (emphasizing the left and right hemispheres as well as the brainstem, limbic system, and cortex). The theoretical assumption follows that an experience that can activate so many parts of the brain must be naturally integrative. Primarily, these authors draw their approach from the research and theories of interpersonal neurobiologists and research on attachment (pp. 7–8). Hass-Cohen and Findlay use the acronym CREATE, which means Creative embodiment, Relational resonating, Expressive communicating, Adaptive responding, Transformative integrating, and Empathizing and compassion as descriptors of the therapist's stance to treatment (p. 1). These six principles are meant to guide directives and how the therapist engages goals with the client.

The actual approach of Hass-Cohen and Findlay appears primarily focused on the use of art experiences to reinforce intellectual, social, and emotional learning. They identify two dialectical forms of learning, concrete and abstract, and use art directives purposefully in order to both build mental models of understanding and grow reflective functioning of the self and others. These authors base their model in part on *experiential learning theory* as proposed by experimental psychologist David Kolb. Kolb (1984) proposed the theory of a four-stage dynamic, cyclical learning approach where knowledge begins formation with concrete experience, leading to reflective observation, then to abstract conceptualization, and finally to active experimentation, and back again (p. 21). The major assertions of Kolb are that learning is a dynamic flow of experience, influenced by subjective reflection and learning styles, not just a process of acquisition, manipulation, and recall of data.

Hass-Cohen and Findlay's approach to art therapy, connecting it with experiential learning strategies, is not new to the field. The idea of integrating learning approaches and creative arts goes back to the beginnings of art as a formal part of therapy with one of the founders, Margaret Naumburg. Naumburg studied with Maria Montessori in Italy before immigrating to the United States. Montessori's approach, which is widely accepted as one of the most effective educational models, integrates sensorial and expressive arts experience into learning curriculum

(Montessori, 1967). Naumburg went on to start the first Montessori school in the United States, *The Walden School* (Naumburg, 1950/1973).

Another theoretical approach in the field of expressive therapy that builds on neuroscience is the expressive therapies continuum (ETC). ETC also incorporates the concepts of learning and information processing as a basis for the effectiveness of art therapy. ETC (Lusebrink & Hinz, 2016), like CREATE, relies on evidence and theories proposed in the field of neuroscience that look at the developmental impact complex childhood trauma has on brain integration. This approach proposes that targeted and specific art experiences have the power to ignite various areas of brain functioning, such as the kinesthetic/sensory, the perceptual/affective, and the cognitive/symbolic. These areas have often been impacted by early developmental trauma (Perry, 2009) and are therefore poorly developed or integrated. The use of expressive art experiences to ignite these areas, such as expressive movement and scribble drawing (kinesthetic and sensory), contour drawing and emotive dance (perceptual and affective), and creating symbols and describing through art (cognitive and symbolic), can increase neural integration and brain growth. Using this approach, therefore, is a means to stimulate healing from developmental trauma by increasing neural integration.

Research on ETC or CREATE as effective trauma treatments still lacks hard evidence as do other neurologically based art approaches. Proving empirically that an art experiences the mechanism of change in a treatment approach is difficult, as there are many variables to consider (e.g., therapeutic relationship, client's feelings about art and expression, client's prior art experiences generally, specific histories of clients and types of traumas, the setting of the art experience). Many subjects as well as control groups would be needed to validate these approaches (as with any research), and replication with accuracy is difficult in the expressive arts. How expressive therapies can strategically be used by being informed by neuroscience is still, therefore, somewhat guesswork. More research on what is happening in the brain during expressive activities over time may yield more defining evidence. Perhaps the field of neuroesthetics will also shed some light on these approaches over time.

Putting aside approaches exploring how an art experience might ignite brain areas, other strategies for exploring the underlying mechanisms of how expressive arts function have focused on similarities that exist with other evidence-based models. Neil Springhan and Val Huet (2018) of the Oxford College of Arts and Therapies advance a biopsychosocial model of art therapy. In a recent paper for the *Journal of the American Art Therapy Association*, "Art as Relational Encounter: Ostensive Communication Theory of Art Therapy," Springhan and Huet assert that what is known from attachment theory and relational neurobiology informs what is most effective between the art therapist and the client. This approach to understanding how art therapy works looks less at the brain and more at what makes any therapy effective. They view art therapy as a kind of interactive approach rather than as a set of art activities that have standalone impact. As these authors propose, art therapy is a kind of "ostensive communication" or "marked mirroring" of another through the created art form. For example, a client creates an artwork that is shared with the therapist. The therapist acts with joint attention to the art form and client and "marks" the creative form, mirroring back to the client a sense of knowing of the form. Similar to the dyadic process between a caregiver and child, the artwork allows for an extended dyadic relational interaction with the client, where the artwork becomes a mentalized aspect of the client's internal world. Because the artwork can be free of the literal, raw aspects of life, the artwork can be playfully distant, operating like play does for the child (Winnicott, 1971/2005).

Dominik Havsteen-Franklin, from Brunel University London, takes this relational approach further by investigating what makes expressive therapy generally effective, whether it be music, dance, visual art, or poetry (Havsteen-Franklin, Maratos, Usiskin, & Heagney, 2016). He does not attempt to create a model or approach but instead looks at how art therapists do their work. His preliminary conclusion and focus of continued research have been that art therapists work in a way that similarly overlaps the guiding principles of mentalization-based therapy (referred to as MBT). MBT is a dynamic model of psychotherapy, which specifically focuses on helping clients develop their mentalization skills for increasing emotional and behavioral regulation, effective relationships, and overall well-being. Mentalization skills are key to emotional regulation and social functioning. As a psychotherapy model for treating trauma, MBT already has an evidence base (Bales, van Beek, Smits, Willemsen, & Busschbach, 2012; Bateman & Fonagy, 1999, 2001, 2008; Lenzenweger, Clarkin, Levy, Yeomans, & Kernberg, 2012). Research on mentalization additionally integrates or is consistent with the fields of relational neurobiology, developmental psychology, psychoanalytic theory, and attachment theory.

If what creative art therapists do effectively mimics MBT, this could shed additional light onto how creative therapies are effective at addressing trauma experience generally. Additionally, if this hypothesis holds, it may unite many of the research approaches taken in the field, including the interpersonal neurobiology theory, neuroscience theories, and experiential learning approach. Furthermore, the conceptualization of expressive therapy as a type of MBT may offer a better way of validating how expressive therapy works, as this approach potentially links to a preexisting evidence base.

Offered subsequently is a description of MBT, and mentalization, to help conceptualize the overlap between the two modalities.

MBT AND MENTALIZATION

MBT is a relatively new therapy model (1999), emerging from developmental research in the areas of Theory of Mind and attachment. Peter Fonagy and his colleague Anthony Bateman, of the Ana Freud Center for Children and Families in London (referred to as "the London School"), are researchers in the field of the Theory of Mind and attachment in children. They have proposed MBT as an approach initially intended to address the difficulties of treating borderline personality disorders (BPDs). However, now MBT is used widely for other diagnoses such as drug addictions, eating disorders, personality disorders, and posttraumatic stress disorder (PTSD; Lorenzini, Campbell, & Fonagy, 2019). The primary objective of MBT is to help build and support mentalization skills so that clients can better regulate emotions and behaviors and make meaningful relationships, therefore increasing their well-being overall.

Mentalization, as Batemen and Fonagy define, is "the process by which we implicitly and explicitly interpret the actions of oneself and others as meaningful on the basis of intentional mental states" (Bateman & Fonagy, 2010, p. 11). Mentalization enables a child to imagine that like themselves, other people have a mental world too, with their own desires, feelings, goals, and preferences. Through this imaginary process, mentalization allows the child to connect to others, feel empathy, and ultimately develop a sense of their own self objectively (seeing themselves through the eyes of others). When this metacognitive skill emerges (typically around 4–5 years of age), a true understanding of empathy, guilt, responsibility, and connection emerges. In addition to taking on another point of view, the child can also develop trust and reciprocity in relationships, making the way for social–emotional learning. Being able to see others as likeminded allows for curiosity of learning from others about self. However, this shared learning is dependent on the child having a trusted other through which they feel safe to be seen. Fonagy describes this trusting relationship stance as *epistemic trust*, which allows for a connected mind state, one not isolated in first-person perspective but utilizing the resources found in connection with the minds of others. This allows for the exchange of knowledge from another's perspective, allowing for more perspective taking and understanding of the self and others more coherently (Fonagy, Gergely, Jurist, & Target, 2002/2004; Fonagy & Allison, 2014).

The development of mentalization skills is disrupted when stress and trauma in childhood impact the child's ability to trust. For example, when a caregiver abuses the child in their care, the child's defensive system is activated, closing off connection in protection of the self. If a child is subjected to chronic abuse, betrayal, or neglect, the epistemic trust, which is reliant upon open connection, is impacted, and *epistemic vigilance* or *mistrust* takes over. This can thwart the development of mentalization skills. Without this skill, which connects the inner world with the larger external social sphere of humanity, the child is psychologically isolated, confused, and without a coherent, objective self-understanding. This isolation and incoherence limit the child's ability to flexibly and effectively interact with others, benefit from the knowledge and connection with others, and feel connected to the world at large (Fonagy et al., 2004; Bateman & Fonagy, 2013).

Ultimately, according to Fonagy, a child experiencing this isolated state under the impact of childhood abuse and neglect cannot maintain this state of isolation and confusion and is forced to "split their ego functioning to maintain dual modes of functioning" (Fonagy et al., 2004, p. 266). In a "split" self, the child finds themselves stuck in either an overly personal and raw emotional state without the benefit of connection and objectivity to make sense of it or a detached dissociated state, cut off from the emotional underpinnings of their experience. Fonagy refers to these two states as *psych equivalent* and *pretend mode* (2004). These two states represent the failure of the development of affect regulation skills that are typically passed on through the attachment relationship with a trusted other. Without the ability to use the attachment figures as a trusted source for learning to regulate, the child splits off from their emotions to cope. These two modes remain underdeveloped and lack integration necessary for digestion of emotional experience. Psych equivalent states represent refractory emotional states where feelings equal reality and take form in primitive, reactive behaviors. These states are evident in the acting out of emotions behaviorally, like the child in a state of meltdown or a teen who uses cutting as a form of numbing in order to shut down emotions. Pretend mode states are detached and emotionally numb, without connection to oneself as an emotionally driven being. These states are manifested when clients seem emotionless and alexithymic when discussing trauma or minimize emotions generally. Because the use of a caregiver to help mediate or resolve the split between dysregulated emotions and dissociated emotions is suspect, the stance of epistemic vigilance and distrust takes over (Fonagy & Allison, 2014). Fonagy and Bateman discuss this as the origin of borderline conditions. They refer to borderline phenomena as part of many disorders and are not referencing the specific diagnosis in the *Diagnostic and Statistical Manual of Mental Disorders* (Fonagy et al., 2004, p. 10).

The lack of perspective taking that goes along with this psychic split further complicates logical reasoning, at least where psychological beings are concerned. Fonagy identifies how the lack of mentalization results in an overly concrete approach to reasoning. Without having a mentalizing stance (a perspective that others have a mental world through which they make decisions, have emotions, and have intentions), what others do is translated solely by the outcome of their actions. Fonagy calls this *teleological mode*. A teleological interpretation refers to believing that the outcome is the reason for the action (Fonagy et al., 2004, p. 223). An example would be the old riddle: *"Why did the chicken cross the road? To get to the other side."* Here, the end point is the rationale instead of an imagined intention on the part of the subject. A mentalizing interpretation might look at whether there is a motivating reason the chicken might want to cross the road, like a food source. With this type of reasoning, "Things have to happen or be done to be meaningful" (Bateman & Fonagy, 2013). This kind of reasoning can function rationally in a matter-of-fact world, but when applied to psychologically minded beings, the teleological mode is missing the necessary data that mentalization skills provide. Teleological reasoning presents as a kind of naive reasoning around the logical understandings of others. Like being stuck in concrete reasoning, using the experiential learning theory model, teleological reasoning is limited and presents as immature (toddlers are naturally teleological in their approach to understanding the world as are those on the severe end of the autism spectrum). However, if trauma of a relational kind is to be worked through, perspective taking is an integral part of the process.

These modes, as Fonagy describes, exemplify the problem with resolving complex states of trauma. Processing the hard edges of reality demands contingency between inner and outer experience, a coming together so that sense can be made of the complexities of reality. The child must reconcile their raw emotions with the facts of the matter. In a healthy attachment relationship, it is the primary caregiver who acts most importantly as the go-between, mirroring and then reframing the emotional experience of the child in an appropriate way, so that the experience is digestible. For example, a parent lovingly explained to their frightened child why grandpa, who has Alzheimer's, was no longer offering hugs or smiles but instead seemed angry and scary, "Grandpa still loves you but is not experiencing all of who he is, including all the loving memories he has about you. He feels lonely and scared because he can't put into words what he is going through. Sometimes he lashes out because he is so scared. But this is not your fault and you are safe." This caregiver in this example gives the child information about an intentional state of the grandparent, whose behavior was interpreted by the child as scary. By doing so, the parent helps the child make sense of their emotional reaction and the facts of the matter. The parent in effect helps the child metabolize the scary experience of their grandparent and thus models to the child the skill of affect regulation through mentalization. Thus, the parent acts as the mentalizing affect regulator between the child's two worlds (inner and outer) until the child's own mentalization skills and knowledge base emerge developmentally as sophisticated enough to take over.

When the child grows up without a caregiver who can act in the capacity as a regulator of the two worlds, but instead dysregulates the child through covert or overt abuse, or neglect, the child is developmentally impacted and traumatized. The developmental impact on mentalization skills increases the complexity of treating trauma effectively with EMDR. Treating childhood relational trauma inflicted by a parent, for example, is particularly reliant on the client imagining an objective point of view (metacognitive), usually with a trusted other (a therapist), where they can see themselves objectively in relation to their perpetrator. These mentalization skills allow for the client/victim to know that they are a child with limited power and the abuse was not their fault but that of the abusive adult. Mentalization skills in this case also allow them to form a trusting enough bond with a therapist to help gain that objective perspective clearly.

Without addressing mentalization deficits, EMDR therapists run the risk of retraumatizing clients who do not have the skills to process through their childhood trauma and could become worse as a result of failure and reexposure to the memory. Theo Ingenhoven from the Center of Psychotherapy, Pro Persona, Lunteren, in the Netherlands, urged caution around trauma processing with a one-size-fits-all perspective, pointing out the differences from simple, or type I trauma, and complex, or type II trauma (Terr, 1991). In his appeal in the *European Journal of Psychotraumatology* (Ingenhoven, 2015), he discusses the complexity of cascading issues proceeding from chronic and early childhood trauma. When defensive responses are employed, namely the fight–flight–freeze responses, mentalization skills shut down. This shutting down of mentalization in the context of chronic childhood stress and trauma results in truncated social emotional skill development over time. In the absence of a secure connection to a caregiver's mind, the child enlists alternate survival-based strategies for managing stress. Survival-based strategies often entail behaviors intended to eternalize emotions through acting out or internalizing in the form of pathological dissociated states. Therefore, the child may come to display aggression toward others, having difficulty owning and controlling behavioral impulses. Alternatively, the child may "act in" displaying self-harm and sematic issues.

A lack of mentalization skills, effectively turned off under triggers or perceived threats, and/or developmentally truncated due to childhood attachment insecurity, presents challenges and risks when processing through trauma. When mentalization skills are lacking, the trauma experience cannot be objectively engaged and is more likely to be experienced as a flashback. The negative cognitive beliefs regarding childhood trauma hang on, defying objective logic, with clients making statements like: "I know I would not believe this for another child, but it still must be true for me." Feelings are felt as if they are the same as external facts, with clients insisting the threats are still real, even when the trauma is long over. Client's actions often seem in the service of "making it real" through suicidal ideation, self-harm, reenactments, and aggressive acting out behaviors. Other clients feel completely detached in pretend mode and can rattle off their history without emotion, holding to only the material facts. They suffer debilitating depression and cannot connect with themselves enough to connect the dots. Additionally, the therapist is often on the receiving end of a client who is locked in a state of epistemic mistrust and suspicion based on early experiences of rejection and betrayal and wanting proof (teleological stance) of caring. These clients can be highly resistant to all efforts made to reach them and act out to push others away.

Children who come to therapy having experienced abuse, neglect, or even an overstressed, overworked parent most naturally embody the limitation of mentalization. Sometimes, with children, this presentation of behavior is dismissed or overlooked as normal or perhaps a bit behind the developmental curve. Children with childhood trauma are by their developmental nature complex clients. Their caregivers often do not provide contingent attunement, having not received it themselves, or are perpetrators of abuse having their own mentalization deficits. Additionally, there are many families that simply are in tremendous states of transition where stress responses prevent mindful attunement. Because traumatized children naturally lack both power in their own life and significant exposure to other minds, they often take longer to form a trusting therapeutic relationship. If trauma processing is introduced too early, and trust is not well established, these children often retreat emotionally or dissociate and detach more. This cycle can build more epistemic mistrust, further complicating treatment.

The use of the EMDR protocol is complicated enough with children who are on track developmentally. Therapists must be creative to help a child learn to identify feelings and beliefs and reflect inward with insight enough to report what the protocol asks for. For those locked in epistemic mistrust, processing cannot move forward effectively and mentalization skills may be lacking to bridge the split. The first step in therapy, therefore, is to help a child feel safe, begin to form connection, and express self in a safe and accessible way.

As expressive therapists are naturally engaging in a nonthreatening way that can increase and support mentalization skills, an integrative approach that capitalizes on this engagement increases the effectiveness of trauma processing in Phase 4 of EMDR. Therefore, expressive therapy, as a type of mentalization therapy, offers a potential to increase EMDR's effectiveness.

Now that MBT and mentalization have been defined, an understanding of how expressive therapies are similar to MBT will further identify the overlap in the two modalities.

EXPRESSIVE THERAPY AS MENTALIZATION THERAPY

Peter Fonagy has been a supporter in the advancement of art therapy research and acknowledges the work that many art therapists do in some of the most challenging settings and with the most complex treatment populations, such as those found in juvenile justice, corrections, substance abuse, and inpatient care. Fonagy (2012, p. 90) writes, "Art therapy has not been well served by research but has served a complex and varied client group arguably better than any other single modality." His belief is that the art psychotherapies hold a possible solution, as he writes, "[A]rt therapy has the key or perhaps a key to our understanding of the mechanisms underpinning change in all kinds of psychological treatments." His view of art therapy's mechanism of healing has to do with how the creative and expressive process unites the psyche's understanding of the external and internal world and externalizes the understanding in a synthesized form:

> The use of art, writing, or other expressive therapies allows the internal to be expressed externally so that it can be verbalized at a distance through an alternative medium and from a different perspective. Experience and feeling is placed outside of the mind and into the world to facilitate explicit mentalizing. (Bateman & Fonagy, 2004, p. 172)

A growing number of researchers in the field of art therapy are beginning to follow the line of reasoning of Fonagy and the research team of Dominik Havsteen-Franklin in London. The approach is to identify the methods the field uses to build mentalizing skills, skills that subsequently support trauma digestion and integration generally. If the overlap between the field of expressive therapy and MBT can be effectively understood, this may help identify some of the key, previously hard-to-validate aspects of expressive therapy that are effective at building mentalization skills (Buck & Havsteen-Franklin, 2013).

Marianne Verfaille, who spent her career working with children with attachment problems in the Netherlands, has been a driving force behind understanding the overlap of MBT and art therapy. In her book *Mentalizing in Arts Therapies* (2016), she proposes recommendations for the art therapist who wants to mindfully engage in facilitating mentalization skills with their clients. Many of these recommendations are discerning what many art therapists naturally do and looking at this through the lens of MBT.

Verfaille begins by noting that mentalizing is "an art, not a science" (p. 119). The mindful therapist in this regard takes a particular stance in relation to their client, not a focus on techniques. The mentalizing therapist works on the premise the client needs to feel understood. The therapist is inquisitive and curious, offers playful interactions, follows the client's pace, and focuses on understanding the client's perspective. The therapist does not challenge a client who is in a state where they are unable to bridge to an objective perspective (namely, in the primitive modes of psych equivalent, pretend, and teleological). Building epistemic trust and seeing the client's point of view are given priority. Verfaille emphasizes vitality and curious openness about the client's process. Equally emphasized is an authentic stance, noticing one's own reactions to the client and the countertransference information. The therapist must be a mindful and honest *mentalizer* of themselves if they are to help their client feel comfortable with opening up. In a stance of attunement with the client, where the therapist is reflecting and marking the connection between the art experience and the client, mentalization is enhanced and modeled.

Much of what MBT recommends might be construed as simply good therapy. Most good therapists provide contingent attunement to their clients along with consistent trustworthy behavior. MBT, however, emphasizes as a part of this attuned engagement an intentional stance of noticing mental states as states and being mindful of the client's mental state over their behavior. In MBT, the mental states are highlighted, and the act of marking and mirroring the client's state of mind takes precedence. MBT values attunement over telling, and collaborative engagement over hierarchical dominance. The mentalization approach takes on the goal of opening up the mental world of the client to both themselves and others, to discover authentic needs, wants, feelings, insights and understandings, and as a consequence, the minds of others by inference. Much of what MBT strives to do pivots on developing a trusting relationship where the client feels truly seen, allowing for epistemic trust to emerge, so that the minds of others can be seen as collaborators instead of threats. With connection to others comes better perspective taking, and a more objective self-understanding.

Art therapy (as a modality of psychotherapy) is naturally focused on the mental world of the client. The artwork is seen as a window into the client's mind as well as an avenue to insight and healing. Art therapists are not art teachers, in this respect. These two disciplines are distinct in that the art therapist's use of art materials is solely for the enhancement of the client's mental health goals, which are internal. An art product is of secondary importance, and not the focus except as it relates to the needs of the client. If a client tears up their artwork and throws it in the trash, it is the stance of the art therapist to notice the client's mental world over the behavior or the object. In this way, the object becomes a part of the process of understanding the internal experience of the client.

Art therapists, as mentalization therapists, prioritize attunement to the client's implicit expressions and behaviors with, and in reaction to, the art media and directives. The mentalizing art therapist's task with the client is to attune, mirror, and mark back the expressive process, making the implicit experiences explicit and seen. Or, by extension to the expressive art object, the therapist stands in contingent alignment with the client, allowing the metaphorical art object to hold the yet-to-be digested experience.

Art therapist works with hands on, tangible processes that align with concrete, teleological mode thinking. Through the technical process of creative problem-solving, the objects and directives can serve to elevate thought processes by creative abstraction of ideas. Linking concepts and forms, the abstract can be symbolized and concretized for easier understanding and integration. For example, when made into an artwork, the often-used *Safe Place* resource exercise can now be represented concretely and physically to help make the concept more real.

Expressive therapy, utilizing the potential of imagery, drama, and creative stories can furthermore allow the client to open their mind to different perspectives. The expressive forms then can stand for what was not experienced but needed to be, or a platform for rehearsing transformation, or trying on new ideas and possibilities. In this way, the art therapist works to expand the client's experiential reach to increase perspective taking.

In art therapy, the expressive form can take on the part of whatever the client may need in the present, such as a resource, symbol for courage, strength, a reparative narrative, a connection, or a mindful experience in the present moment, to help stay grounded. The art object alternatively can act as a mirror revealing parts of the self yet to be integrated and affect that is still hard to verbalize. Furthermore, art expression used metaphorically has the potential as an actor on stage to distance psychic reality and make it safe for true digestion. In these ways, art expression serves to connect the client to skills and aspects of their psyche needed for digestion of traumatic experience and has the potential to bridge to the power of EMDR Phase 4.

EMDR, ART THERAPY, AND MAXIMIZING MENTALIZATION FOR PROCESSING

As outlined earlier, expressive arts therapy holds the potential as a special form of mentalization therapy that can enhance a client's metacognitive skills and open them to reflect on themselves and others and help bring traumatic experience into a form for digestion. The question becomes how can the creative therapist best utilize their vocation to maximize these potentials for increasing readiness for EMDR processing?

The following section outlines approaches, with emphasis on the stance rather than the technique. However, as creative therapists, techniques are a part of the material work. Actual hands-on actions happen as a part of the therapy. Therefore, in this discussion, a balance of emphasis is on the therapist's stance in relation to the materials and methods as an unfolding experience. The methods used subsequently are discussed within a therapeutic case study following the phases of EMDR. The intention for the therapist is to build metacognitive skills, reflective insight, and trust while maintaining contingent attunement to the client's mental state. This approach requires that the therapist take a flexible stance that defaults to the needs of the client in the moment rather than prioritizing the activity. Therefore, the case example given later cannot be viewed fully outside of the therapeutic relationship. Clinical judgment and knowing one's client are paramount to making the call as to when to continue with an activity and when to diverge on the assumption that the client is struggling too much. After all, part of the process of creativity is meeting a challenge that can easily flip to a burdensome task or frustration. The job of the therapist is to know that tipping point and keep attunement to the client while holding the larger frame.

With this in mind, caveats for non-art/expressive therapists working with specific media and directives should be understood. Expressive and arts therapists undertake special training to understand the nature of the experience of utilizing a particular media and directive. This training allows for safety and attunement to be held with clients, as the trained therapist can account for the possible pitfalls as well as hold the experiential mirroring, being able to mentalize the experience the client is having with the art media. The non-art therapist, who chooses to take advantage of the potential of expressive therapy, still needs training in a media and directives to safely administer to complex clients. Those who are untrained in an expressive modality run the risk of not holding attunement while offering what might be to the client a challenging or risky art directive. Therapists who naively offer paint, for example, without knowing the potential risks for their client (such as triggering a regressive state, frustration for not meeting internal expectations, or potential sensory flashbacks) may destabilize their client in session. All media present unique technical, sensory, and emotional experiences. Where necessary, the untrained therapist would be well advised to seek consultation from an art or expressive therapist as well as specific training in the media they use.

In the next section, I describe a case study outlining the integration of creative arts with the intention of strategically increasing readiness for trauma processing. I follow the phases of EMDR therapy, but with the understanding that mentalization skills need support and development for safe processing to occur. This case demonstrates my thought process regarding building the scaffolding needed to work through complex trauma using EMDR.

INTEGRATING CREATIVE ARTS AND EMDR: THE CASE OF ELLA

Ella is a 13-year-old girl referred by her mother due to separation anxiety, flashbacks, panic attacks, somatic issues, and a history of sexual abuse by her father. Following discovery and indictment of Ella's father for his involvement in child pornography 2 years prior, Ella received counseling by several clinicians to address the abuse history that appeared to extend as far back as early childhood. Counselors, according to Mom, had expressed after a handful of sessions that Ella was remarkably resilient, and the abuse did not seem to have affected her too much. Mom also received the advice that she was too enmeshed with her daughter and needed to let her "move on."

Ella, who disclosed the abuse after pictures of the abuse were found on the father's computer, presented nearly always with a big smile and seemed upbeat to those around her. Ella's cheery demeanor was charming, and her care for others was interpreted as a part of her astounding resilience. Additionally, Ella expressed she was happy and seemed full of almost manic energy to involve herself in social activities with others. By all surface accounts, Ella presented as an energetic and happy young teen.

Ella's mother openly disclosed to Ella's counselors that she had her own abuse history and was in counseling for it. Mom demonstrated "enabling" behaviors toward Ella, such as helping her daughter articulate her experiences by speaking for her, often finishing her sentences, and homeschooling Ella. It was easy to see how counselors could interpret Mom as an enmeshed parent who had her own mental health challenges.

When I first met with Ella's mom, I presented her with this theory of enmeshment as a part of an attachment evaluation in preparation for working with her daughter. Ella's mom was quick to express that her enmeshment with her daughter has been her concern for years (well before the abuse was disclosed) and recounted her failed efforts to help her and her daughter become less fused. Mom discussed a memory she had of Ella when she was 17 months old where she observed that Ella seemed to have "switched" overnight from a normal acting toddler into a highly anxious, but seemingly cheery one. At that time, Mom recalled, Ella also shifted from being a relatively good sleeper to needing to sleep with her nearly every night. With feelings of both guilt and shame, Mom recounted her unsuccessful efforts trying to help her daughter self-regulate. Mom expressed knowing her behaviors were enmeshed, but also that when she has consistently held herself back, Ella plummeted into somatic illness and complaints that were frightening for both of them.

Following my meeting with Mom, Ella reluctantly agreed to come in for another attempt at counseling. Upon assessing Ella, with Mom present as this was the only way Ella would agree to come, the immediate impression was that Ella looked developmentally like a toddler might with her mother. Ella was hyperfocused on her mother's face, frequently asking for help understanding her experiences, physically clingy, and constantly fidgeting. For example, during the history-taking, Ella would stall over and over and look to her mother with a big wide smile, as if to say, "Please say what I can't find words for." Mom, in sync with her child, would recount the trauma experiences Ella had disclosed, in headline form, along with related data to help with the history-taking. When Mom was asked to reserve her response and allow Ella time to work out her own way of expressing herself, Ella would stall out, laugh, and repeat, "I don't know, I don't know . . ." or "Happy, happy, happy" over and over. Her body would follow with a bouncing motion, appearing pleading and toddlerlike. When taking the distress ratings (Subjective Unit of Disturbance Rating Scale [SUDS]) for the target memories, again Ella was unable to pick a number, could not identify a feeling out of her own head (even with a chart in front of her), and looked to her mother with a wide questioning smile. Mom would offer data about how upset Ella had been in the past when she had a flashback or how she struggled with reminders of the trauma.

Without Mom's detailed observations and recollections, an understanding of how Ella was affected by her trauma would not have been possible. It was as if Ella utilized her mother, even at 13, to mentalize her emotions and make sense of her experiences. While her mom could recount her flashback experiences, sleep issues, panic attacks, somatic complaints, and shutdown states, Ella could only recount the very surface of the narrative. It was quickly apparent in the assessment phase that Ella was stuck in a pretend mode, sequestered away from emotional information with only the acknowledgment of facts. Her only engagement emotionally was described by her as a "happy part" that always wanted to take care that she stays "happy." While in states of emotional trigger, as Mom described and later as work evolved, it also appeared Ella was not able to articulate her internal experience other than the feeling of needing to be rescued and feeling overwhelming panic, a probable psych equivalent mode. In this mode, she would cling to mom, phone her in a state of needing rescue if she was not with her, or hide. Ella appeared to present, as the history was told, to be either in a primitive all emotion state or unable to cognitively label her emotions and connect inward. Ella also experienced somatic symptoms frequently. She would become sleepy and/or develop headaches or stomach aches to the point of throwing up.

As can be imagined, a young child experiencing sexual abuse from a caregiver is in a double bind. When a child lacks power and the ability to resolve, an adaptive response is to avoid reflecting inward, to dissociate from emotional messages, and to seek whatever secure attachment base that can be found to stabilize. In the case of Ella, she appeared to have locked herself into a strategy of disguised dissociated happiness, except to her mother, who could hold her mind in mind and keep her system in a state of relative homeostasis, much like a mom and infant dyad. In fact, it appeared that Ella and her mom were locked in time from the observed 17-month-old Ella to the present. Ella therefore needed her mother as a bridge to connect her inner and outer realty much like a young child.

When mom withdrew and attempted to leave Ella to figure it out, Ella, lacking the internal skills to name her feelings and digest mindfully, became hyper, anxious, and physically symptomatic. As found by the research team of Sergi Ballespi in Barcelona as well as Fonagy and the London School, "Somatization processes are usually associated with a lack of insight or with emotional unawareness, especially in adolescents where the ability for self-reflection is beginning to mature" (Ballespi et al., 2019, p. 1). Ella presented habitually with somatic symptoms, which Mom expressed were the most frightening part of her reactions to stress: severe headaches and throwing up with stomach aches. When Ella was presented with stressful situations unfamiliar to her or triggering the past trauma, Ella would decompensate and present as overwhelmed by these symptoms. Ella's inability to name and comprehend her emotional states left those emotions in a primitive form that was often expressed physically in somatic symptoms. The inability to cognitively link emotions and body sensations has been found as a key component of somatization issues in traumatized clients. Ballespi and colleagues write:

> [M]entalizing (or reflection on) of emotional states prevents somatization because comprehension plays a role in the emotional metabolism, while the non-mentalization of emotional states fosters somatization, especially when emotions are detected but not understood. This is consistent with the idea that when people cannot "digest" what they see, not paying attention to that content can be a better option. This is consistent with the popular advice "out of sight, out of mind", as well as the use of distracting CBT techniques to reduce suffering. However, since current results highlight the internal process of "comprehending" as an important step towards "true insight", implications for mental health should be considered. (Ballespi et al., 2019, p. 10)

Ella's options as a child whose father was the perpetrator and who had not developed a cognitive understanding of her emotional states at the time when abuse began was to naturally adapt using the "out of sight, out of mind" option. This provided Ella the ability to manage her homeostasis, with the help of her mother, while still living with her father. However, putting her emotions out of sight stunted her skills for identifying her feelings and digesting her experiences in the long run. At 13, Ella still presented with the emotional regulation skills of a young child in relation to her trauma memories.

What follows are descriptions of the creative therapy activities, interventions, and the general therapist stance used to address Ella's developmentally stuck mentalization skill development, where she seemed unable to read her own feelings, needs, and wants, to know her own mind, and was stuck relying largely on the mentalization of her mother. I follow the phases of EMDR, beginning with history gathering, psychoeducation, resourcing, and skill development (Phases 1 and 2 of EMDR), through play and expressive supported processing (Phases 4–7), and finally, to the integration for future challenges.

The first task of therapy is developing with the client a framework of what treatment should look like. I use a collaborative approach where the clinician is upfront about theoretical orientation as well as the specific understanding of the client's case. The collaborative approach models a mentalizing stance, where the therapist is open and honest about their mental process and collaborates with the client as a partner and the ultimate agent of change. This approach supports the building of epistemic trust and limits over- or underreliance on the therapist (Greenwald, 2005; Boon, Steele, & Van Der Hart, 2017). Clients express investment in treatment, knowing what their therapist is up to mentally, feeling respected for having been offered theoretical understanding, encouraged by the openness to question choices, and oriented to their role as an ultimate agent of change.

With both Ella and her mother, I therefore began the process of therapy with an open discussion about my own theoretical approach and initiated the process of information gathering. As a part of this process, I began with metaphors and expressive techniques to help Ella manage the process. History-taking can be very challenging for traumatized clients. Every exposure to memories has the potential to retraumatize, especially with children and complex trauma generally, where mentalization skills and resources may not be robust. Therefore, our discussion began with how to go about this process safely.

Ella was particularly anxious in her presentation, looking nearly all the time to her mother. Mom was able to set up a plan with Ella in advance that included special treats as the days went. As our therapy model was primarily intensive (full- and half-day sessions with frequent breaks), this worked well as a motivator. Additionally, Ella and her mom identified positive soothing skills, some of which Ella had already used to help herself. Making these skills more understood and appreciated was discussed to help build Ella's confidence in her ability to help regulate herself. This discussion also was focused on reflecting on what Ella's internal wants, needs, and feeling states are, a beginning of self-understanding.

Ella discussed enjoying walking, playing with clay, reading the Harry Potter books, and acting. The discussion of Harry Potter, plays, and props led to ideas of how to create a unique timeline. When taking a history with children or complex clients, a timeline can often help structure the information outside of the client's head. Since with complex trauma, events often feel disorganized, a timeline adds order to disorder. Moreover, a timeline also offers orientation to the present as opposed to the past. This can decrease the client's vulnerability to go into a flashback by being able to concretely see the past as opposed to the present. With complex trauma and with children who lack a good comprehension of time, time-orientation strategies should be used frequently to help the client connect to the safe and present moment (Martin, 2016).

In collaboration with Ella and her mom, we developed the idea of a *timeline scroll*, similar to what Dumbledore might have had in the Harry Potter movies. This metaphor was unique, with some special qualities built in, such as some parts of the timeline could be hidden under the curl while other parts were available for view. This allowed for another way to limit exposure, metaphorically. Additionally, this seemed a fun element to the process of history-taking, enlisting creative expression and formation of a metaphor (Figure 6.4).

The *scroll of life*, as it came to be known, was filled year by year from birth to the future. Each year, Mom helped Ella identify positive experiences as well as the traumatic ones, giving only the headlines to limit triggering trauma memories. This titrated approach helped to balance the stress that Ella was experiencing.

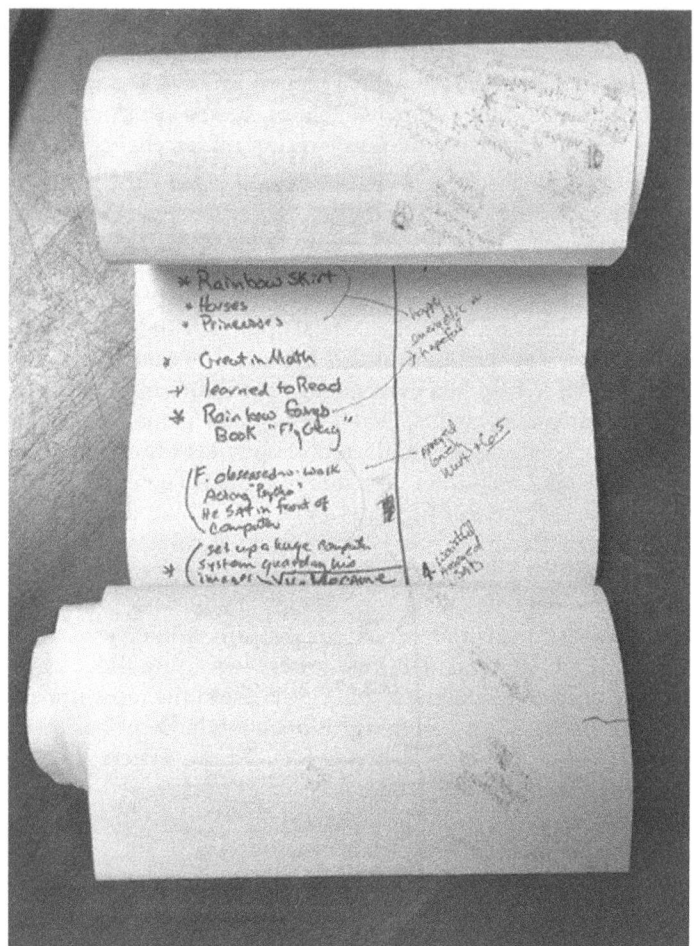

Figure 6.4 *Timeline Scroll for History-Taking*

At times, a good memory was discussed in full while taking the history. At the end of this process, a metaphorical object was created, a scroll of life, which could function as time orientation, contain the facts, enhance the coherence of understanding the past, and increase reflective self-understanding, as well as hold a fun association. This scroll aptly demonstrates the power of a metaphor in therapy to help hold meaning and structure.

With the scroll completed, the territory that would be covered with EMDR was better understood. Also more clearly understood was Ella's tolerance for exposure to the memories, her ability to regulate herself with and without Mom, and her limitations for cognitively reflecting on the past. Discovered through this process was Ella's inability to place an SUDS on the traumatic memories. Mom was able to describe Ella's response at the time the memories emerged. Ella, appearing in pretend mode, was unable to access the emotional content that the memories harbored. At times in the process, she became very tired, and at one point, she developed a headache. At these times, it was assumed her tolerance for the process was exceeded, and the conversation and activity shifted to light and fun with walking and breaks woven in.

Following history-taking and formulating the approach to treatment, focus shifted to psychoeducation, which had begun earlier at the outset of treatment with a discussion of trauma, window of tolerance (WOT), complex trauma, and mentalization. Working with children and/or complex trauma, psychoeducation needs to be a part of the treatment journey. Understanding attachment, how trauma affects the brain, nervous system, emotional regulation, beliefs, the body's embedded responses to trauma triggers, defenses or ego states, what is normal, and so forth are topics that help the client understand their own experiences and make sense of them. Education also provides the often-missing adaptive information, particularly around what is normal and healthy (Steele et al., 2017).

The therapist's task in the process of psychoeducation is to offer the client a model for understanding themselves and feeling recognized, or mirrored. Essential to this process is the client feeling seen or mentalized correctly (Lorenzini et al., 2019). This aspect of mentalizing the client's experience through learning and teaching can help increase epistemic trust, lower defenses, and begin to build a cognitive framework that primes the brain for processing the traumatic experiences. Psychoeducation, additionally, also overlaps skill building and resourcing. With an understanding and framework of symptoms comes a way to manage and regulate better.

The creative process here can greatly enhance the process of learning. As noted earlier, learning through creative, hands-on approaches allows for richer understanding. When teleological or concrete thinking is dominant, this approach may scaffold a client into a more elevated and objective option through the use of metaphoric props. Expressive therapy used in this way can increase digestion of concepts and make learning them more appealing.

To begin to understand how panic and somatic symptoms are triggered and how to help manage them, I engaged Ella in a fun way of exploring the concept of *WOT*. WOT is a metaphor proposed by neurobiologist and psychiatrist Dan Siegel (1999) to help explain the way the brain and nervous system reacts to stress. This concept has become a very useful tool in trauma treatment, as it helps the client understand their nervous system reactivity around triggers. In what follows, I offer a simple sample script for older children, such as Ella, for how to discuss WOT. I use this kind of language in combination with drawing a WOT on a whiteboard and using a brain model.

> *We all react to stress a little differently and have our own comfort zone, or Window of Tolerance, "WOT" for short. Inside our WOT, we feel pretty good, as we can think clearly and relate to others and our life feels manageable. When we are too stressed, frightened, or threatened, however, we can go out of our WOT. When this happens, our brain switches gears and tunes out the smart thinking part (prefrontal cortex [PFC]) and tunes into our emotional brain more (limbic brain and brainstem). At this point, your smart thinking brain is no longer fully online, and you may feel strong emotions, like fear, anger, or panic.*

> *When our emotional brain takes over, we are in what's called survival mode. In survival mode, our brain and body act to save us from immediate danger. It tells us to either fight, flee, freeze, fawn, cry out, or in some cases shut down all together. Survival mode helps us survive when overwhelming, life-threatening events occur. Going into survival mode is often triggered by real danger in the immediate environment.*

Examples from the client's experience should be offered here, or something general.

> *For example, if you are walking on the street and you see a car coming directly at you, you don't stop to think about what to do. You jump out of the way. Afterward, you may notice your heart beating fast and feeling fear. That is your survival brain taking over. Later, you may think to yourself, wow, that happened so fast I didn't even have a chance to think. These responses are mostly out of our conscious control. That is because your emotional brain works fast, before you can even notice consciously. Thankfully, our brain has the capacity to go into survival mode and make quick, life-saving decisions, as our smart brain takes too long to decide, and we might not survive if it was in charge.*
>
> *If we have experienced a lot of stressful and overwhelming events in our lives, in other words, been outside our WOT often, we can become overly sensitive. We may notice we don't have patience for what we used to, or we may feel less adventurous, more anxious, or depressed. This happens because reminders of overwhelming events that we have not fully worked through are signaling survival mode to take over and/or narrowing our WOT, causing us to withdraw and take caution to avoid reminders. These reminders, called triggers, are not actually life threatening but are perceived by our brains as being too similar to overwhelming stuff from the past and are therefore dangerous. These triggers cause us to overreact and/or keep us from living to our fullest potential. As a result, we may avoid more and more places and experiences that might remotely remind us of the past. For example, do you know anyone who fears dogs or water or is afraid to be alone or in the dark?*
>
> *Triggers can get larger over time if we don't work through the overwhelming experiences from our past. This is because the more we go into survival mode, the more our brain tells us we are in danger and need to be on alert. Like a snowball getting bigger and bigger as it rolls downhill, our triggers and reaction to them can get bigger and bigger the more they misfire and send us into survival mode.*
>
> *Depending on the past, some people are triggered into shutting down, while others into freeze, flight, fawn, crying out, or withdrawing. Still others may get angry in a flash and go into fight. Triggers seem to have a pattern of sending off a particular response in our systems. Knowing how your triggers send you into survival mode can help you become aware of how to calm down and bring your whole brain back online.*

With an explanation such as the one given earlier, I worked with Ella to begin to imagine how she experiences her WOT. To explore this playfully and encourage curious openness to self-reflection, I offered an expressive therapy directive (given subsequently). Directives in art therapy are always given with a choice to engage or not in the activity. Ella was interested and excited to explore and was given an array of art materials as options.

> *I have a fun way to explore your WOT. Do you want to give it a try?* [If yes], *Recall a recent situation where you struggled to keep calm or stay present. This may have been a situation where you think you may have been triggered and felt your body and brain go out of your WOT.*

Here, the therapist should use caution to not pursue a memory that still feels out of the client's WOT. I then briefly discuss with the client the experience, asking questions.

> *How did your body react to the experience? What emotions did you notice? What thoughts did you have about yourself and others?*

Now, I invite the client to draw their own creative version of their WOT.

> *Now draw the way you felt in this situation. You may want to draw a body outline, or an actual window like the one I showed you.*

If the client needs a menu to get started, add the additional explanation.

> *You may have your own symbol or image that portrays how you experienced this triggering situation. There is no right or wrong way to do this. Whatever you come up with is okay.*

This approach to creatively exploring WOT encourages reflective functioning while framing the activity in a curious and expressive way. Ella was able to explore her window using markers and drawing of a body outline. She recalled the memory of feeling overwhelming panic at a social event triggered by the feeling and belief of being excluded and rejected by her peers. In this drawing seen in Figure 6.5, she depicted feeling small and helpless, not owning her full size, wanting to hide and run away, which she did.

This directive is not complete without a second part. As a directive focused on the feeling of the trigger, the next step is noticing how one emerged from it. Care should be taken here to be open to all choices the client may have made even if these are deemed negative (e.g., cutting, binging, drinking) without judgment or shaming the client.

> *Now add to your drawing (or create one on another sheet of paper) what you did to try to get back into your WOT. You can use words, colors, or symbols.*

In Ella's case, she phoned her mother and frantically asked to be picked up. Ella's second drawing depicts her outreach to Mom. She notes her mother's possible irritation at being needed as well as her own relief in making contact. Both of these expressions are a sign of mentalizing, in retrospect, what she and her mom

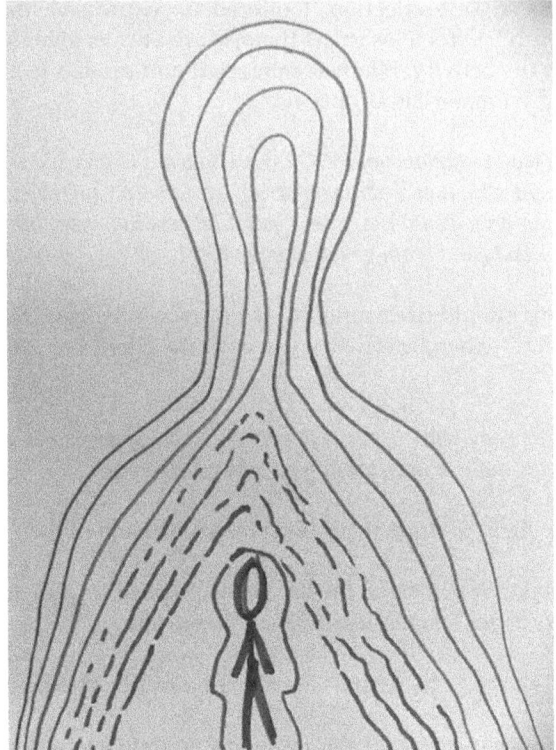

Figure 6.5 *Window of Tolerance, Part 1*

might have experienced. This aspect of her drawings was highlighted to draw attention to her and her mother's mental states (Figure 6.6).

Although these drawings appear expressive of anxiety, Ella was only in her "happy" part, as she called it (pretend mode), throughout the process. These drawings, much more graphically than Ella's words, deliver the understanding of her emotional experience. This art expression allowed for her emotional experience to be more accurately mirrored and "marked" back to her encouraging her reflection on the part of herself that felt panic and separation, the psych equivalent part. As the drawings were discussed, the gap between the psych equivalent and pretend mode was able to be explored with curiosity. Furthermore, Ella's mental world was explored and supported by the mirroring and marking of her artwork.

This gap was similarly explored in another directive, "inside/outside self." In this directive, Ella was offered paint and a paper mâché mask to depict her *social self* on the outside and her inner *private self* on the reverse side. On the outside, Ella coated the mask with multiple layers and tones of blue paint without details of a face. On the inside, Ella depicted bright orange, red, and yellow in an explosion of disorganized chaotic color. Discussion of the two sides of the mask was explored. Initially, staying within the metaphor is useful as the art expression allows for distance and curiosity that may make the exploration safe (Gil, 2015, p. 161). As in play therapy, the art allows for the extension of the feelings without the burden of

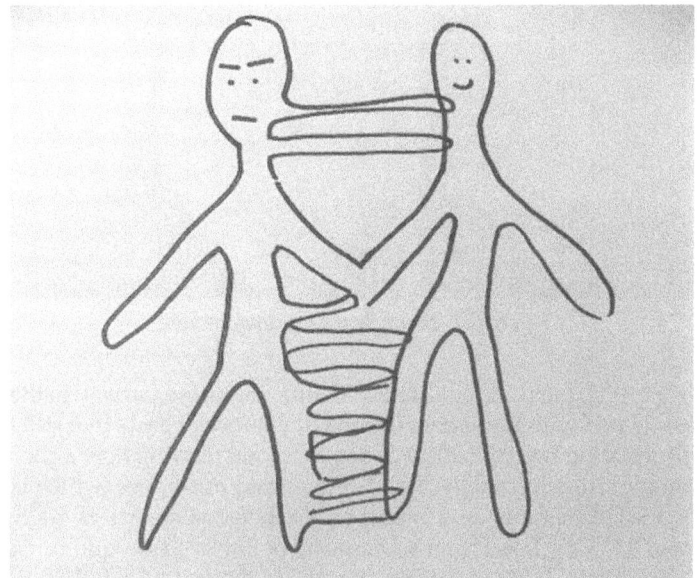

Figure 6.6 *Window of Tolerance, Part 2*

direct reference, which might lead to overwhelming or defensiveness. Over time, Ella was able to explore this more and more directly and notice her two states more objectively.

Along with WOT, many parts of psychoeducation and skill building can be approached using expressive exploration. Ella also used a box as a metaphor for a container. This directive is a literal interpretation of the container exercise commonly used as a resource in EMDR therapy. Making the container a literal container, rather than just an imaginary one, helped Ella's more concrete thinking process make sense out of the container resource exercise.

Play therapists and art therapists trained in EMDR commonly use concrete metaphors of this type with young children (Adler-Tapia & Settle, 2008; Gomez, 2013). This seems natural as children are still developing out of concrete reasoning into more abstract ways of thinking. Given that mentalization skills are often lacking in traumatized adults as well, leaving adults or parts of adults limited in teleological reasoning modes, using these strategies with complex adults can also enhance the effectiveness of the skills.

Ella, upon surveying the choices of boxes (which consisted of various recycled boxes), chose a heart-shaped valentine box as her container. Some single words and headlines of traumas were then written down, and Ella placed them in the protection of the "Heart Box." She was able to express the feeling that the memories seemed "really put away and cared for." Being able to literally put the memories away may seem to make the process real (Figure 6.7).

Moving away from directly referencing trauma memoires, in Phase 2 of EMDR therapy, Ella was invited to engage in an exploration of a "Parts of Self" exercise based on the concept of Fraser's Dissociative Table Technique (Martin, 2012). The Dissociative Table Technique is a guided imagery exploration used for

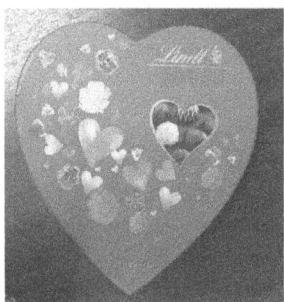 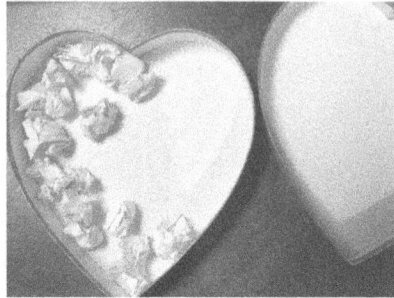

Figure 6.7 *Heart Boxes for Containment*

identifying aspects, parts, or ego states. Identifying these parts, whether they be defenses associated with managing trauma or emotional parts that still hold maladaptive information (Martin, 2012), is key to understanding how a client is managing traumatic stress internally. The directive and procedure (which is outlined in detail by EMDR therapist and expert on dissociative disorders, Kathy Martin, in her paper "How to Use Fraser's Dissociative Table Technique to Access and Work With Emotional Parts of the Personality" in the *Journal of EMDR Practice and Research* [2012]), guides the client through a visualization where the client then invites various aspects of themselves into an imaginary meeting space. Once the parts of self are identified in the imaginary space, the therapist works with the client to explore the relationships between the parts, identifying various aspects of the internal self-management system (e.g., feeling, body sensation, "name," role or function, alliance, beliefs). The client's self-organization is then explored looking at dynamics and clues for how to work with trauma memories effectively, without increasing symptoms while accessing necessary neural networks.

This exercise, although especially intended for work with clients who dissociate significantly, can be useful for any client to increase general self-awareness. When the reflective functioning of a client is low and inner experience is largely avoided, this imaginary exploration can often help increase a client's metacognitive awareness about themselves in a playful way, helping to develop a better sense of inner structure. Additionally, and in the case of Ella, this exercise can help identify the emotional parts that a client presenting in pretend mode might be avoiding, that is, emotional parts that are isolated. This can help the client begin to develop access to them in a safe way for future processing.

When working with Ella, or children generally, I frequently call the exercise "Creative Meeting Place" to get away from what sounds odd to a child (Fraser's Dissociative Table). I also include an art activity using either drawing or clay to help the child create a more concrete sense of their imaginary parts. Not unlike the "part" characters from the Disney movie, *Inside Out*, the child is invited to make a creative rendition of their inner aspects of self.

Ella was excited to participate in the visualization and chose to use polymer clay to create renditions of her "parts." She imagined her parts meeting in an elaborate hamster tube playground. Her main part she identified as a "Koala" that just wants to feel "happy and exuberant" and says "I don't know" to keep bad thoughts away. She also identified a kale and sugar eating part named "Ahhh"

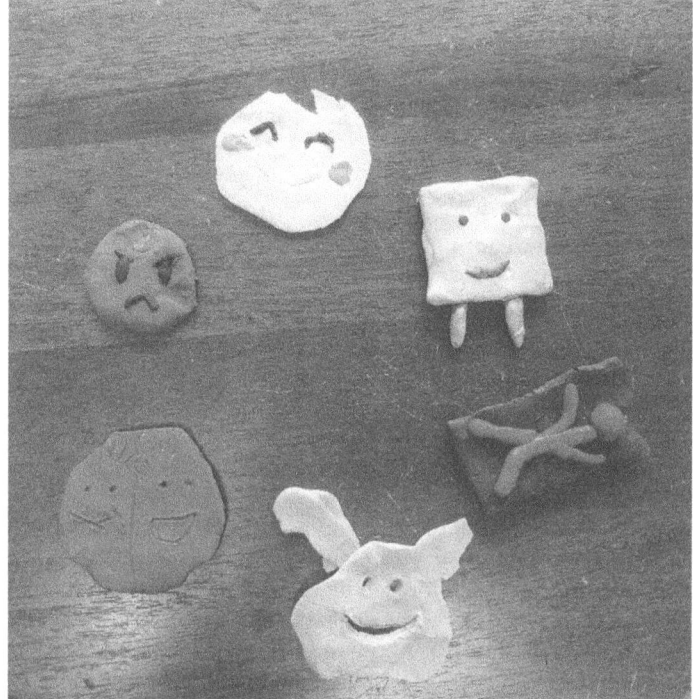

Figure 6.8 *Parts of the Self in Clay*

that just wants to feel good, a "What!!!" angry part that gets sad and has to "Deal with being upset," a "Brain shutting down" part that wants to sleep, an organization "Droid" part that gets things done, and a part that keeps joking, not allowing the self to be sad, which she depicted like a comedy/tragedy theater mask (see Figure 6.8).

As the therapy process moved forward, Ella now had a tool for accessing her inner experience in a new way in order to communicate and begin to notice more. Ella used these imaginary renditions of her inner experience as portals to help her increase self-awareness as well as communicate more meaningfully in therapy. When topics were brought up, a quick "check in" with Ella's imaginary crew gave her a way of noticing if the discussion felt okay. Additionally, through the process of dialoguing with the parts, time orientation and exploration of how these strategies might need an update could be addressed.

With this tool to enhance metacognition and self-reflection, therapy began to focus on increasing access to, and adoption of, adaptive information. Children may not have adaptive information due to limited examples of what is healthy and normal. Often, considerable effort and attention in therapy need to be given to establishing what healthy normal boundaries are, healthy attachment, and addressing pathological attachment to the offending caregiver. Fortunately, Ella had a secure attachment to a mother who was vigilantly protective. Additionally, her perpetrator father was in prison, and her life had dramatically improved. These factors greatly increased the likelihood that EMDR therapy could go

210   I. MODELS FOR INTEGRATION

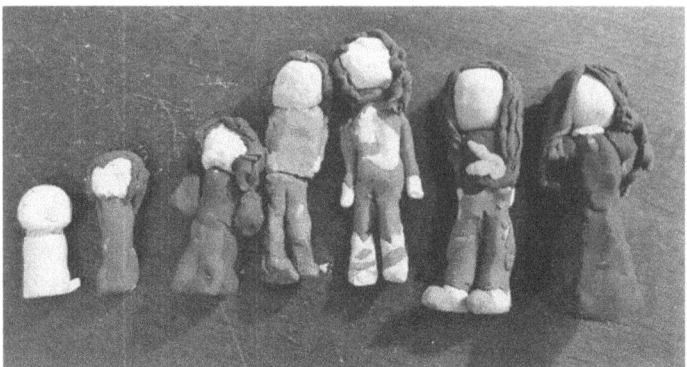

Figure 6.9 *Self Through Time (Clay)*

forward on pace safely, and developmental defenses could be updated with increased mentalization.

Toward this goal, Ella was offered another directive (given later), again utilizing polymer clay (although several media options were given, this was Ella's preference). The directive was embraced by Ella, who expressed a feeling it would be "fun and cool to try." Ella's mother was invited to participate as a biography expert on Ella. If Ella's mother was not securely attached to Ella, then this activity could be used to increase secure attachment and help repair lost connection (if the parent is currently in a good place to offer the repair).

> *Sculpt yourself through time, starting at birth to the present. At each age, offer yourself gifts and symbols of what you think you might have wanted, needed, or anything that helps that age of you feel happy, healthy, and safe. You can ask for help from your helpers* [myself and in this case Mom] *to create all that you need and want.*

Notice that the emphasis is not on accessing the trauma memories at the various ages, but to talk about what each age needs/wants to be happy and healthy. This directive is always done with great care to the risk of triggering early traumatic memories out of the WOT. However, due to how Ella was navigating discussion around various ages of her life, and her mother's ability to offer some regulation and direction in this exercise, this directive appeared on target strategically for increasing adaptive information (see Figure 6.9).

Ella elected to create seven figures of herself, making each about 2 years apart. Working with her mom, they engaged in a playful discussion regarding what Ella was like as a child, her favorite toys, books, friends, and movies. This activity served also to help Ella orient her biographical timeline. Connecting to these parts of herself, Mom discussed how she wanted to care for Ella, what she wished she would have done more of, and her pride and love for Ella at each stage.

In her most recent figure, her 13-year-old self, Ella depicted a "dark" princess, emerging from the "evil" in her past. She then created a figure to represent the police officer who helped her as well as a magical butterfly. Discussion around the dark princess brought up the differences in her life in the present as opposed to the past. Her expressive rendition of her present self was that of being powerful and aware. When discussing this present self, Ella was able to embrace her bravery and strength as well as how much she has overcome. However, it is curious to note that in this figure, Ella omitted her arms, as is the case in some of her younger figures. Often art offers the opportunity to express the vulnerable aspects of self that are not ready to be known consciously. Ella still struggled at this point to acknowledge herself as a child who had been victimized. Her figure offered a possible window into that part of herself that was still isolated and helpless, having emotional connection with the trauma experience.

The creation of these figures offered Ella an opportunity to safely reflect on herself through time as a child growing up with needs, wants, and experiences. She was able to lean into the sensory and creative aspects of the directive to enjoy and play with these ideas and understandings. Additionally, she mirrored through her art what her experiences, needs, and wants might be like. She also was offered the support of helpers in this journey, eager to offer assistance in her creative vision of her selves. The helper figures were installed using tapping as a part of resource installation.

The expressive activity was used strategically to build and reinforce a knowledge base around what was healthy and normal. One conflicting fact that Mom had discussed with Ella, and had emerged as the abuse was discovered, was Ella's belief (based on what her father told her), that "all fathers do this with their daughters," and her need to be "silent or she'd break up the family and they will all be poor." Although at this point, Ella was aware that her father was manipulating her from the information acquired in prior counseling and the interviews with detectives, this hands-on review of normal and healthy helped to concretize this, potentially engaging the adaptive information for future processing.

In addition to the earlier given expressive directives meant to increase metacognitive awareness, self-knowledge, and adaptive information, Ella worked with this therapist substantially on learning to identify feelings internally. Initially, Ella presented as blocked, only identifying "happy." Using a feeling chart, "Bothering Scale," "Truth Scale," and "Stop Sign" in sessions and for homework as practice, Ella practiced at inward reflection and noticing. These props in Figure 6.10 were created for the express purpose of making the exploration of feelings easier and more playful, in preparation for EMDR Phases 3 through 7. Although a simple exercise, it is meant to increase the frequency and feeling of safety in order to notice self-states while making them more conscious and cognitive. These strategies work on the premise coined and often said by neurobiologist Dan Seigel (2012), "Name it to tame it." In addition to these strategies, Ella and Mom also created a feelings notebook and games to increase feeling literacy at home.

Although effective tools, props may not go deep enough, and concepts can remain with only a surface level of understanding. In order to help Ella connect as authentically as possible to herself, the use of expressive therapy for feelings literacy was also used to help define and explore those difficult to categorize or rate states.

One of the great benefits of expressive therapy lies in its power to reach beyond words, to that yet-to-be-defined zone. As stated by Fonagy earlier, "Expressive therapies allow the internal to be expressed externally. . . . Experience and feeling is placed outside of the mind and into the world to facilitate explicit mentalizing"

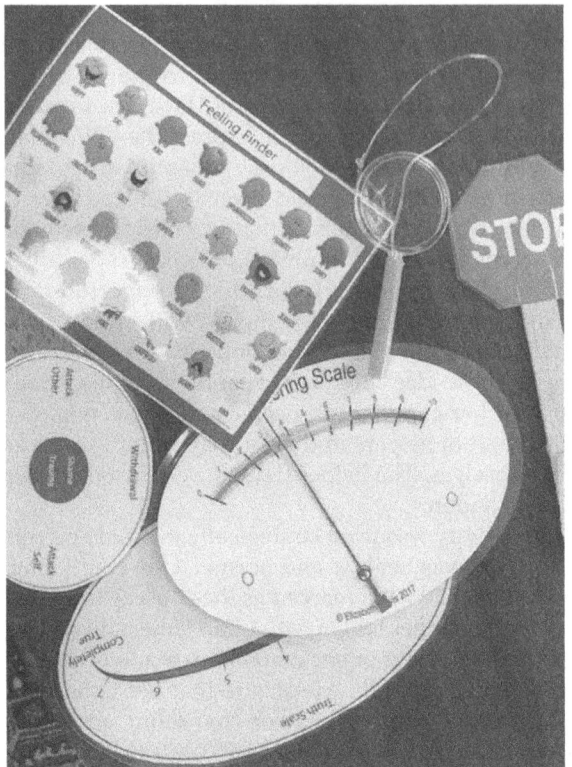

Figure 6.10 *Props for Eye Movement Desensitization and Reprocessing Processing*

(Bateman & Fonagy, 2004, p. 172). The process of expressing feelings through creative imagery in this way helps to connect with emotional states and parts that may otherwise remain primitive and out of conscious awareness.

Ella was invited to use art materials to create different ways she felt in different situations. We began with "happy," as she most identified with this state. Her depiction of "happy" in Figure 6.11 shows this "happy" with large vigilant, pointed eyes and high brows and appears anything but happy.

As Ella drew and reflected on her piece, she was able to note this discrepancy. Initially, she added the heart, as if to try to fix the image back into a state of happy, away from the more maniacal, or as Ella later expressed, "evil" look. This simple exercise of drawing this feeling was able to seemingly connect her with its opposite. This opened the discussion about the usefulness of anger and the need to get those feelings out and listen to them.

Work on boundaries was also explored using props, the "stop sign," and expressively through art. Ella and her mother had previously discussed her fear of telling anyone but her mother "no" and described how she had frozen, withdrew, or just went along with what others wanted in the past. Children who have had their boundaries violated often do not fully develop them intact. The belief that they have the option to say "no" can be compromised by the trauma of the parent's betrayal and violation. Children may wall off into a state of epistemic

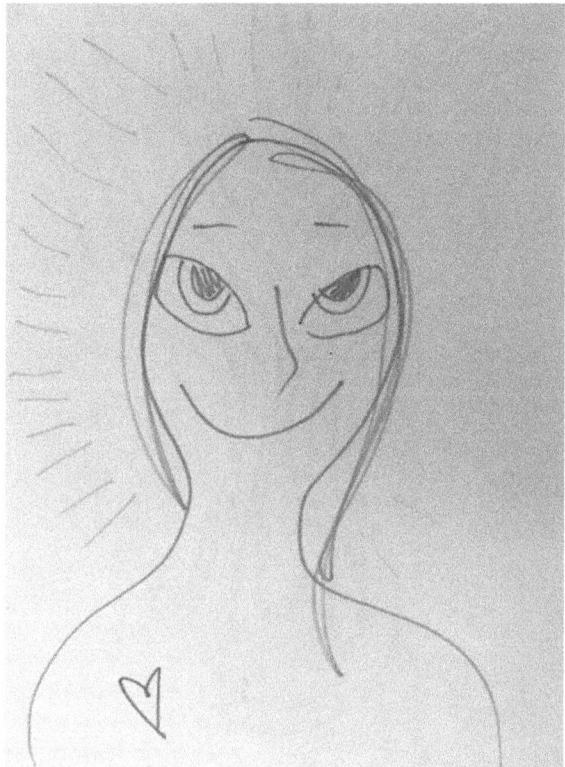

Figure 6.11 *Happy (Example of Drawing Feelings)*

distrust following a traumatic violation by a parent (Fonagy, 2004), not integrating and updating information, but isolating that part of the self in a state of shame. In these cases, the objective, or meta-perspectives that hold the clarity of responsibility and ownership, is not fully integrated into their knowledge base. So even as adults, a client may express believing the trauma was their fault because they were "bad" or asked for it. These stuck scripts can collapse the client's esteem in triggering situations, impacting the client's ability to hold their boundaries in balance with others. In the case of Ella, defenses that at one point served as a submissive and protective strategy needed updating and reorienting to the present to become an effective stance of holding her own space and believing and feeling the right to do so.

Discussions of boundaries began with Ella by reflecting on her "dark" princess figure and how that figure lacked the ability to push others away or hold up a stop sign, having no arms. Mentalizing what it would be like to be in that figure was explored, with Ella noticing seemingly for the first time the lack of arms on some of her figures. Following this exploration, Ella decided to paint an updated version of her "dark princess" self. In this version, she depicted herself with strong arms and hands. Ella's demeanor seemed to follow suit as she painted. She emoted the feeling of power and held her arms up showing off her muscle (Figure 6.12).

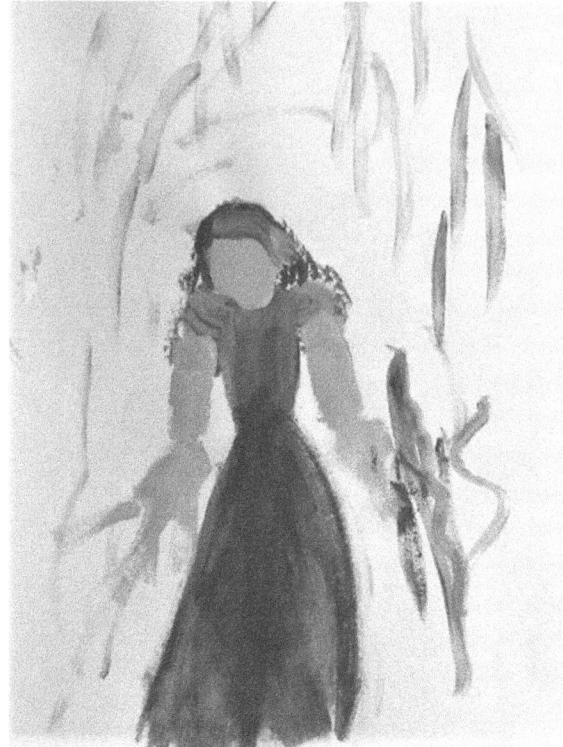

Figure 6.12 *Dark Princess (Example of Self-Drawing)*

Over time, these skills became easier for Ella, who expressed pride when talking about how she told a peer, "no," and even disagreed with the directive of an adult who was making a questionable decision. She was also able to discuss what feelings she had when her boundaries were crossed and how she believed others felt in the situation, a sign of more robust mentalizing skills.

Having acquired the skills to both identify feelings in the body and feel entitled to say "no," Ella possessed prerequisite skills for effective and safe processing using EMDR. Safe processing requires that the client can both feel empowered enough to say stop when the processing feels overwhelming (Greenwald, 2005) and to be able to engage their internal experience enough to know how much distress they are feeling. In other words, the gap between raw emotion, and the cognitive skills to identify and manage it, needs to be close enough so that the emotional content does not become overwhelming (psych equivalent mode) or disconnect altogether, in a (pretend mode). Ella's go-to strategy had been to wall off her emotional knowledge and experience and maintain a state of happy pretense. With more connection to her feelings, and tools to recognize, name, and manage them, she was more aware internally and had the skills to attempt processing trauma.

A longer intensive session was set aside to begin EMDR Phases 3 to 7 processing. Ella's scroll of life was revisited, and a test memory was chosen. Ella agreed to work on an experience of having a panic attack at camp. She was able to identify an SUDS rating, a belief, and to notice "sad and scared" in her stomach. This memory seemed also remote enough from the content of her father's abuse that the processing could be contained if necessary.

Ella was offered the sand tray as a place to tell the story, rather than just verbally. Ella still struggled to talk more than a few words about her past without deferring to her mother as biographer. Playing out the experience using sand tray figures allowed her another less threatening way to communicate. Ella could have also elected to just think about the memory. However, given her struggle to connect consistently with memories previously without a "part" of herself distracting, fidgeting, or changing the subject, the sand tray offered a way to focus and structure the processing. Additionally, the figures externalized the story from inside her head to outside in a space to explicitly work them through.

As Ella was going to be moving figures and working in the sand tray, tappers were used for bilateral stimulation (BLS). Ella elected to use the weighted lap blanket with the tappers in pockets over each knee. This is a very grounding way to offer BLS, if available.

Poised at the sand tray, with blanket, tappers, and tray figures, as well as resources, Ella processed the memory of the panic attack at camp using the standard protocol. She played it out as a performance but was able to connect with emotions and resolve feelings of embarrassment, fear, and sadness as well as not believing she was safe. This memory also helped her to connect her feeling of panic to the trigger of being alone with her father in the past. The interweave of bringing her now-empowered "dark princess" self in to help her was used as a resource during part of the process.

With success processing this memory, Ella expressed readiness to begin to address memories related to childhood abuse with her father. There were many abuse memories beginning as early as she could remember and with weekly frequency through periods of her life. Fortunately, her life was also full of positive experiences and connection to others along the way.

My approach in these cases varies depending on many factors, including the degree of distress and the accessibility the client has to their memories. For most of her memories, Ella expressed feeling they ran together and were hard to separate one from another. While generally I approach processing from a chronological strategy by cluster, most or all of Ella's identified traumas were within this one cluster and felt the same to her in time. After considering the list and options, I decided, in collaboration with Ella and her mother, to begin with a memory that felt most distinct, hoping that the emotional content would be more solidly accessible if paired with the sand tray approach.

What follows is an account of the processing through of one target that appeared to help clear and orient the others significantly. Because this memory seemed to shift her perspective, the other memories processed more quickly. When memories feel so similar, sometimes this strategy works, essentially beginning with an iconic memory that stands out, and is a strong example for the others.

To this session Ella came armed with her resources (figures and art pieces that recall strengths and supports), developmental self-sculptures, as well as her "parts." She had picked out sand tray figures to represent her father (a snake and a small human figure) and herself (a rabbit and her clay figure that represented the age of this experience). Ella was 6-years-old when her father took her to a park, photographed her in various ways, and molested her. Much of the details of this event were known by Mom due to her having to review evidence in the criminal investigation. This memory in particular also had come up in flashbacks in the past. In these instances, Ella was able to talk it out with her mother, spilling out some of the details before reorienting to the present.

Ella began the session by identifying her helpers for this memory and any resources she might need just in case. Chosen resources were her favorite police officer, her princess self, her mom, and her brother. Ella was encouraged to play with the memory narrative in the sand tray using her resources ahead of time, acting out the way she would want the events to go. Offering Ella permission to play with the memory can help break the trance power that memories like this often have. Just like playing with the fast-forward or slow-motion button on a remote control, the memory is recognized more as just a memory, not a real event happening.

Ella had not played with her memories before in this way. In fact, Ella did not play with toys much growing up, as Mom observed, but always seemed oriented toward people. Now, she seemed to enjoy setting up the scene and playing out "revenge" and "justice" in the sand tray. Fortunately, in Ella's case, her father was incarcerated, which allowed her to feel that some justice was served.

As the memory was set up for processing, Ella was able to use the figures and play the events out as she recalled them in the memory. She was observably emotional but seemed focused and determined. During some sets, she played out the memory differently and used the figures to express her feelings, such as anger and outrage (the "what!!" part seemed to get a voice here), once stomping her father into the sand and burying him with protector figures on top. The sand tray approach offered her a way to extend herself to her emotional parts, where figures could play what was so hard to feel directly in her body. At the end of the session, following installation of "I am strong" and "I am safe now," Ella expressed feeling different, accomplished, and proud of herself. Overall, the session seemed cathartic for Ella.

When Ella returned for the next session, the memory was revisited. Ella had expressed feeling the SUDS was low, a 2, where before it had been an 8. With the weighted lap blanket and the tappers, Ella was offered art materials this time as a way to revisit the memory. Ella quickly drew herself as the "dark princess" in the park hitting her father with a boat "paddle." She was able to directly feel anger at her father. With this emotion active in her body, Ella was invited to throw some clay at a target in the playroom as a way of processing through the body sensations empowering her to express her feelings (Figure 6.13).

Used as an interweave, addressing the need to defend herself by offering her the opportunity to physically act out a protective behavior accelerated processing and increased access to the parts of self that wanted to fight. Ella seemed excited and seriously aggressive throwing clay at a target. At times, she imagined it was her father and enlisted our attention at how hard she could throw the clay. Additionally, she asked me and her mother to help her throw the clay as hard as possible.

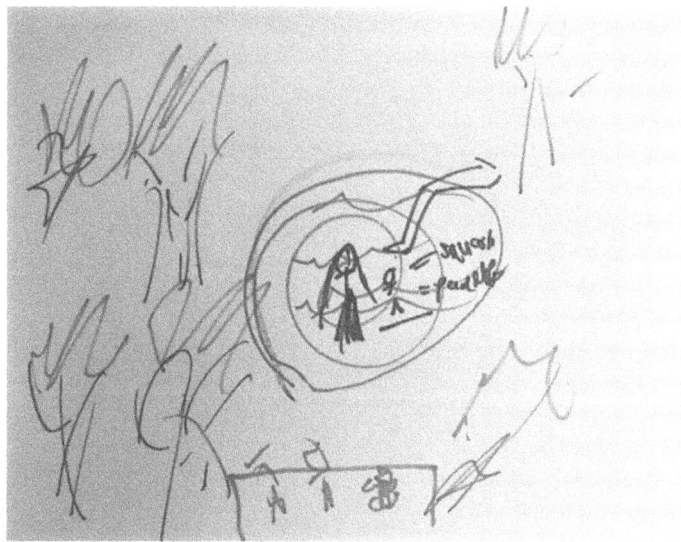

Figure 6.13 *Dark Princess With Paddle*

Following this interweave, regular processing with BLS was resumed. The positive belief "It's over" was installed, and Ella expressed feeling strongly that it was true. She described the experience of the memory seeming to be more distant and "flat." Following this session, other memories were addressed in relative order. These seemed to resolve more quickly.

In follow-up from the processing sessions, Mom and Ella expressed that she had remarkably improved. Somatic symptoms had disappeared by all accounts; anxiety was present here and there but no panic attacks. Ella was regularly talking about feelings and expressing herself in a more age-appropriate way. Mom had also noticed that Ella had moved through some unfamiliar challenging situations without panic or meltdowns. These developments appeared to be good confirmation that the processing was indeed successful.

However, Ella remained nervous about some important future challenges. Most notable was an upcoming court testimony she would likely have to give. As part of the eight phases and three prongs of EMDR, the future template was the next step in treatment. What was targeted next was the future experience of testifying.

Ella identified being nervous but not terrified or overwhelmed by the thought of seeing her father in real time. But as Mom was quick to point out, saying that and then really seeing and hearing him are too different things. To aid in the processing of the future template and to connect with more of a real experience of seeing him, Ella was invited to paint a rendition of her father to look at and practice with.

Ella took the paint and quickly threw together a funny caricature of her father. Seeing a symbolic representation staring back provided an opportunity

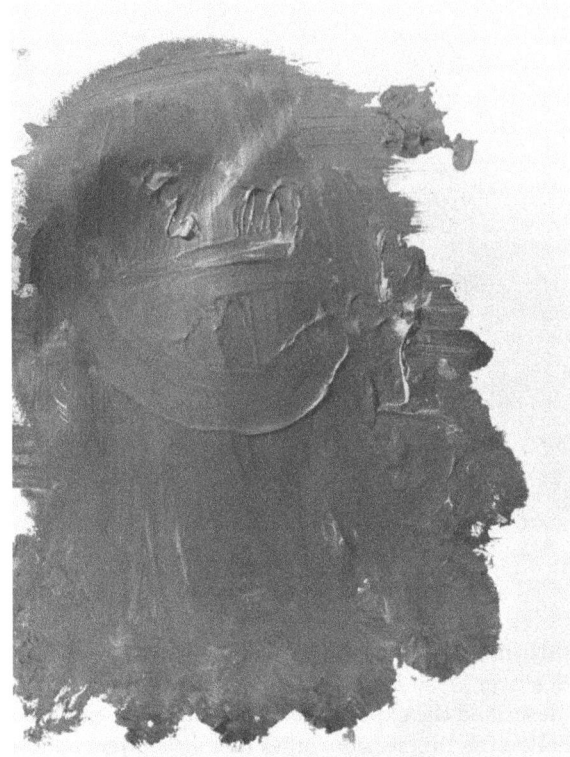

Figure 6.14 *Painting of Father*

for Ella to get some feelings. She played with the image, exaggerating the features and laughing with her mom. Eventually, Ella played with her power to distort and destroy the image altogether by smearing it with gray muddy paint. She then redrew the face impression as seen in Figure 6.14.

Following this expressive activity, Ella easily processed the future target of testifying. She stated having done the art helped her feel powerful over his gaze. Although she acknowledged that his face and voice might still be very shocking, she practiced imagining hearing him and seeing him in the courtroom while she is painting over his face. She expressed knowing she was strong now helped her in the face of this future challenge.

Follow up with Ella later revealed her resilience and ability to move through the stress of court. According to her and her mother, she was able to manage the process without a panic attack maintaining connection to her supports and resources.

Creative and expressive art therapy integrated into the eight phases of EMDR therapy improved Ella's ability to move through the phases by supporting and helping her build the self-reflective skills necessary to process trauma. Ella began therapy locked in a childhood adaption of regressive dependence on her mother in order to mentalize her emotional experience. Walled off from her feelings, needs, and wants as a way to avoid the trauma experiences inflicted by her father, Ella utilized her mother for translating her emotions and disturbing experiences. Ella's body, in turn, somatically expressed what her mind could not in the form of panic, headaches, and gut-wrenching pain.

The integration of arts therapy used mindfully and strategically to increase mentalization skills for self-knowledge and perspective taking helped Ella safely begin to reconnect with her emotional experiences. The distance offered in the expressive arts space allowed Ella to extend to her emotional parts of self through the expressive use of clay, drawing, and paint. This allowed for marked mirroring of her inner emotional experiences, reflection, and insight. These expressive activities allowed for a reconnection to feelings.

The special qualities inherently carried by expressive arts therapy helped to enhance and develop skills critical to the success of EMDR, such as the ability to recognize and identify feelings, exert boundaries regarding self needs, and connect effectively with resources. Ella's expressive creations also helped elevate her concrete thinking to engage a more metacognitive perspective on herself and her trauma, allowing the responsibility of the traumatic experience to be understood.

CONCLUSION

This case example illustrates the power of expressive arts therapy, as a type of mentalization therapy capable of extending the reach of EMDR therapy. In cases of complex trauma, where mentalization skills have been compromised, expressive therapy offers a modality that can help build the way for processing safely and effectively.

Complex trauma or complex posttraumatic stress disorder (CPTSD), a term proposed by the World Health Organization for International Classification of Diseases 11th Revision (Brewin, 2019), is a rapidly growing problem. In a recent study published in the *European Journal of Psychotraumatology* (Karatzias et al., 2018), researchers confirm what many trauma therapists have long suspected, CPTSD is more common than PTSD. Studying the clinical samples, researchers also point out that it is not only more common but also more debilitating. With childhood abuse and the subsequent developmental impact being at the core of most cases of CPTSD, effective treatments need to begin to address not only effective trauma resolution methods but how to help clients navigate to a point in treatment where they can take advantage of them.

Expressive arts have long been a part of our instinctual process of digestion and healing. Expressive arts as a form of psychotherapy draws upon this ancient instinctual wisdom. In an age where CPTSD is on the rise and most treatments are marginally effective, one of the most versatile, accessible, and tried-and-true approaches is heavily underutilized and underappreciated. By highlighting and promoting an increased understanding of the underlying mechanisms that make expressive therapy an effective trauma treatment, this example illustrates how expressive arts therapy can be used within phase model trauma treatment strategically, to help support the power and potential of EMDR processing.

REFERENCES

Abbing, A., Ponstein, A., Van Hooren, S., de Sonneville, L., Swaab, H., & Baars, E. (2018). The effectiveness of art therapy for anxiety in adults: A systematic review of randomised and non-randomised controlled trials. *PLoS One, 13*(12), 1–17. doi:10.1371/journal.pone.0208716

Adler-Tapia, R., & Settle, C. (2008). *EMDR and the art of psychotherapy with children.* New York, NY: Springer Publishing Company.

Anderson, F. (1978). *Art for all the children: Approaches to art therapy for children with disabilities.* Springfield, IL: Charles C. Thomas.

Bales, D., van Beek, N., Smits, M., Willemsen, S., & Busschbach, J. V. (2012). Treatment outcome of 18-month, day hospital mentalization-based treatment (MBT) in patients with severe borderline personality disorder in the Netherlands. *Journal of Personality Disorders, 26,* 568–582. doi:10.1521/pedi.2012.26.4.568

Ballespi, S., Vives, J., Alonso, N., Sharp, C., Ramırez, M., Fonagy, P., & Barrantes-Vidal, N. (2019). To know or not to know? Mentalization as protection from somatic complaints. *PLoS One, 14*(5), 1–20. doi:10.1371/journal.pone.0215308

Bateman, A., & Fonagy, P. (1999). The effectiveness of partial hospitalization in the treatment of borderline personality disorder—A randomised controlled trial. *The American Journal of Psychiatry, 156,* 1563–1569. doi:10.1176/ajp.156.10.1563

Bateman, A., & Fonagy, P. (2001). Treatment of borderline personality disorder with psychoanalytically oriented partial hospitalization: An 18-month follow-up. *The American Journal of Psychiatry, 158*(1), 36–42. doi:10.1176/appi.ajp.158.1.36

Bateman, A., & Fonagy, P. (2004). *Psychotherapy for borderline personality disorder: Mentalization-based treatment.* Oxford, UK: Oxford University Press.

Bateman, A., & Fonagy, P. (2008). 8-year follow-up of patients treated for borderline personality disorder: Mentalization-based treatment versus treatment as usual. *The American Journal of Psychiatry, 165*(5), 631–638. doi:10.1176/appi.ajp.2007.07040636

Bateman, A., & Fonagy, P. (2010). Mentalization-based treatment for borderline personality disorder. *World Psychiatry, 9*(1), 11–15. doi:10.1002/j.2051-5545.2010.tb00255.x

Bateman, A., & Fonagy, P. (2013). Mentalization-based treatment. *Psychoanalytic Inquiry, 33,* 595–613. doi:10.1080/07351690.2013.835170

Boon, S., Steele, K., & Van Der Hart, O. (2017). *Treating trauma-related dissociation.* New York, NY: W. W. Norton.

Brewin, C. R. (2019). Complex post-traumatic stress disorder: A new diagnosis in ICD-11. *BJPsych Advances,* 1–8. Cambridge University Press. doi:10.1192/bja.2019.48

Buck, E., & Havsteen-Franklin, D. (2013). Connecting with the image: How art psychotherapy can help to reestablish a sense of epistemic trust. *Art Therapy Online, 4*(1), 1–24. doi:10.25602/GOLD.atol.v4i1.310

Dewey, J. (1980). *Art as experience.* New York, NY: G. P. Putnam's Sons. (Original work published 1934)

Fonagy, P. (2012). Art therapy and personality disorder. *International Journal of Art Therapy, 17*(3), 90. doi:10.1080/17454832.2012.740866

Fonagy, P., & Allison, E. (2014). The role of mentalizing and epistemic trust in the therapeutic relationship. *Psychotherapy, 51,* 372–380. doi:10.1037/a0036505

Fonagy, P., Gergely, G., Jurist, E., & Target, M. E. (2004). *Affect regulation, mentalization, and the development of the self.* New York, NY: Other Press LLC. (Original work published 2002)
Gil, E. (2015). The creative use of metaphor in play and art therapy with attachment problems. In C. Malchiodi & D. Crenshaw (Ed.), *Creative arts and play for attachment problems* (pp. 159–176). New York, NY, and London, UK: Guilford Press.
Gomez, A. (2013). *EMDR therapy and adjunct approaches with children.* New York, NY: Springer Publishing Company.
Greenwald, R. (2005). *Child trauma handbook.* New York, NY: Routledge.
Hass-Cohen, N., & Clyde Findlay, J. (2015). *Art therapy and the neuroscience of relationships, creativity, and resiliency: Skills and practices.* New York, NY: W. W. Norton.
Havsteen-Franklin, D., Maratos, A., Usiskin, M., & Heagney, M. (2016). Examining arts psychotherapies practice elements: Early finding from the horizons project. *Approaches: An Interdisciplinary Journal of Music Therapy, 8*(1), 50–62.
Ingenhoven, T. J. (2015). The place of trauma in the treatment of personality disorders. *European Journal of Psychotraumatology, 6,* 27629. doi:10.3402/ejpt.v6.27629
Kandel, E. (2012). *The age of insight: The quest to understand the unconscious in art, mind, and brain.* New York, NY: Random House Publishing Group.
Karatzias, T., Cloitre, M., Maercker, A., Kazlauskas, E., Shevlin, M., Hyland, P., . . . Brewin, C. (2018). PTSD and complex PTSD: ICD-11 updates on concept and measurement in the UK, USA, Germany and Lithuania. *European Journal of Psychotraumatology, 8,* 1418103. doi:10.1080/20008198.2017.1418103
Kolb, D. (1984). *Experiential learning: Experience as the source of learning and development.* Englewood Cliffs, NJ: Prentice-Hall.
Lenzenweger, M. F., Clarkin, J. F., Levy, K. N., Yeomans, F. E., & Kernberg, O. F. (2012). Predicting domains and rates of change in borderline personality disorder. *Personality Disorders: Theory, Research, and Treatment, 3*(2), 185–195. doi:10.1037/a0025872
Lorenzini, N., Campbell, C., & Fonagy, P. (2019). Mentalization and its role in processing trauma. In B. Huppertz (Ed.), *Approaches to psychic trauma* (pp. 403–422). Lanham, MD, Boulder, CO, New York, NY, and London, UK: Rowan & Littlefield.
Lusebrink, V., & Hinz, L. (2016). The expressive therapies continuum as a framework in the treatment of trauma. In J. King (Ed.), *Art therapy, trauma, and neuroscience* (pp. 42–66). New York, NY: Routledge.
Martin, K. (2012). How to use Fraser's Dissociative Table Technique to access and work with emotional parts of the personality. *Journal of EMDR Practice and Research, 6*(4), 179–186. doi:10.1891/1933-3196.6.4.179
Martin, K. (2016). *EMDR and structural dissociation theory webinar series.* Webinar, January–March, 2016. Retrieved from http://www.kmccs.com/webinar.maml?page=webinar_winter_2016
Montessori, M. (1967). *The absorbent mind.* New York, NY: Henry Holt.
Naumburg, M. (1974). *An introduction to art therapy: Studies of the "free" art expression of behavior problem children and adolescents as means of diagnosis.* New York, NY: Teachers College Press and Columbia University. (Original work published 1950)
Perry, B. (2009). Examining child maltreatment through a neurodevelopmental lens: Clinical applications of the neurosequential model of therapeutics. *Journal of Loss and Trauma, 14,* 240–255. doi:10.1080/15325020903004350
Perry, B. (2015). Forward. In C. Malchiodi (Ed.), *Creative interventions with traumatized children* (2nd ed.). New York, NY: Guilford Press.
Schouten, K., de Niet, G., Knipscheer, J., Kleber, R., & Hutschemaekers, G. J. (2015). The effectiveness of art therapy in the treatment of traumatized adults: A systematic review

on art therapy and trauma. *Trauma, Violence and Abuse, 16*(2), 220–228. doi:10.1177/1524838014555032

Shapiro, F. (2018). *Eye movement desensitization and reprocessing [EMDR] therapy* (3rd ed.). New York, NY: Guilford Press.

Siegel, D. (1999). *The developing mind: How relationships and the brain interact to shape who we are.* New York, NY: Guilford Press.

Springham, N., & Huet, V. (2018). Art as relational encounter: An ostensive communication theory of art therapy. *Journal of the American Art Therapy Association, 35*(1), 4–10. doi:10.1080/07421656.2018.1460103

Terr, L. (1991). Childhood traumas: An outline and overview. *American Journal of Psychiatry, 148*(1), 10–20. doi:10.1176/ajp.148.1.10

Van der Kolk, B. (2015). *The body keeps the score: Brain, mind, and body in the healing of trauma.* New York, NY: Penguin Books.

Verfaille, M. (2016). *Mentalization in arts therapies.* London, UK: Karnac Books.

Winner, E. (2019). *How art works: A psychological exploration.* Oxford, UK: Oxford University Press.

Winnicott, D. W. (2005). *Playing and reality.* London, UK, and New York, NY: Routledge Classics. (Original work published 1971)

7

Playful and Creative Approaches for EMDR Therapy With Latinx Children

VIVIANA URDANETA AND VIVIANA TRIANA

INTRODUCTION

The Latinx population is growing in the United States, and it is imperative that therapists provide culturally sensitive services to this population. In this chapter, we highlight important cultural and clinical considerations when utilizing eye movement desensitization and reprocessing (EMDR) therapy with Latinx children and teens through the lenses of three main principles: (a) Follow the child's lead and interest; (b) be curious, ask questions, and maintain an open attitude; and (c) utilize and emphasize cultural and individual strengths. It includes playful and creative interventions that have been helpful during the different phases of EMDR therapy with this population in order to make their treatment more culturally attuned and developmentally appropriate.

BACKGROUND AND LATINX TERM CLARIFICATION

In general terms, working with children in a therapeutic context can be a learning experience for both new and seasoned therapists since each case/story brings its own nuances. However, it might be especially challenging if the cultural backgrounds of the therapist and the client are different. Often, counseling programs require students to take a one-semester multicultural sensitivity course to get them ready for their therapeutic work with clients from different cultures. However, academia can provide only a small window of general knowledge that sometimes can lead therapists to generalize the experience of groups, which might differ from the individuals' own experiences. Also, when the therapist is from the same ethnicity or cultural background as the client, it is important to avoid generalizations based on personal experiences and have one's eyes and ears ready to experience the child with genuine interest and care. The challenge is to be able to expand our knowledge about working with children from different cultures in a practical and culturally sensitive manner in the therapy room.

We were both born and raised in Colombia, South America, and immigrated to the United States in pursuit of our educational goals. Our therapy practice has been influenced by our cultural values, immigration experience, race, acculturation process, and experiences of being a part of a minority group in this country. As Latinx immigrant women of color, our upbringing has facilitated using appropriate tools and information to connect with clients who share our cultural background. At the same time, our experiences have made us aware of further areas of growth, given that not all Latinx look, act, and share the same values and this is true of any culture. We emphasize a strengths perspective approach and the importance of seeing our clients as people within an environmental context that sometimes invites them to grow and thrive and, at other times, is the cause of oppression and prejudice.

The makeup of the United States society is continually changing, and the rapid growth of the Hispanic/Latinx community is evident. According to the U.S. Census Bureau, as of July 1, 2017, the Hispanic/Latinx community made up 58.9 million of the total U.S. population, making people of Hispanic/Latinx origin the nation's largest ethnic or racial minority. Also, the Hispanic/Latinx population is projected to grow to 111 million by 2060 (U.S. Census Bureau, 2018). This remarkable growth makes it very likely that most therapists will work with Latinx children and their families at some point. Due to this growth in population, it is imperative and relevant that Latinx clients receive counseling services that meet their cultural needs.

We would like to clarify the term Latinx in use throughout this chapter. Even though there is an overlap between the words Hispanic and Latinx and many people believe they are the same, they are not. Hispanic refers to people who speak the Spanish language. On the other hand, Latinx is more general than Hispanic and includes anyone who can trace his or her ancestry to a Latin American country (Samovar, Porter, McDaniel, & Roy, 2017). Latinx includes people who do not speak Spanish but are descendants from Latin American immigrants. The x in Latinx allows the inclusion of people from all genders who might not identify in binary terms (LGBTQ). In this chapter, we use the term Latinx as it is more inclusive and gender-neutral. However, there are some authors who opposed the term Latinx because it is not part of the Spanish language and argue that Latinos is already an inclusive term. Finding common language about culture in general and about a group specifically is challenging because it is impossible to get it "just right." Nevertheless, it is important to make efforts to use language that is respectful, understandable, inclusive, and acceptable (Nickerson, 2017). Another important note for this chapter is that all the client's names are pseudonyms and that case information has been altered to protect confidentiality.

CULTURE AND CULTURAL COMPETENCE

Culture is a set of humanmade elements that are passed from one generation to the next. It is not innate but is shared and learned. It becomes internalized by the members of each culture (Samovar et al., 2017). As EMDR therapists, we need to increase our intercultural competence in order to provide treatment that supports healing among people from all cultures. The therapist must recognize their own culture and the role that it plays in the therapy room and also acknowledge and celebrate the client's culture in order to provide an experience of therapy that promotes empowerment and emotional safety.

"There is a consensus that a first step in becoming cross culturally competent is for a therapist to develop an understanding of his or her own ethnic identity and cultural values" (Gil & Drewes, 2005, p. 5). Therapists have a responsibility to understand how their culture is impacting the therapeutic process. It is impossible to practice therapy without paying attention to cultural issues because therapists bring themselves as part of the therapeutic process and form a relationship with the client that is based on the therapist's and client's culture. One of our goals is to discuss how it is relevant to include a perspective of cultural awareness, sensitivity, and humility in the therapeutic process in order to be effective in the work with Latinx clients given that "a major obstacle is that many people don't even realize that they have culture, they think that they are standard-issue humans that they are normal, natural, and neutral … so instead of sweeping culture under the rug, we should embrace it, understand it, and most important, mobilize it for good" (Markus & Conner, 2014, pp. xxii, xxiv).

Practicing therapy from a culture-blind perspective minimizes other people's experiences and overemphasizes the therapist's power and privilege. This issue of power difference is even more relevant in play therapy because children and teenagers have less power in family and society, so in order to provide an adequate therapeutic relationship, we need to give the power back to the child, including acknowledging, appreciating, and embracing the child's culture. This chapter is a call to consider interventions that acknowledge, value, and celebrate the culture of our child clients. "Embracing our diversity can lessen racial and ethnic tensions, while pretending that race and ethnicity don't matter may actually deepen culture divides" (Markus & Conner, 2014, pp. xxii, 64).

Multiple studies show a usual pattern that people in minority groups generally include their race or ethnicity in their self-descriptions, while those in the majority hardly ever do that. A 2013 survey of a representative sample of Americans found that while 50% of Whites never think about their race, only 12% of Blacks report that their race never crosses their mind. When someone is part of a minority group in terms of ethnicity, race, or identity, they might tend to be more self-conscious about what makes them different from the majority group (Markus & Conner, 2014). For example, when we were living in Colombia, although our country had different races such as Black, White, indigenous, and mestizo, we did not think about our race or ethnicity because we were part of the majority and considered ourselves just Colombians. However, when we moved to the United States, we began to be recognized by our Latinx background. When we moved to Texas, people identified us as Hispanics, and when I (Viviana Urdaneta) moved to California, people began to see me as a "person of color." So, we definitely have noticed more of our differences and that we stand out because of our looks, our names, and the way we speak in the U.S. context.

When Latinx clients come for therapy, they will be more likely to be thinking about their race, ethnicity, and culture as an important factor whether consciously or unconsciously. For this reason, developing interventions that highlight the child's culture becomes an essential part of doing therapy, and this becomes even more important when doing trauma work due to the sensitive material that will be part of the sessions. For example, when asking a Latinx teen client about the song he hears the most at home, he talked about *La Jaula de Oro* (The Golden Cage) by los Tigres del Norte. This popular song talks about how sometimes immigrants call the United States "the golden cage" because even though they are doing better financially, they feel like "prisoners" because they cannot go back to their country of origin. This information allowed us to work on the teen's feelings of guilt because he hears his parents saying very often that they were inside this "golden cage" for his well-being so he could get the education and opportunities he could not get in their native country.

It is important to highlight that the acknowledgment, celebration, and embracement of our clients' culture begins not just from the moment we meet at intake, but it begins from the moment a family or client calls to make an appointment or visits a website to learn more about therapy services. Oftentimes, the verbal and written messages we as therapists communicate could open or close doors for the treatment of clients who belong to a minority group. For example, if a Latinx family is seeking services, and parents are not completely fluent in English and are unable to read information or talk about services in their own language, they might feel apprehensive about moving forward with services. Therefore, it is imperative that when engaging in the work with clients who belong to a minority group, we find ways to facilitate written or oral information in their own language and furthermore look into providing a physical space that communicates acceptance and inclusion. For instance, it would be important to consider finding ways to design the therapy room and office space with the multicultural community served in mind. They might include images of people from diverse backgrounds in their office space and website, have magazines or books in different languages, and have all paperwork, including consent and intake forms, in different languages other than English. In this way, we are communicating being culturally aware and inclusive to our clients who belong to a minority group right from the beginning and in turn setting the stage for greater therapeutic success by decreasing potential barriers due to differences in language and culture during their treatment.

As bilingual and bicultural therapists, we recognize the challenge that our profession and professionals in our field face when needing to serve families who have a different language and culture. Although in most cases there is an acknowledgment of this principle in the therapeutic process, linguistic resources to mitigate language barriers could be very hard to find making treatment more challenging. When working with Latinx second- or third-generation children whose parents might not be fluent in English, it is not uncommon to use the child as translator during parent consultations, school meetings, or doctor's appointments; therefore, language barriers can pose a challenge and potentially an ethical dilemma in treatment. Although it might be very hard to find ways to communicate in the same language of our clients or their families without using a person in the family unit who is able to speak both languages, foreign language interpreting should be offered outside of the family unit in order to avoid any triangulation or potential ethical dilemmas in treatment.

In our context of practice and when providing consultation and support to our colleagues who are not fully bilingual, but are working with Latinx families, we have suggested to network with bilingual providers in order to contract with them and use them as resources to help navigate linguistical challenges. Although it is not ideal, therapists can make use of language lines or find someone else at their workplace who is bilingual, even if this individual is not a therapist, to help with translation services as needed during treatment.

GENERATIONAL DIFFERENCES AND ACCULTURATION LEVELS

Within the Latinx community and in general when working with immigrants, it is very important to understand how individuals identify generationally. Several authors agree that the level of acculturation must be considered when working with the Latinx community. Acculturation has been defined as "the steps by which ethnic minorities ascertain world views and cultural or social values of the dominant group and adapt their cultural patterns" (Pradilla, 2007). When we discuss the clinical implications of working with Latinx children and teens from different generations and acculturation levels, we refer to first/foreign-born as the generation for those individuals who are not U.S. citizens at birth and whose parents are not U.S. citizens; second generation as those individuals who are U.S. citizens at birth, as well as those born elsewhere to parents who are U.S. citizens, with at least one first-generation parent; third or higher as those individuals who are U.S. citizens at birth with both parents being U.S. citizens at birth.

When working with first-generation children and teens, it would be important to consider their immigration history and acculturation process, as both of these factors could bring challenges and strengths (Fry & Passel, 2019). Often, when engaging in treatment with first-generation/foreign-born clients, there is a high likelihood that some of them might be undocumented, meaning not having the authorization to legally reside or work in the United States, making resources limited due to legal status and language barriers. Families that have members who are undocumented might be concerned about seeking help due to fear of being reported to Immigration and Customs Enforcement (ICE); therefore, the therapist needs to be sensitive when trying to engage this population in treatment. Often, once the child and family feel safe and can trust the therapist, they tend to invest themselves in the therapeutic process and try to get as much out of it as possible. With this population, a therapist would benefit from researching common games and songs in the client's country of origin to be used as interventions. For example, we have used the Colombian version of "hot potato." In this game, one person says the words "tingo tingo tango," while the other members of the group pass an object to one another. This game is great to play during the preparation phase of EMDR therapy with families or groups in order to find and build resources. The person that gets the object/hot potato will identify a resource such as a skill, a time in the past, a person or friend they admire, or a symbol that reminds them about their strengths.

Often second-generation Latinx children have mixed statuses in the family, as some members are U.S. born and others might be in the country undocumented.

For example, a 13-year-old came to therapy and was hesitant to talk at first. Later, when she began to trust the therapist, she disclosed that she was afraid to talk with any professionals because her aunt was undocumented. She said that her parents and siblings had legal documentation or what is commonly referred as green cards in the United States, but her aunt who lives with them did not. This teen disclosed that she was afraid that her aunt could be in trouble if anyone outside of her family knew her aunt's status. Another typical scenario that can happen when working with second-generation children relates to tension and prejudice among family members due to the different legal status family members hold. The Sanchez family came to therapy due to difficulties between their teenager children. Their 18-year-old Andres was born in Mexico and was undocumented, but their 16-year-old Jose was a U.S. citizen. Jose minimized Andres and called him "wetback" (*mojado*, a pejorative term for people who do not have legal status in the United States) and was constantly bullying his brother to the point of physical aggression. As a result of this experience, it was important to help Andres process during EMDR therapy his negative cognition "I am not good enough" and "I am not valuable" as the lack of proper documentation in the United States had made a profound impact in the way he saw himself and the way he perceived others would see him.

Second- and third-generation Latinx children and teens also might encounter different challenges as they might struggle with a sense of belonging (Hovey & King, 1996). It is common when working with Latinx teens to hear them making statements like "I don't fit in here nor there." There is a divided sense of loyalty to their roots but also to the cultural norms outside their home environment. Therefore, at first, treatment might need to focus around negative cognitions such as "I don't belong," "I am different," or "I am a fraud," especially as they are trying to complete major and expected milestones such as finishing high school and getting into college. Families might have different expectations about education according to their acculturation process. In some families, it might be expected that children and teens do well because they are the first generation getting higher education and so they have to take advantage of this opportunity. This puts a lot of pressure on the children. In other families, the expectation is that the teenager needs to work as soon as possible to contribute to the financial situation here and back home. So, when a teenager wants to go to college, they might encounter lack of support from their parents.

Another important factor connected to the acculturation process is the use of Spanish during the therapeutic process. According to research, even Latinx fluent in English may find it easier to recount stories and talk about their feelings in Spanish. Some research also suggests that switching to English (if Spanish is their first language) in the middle of a therapeutic session might mean that the client wants to distance themselves from their emotions. So, it is important to realize as therapists that language switching has a logic to it (Dingfelder, 2005). We have utilized in therapy both English and Spanish and a mixture of both (Spanglish) as a way to support client's expression of this part of their identity. We use the language that the child feels most comfortable with, and we switch if they decide to do so. This is relevant for Latinx children, since a 2003 study published in the *International Journal of Bilingualism* found that individual words to bilingual people may have richer meanings in one language than another (Dingfelder, 2005). For example, a 10-year-old boy who was separated from his mom when he was 4 years old would speak primarily English during most of his sessions, but whenever we were using EMDR to target his experience of being separated from his mother and culture when he came to the United States with his dad, he would switch to Spanish to report what he was noticing between sets of bilateral stimulation (BLS). Therefore, it is important to consider that although there might be a dominant language for a child, experiences or feelings in bilingual children might be clearer in the other language depending on when and where those events happened.

INTEGRATING PLAYFUL AND CULTURALLY RELEVANT INTERVENTIONS THROUGHOUT THE EMDR PHASES

In this section, we present playful and creative interventions that have been helpful during the different phases of EMDR therapy with Latinx children through the lenses of three main principles: (1) Follow the child's lead and interest; (2) be curious, ask questions, and maintain an open attitude; and (3) utilize and emphasize cultural and individual strengths.

FOLLOW THE CHILD'S LEAD AND INTEREST

In order to provide an environment of safety and trust, it is important to meet our clients where they are. We would like to offer different playful child-centered interventions that we have found useful when working with Latinx children and their families during the different phases of EMDR therapy.

During the initial phase of EMDR, the therapist gathers information about the client's history and their goals for treatment and begins the assessment of both possible resources and traumatic events to process. It is useful for the therapist to talk first with the parents (without the child present), then with both, parents and child together, and finally, the child alone (without the parents present). This three-step process may allow the parents and child to speak freely without the presence of the other and may give the child a sense of being special when the therapists listen to him or her exclusively (Shapiro, 2018). Special arrangements when working with Latinx clients may be needed related to language, since the parents might feel more comfortable speaking Spanish and children might feel more comfortable speaking English. It is possible that there might be a mix of languages (English and Spanish) during the meetings.

As we keep in mind our principle of following the child's lead, during the history taking and treatment-planning phase, the therapist can be creative and utilize what the child likes as a resource to gather information. For example, the therapist can ask the child/teen to imagine they are creating a YouTube channel or a playlist in which they will identify songs that represent their family in different stages including the times before that they came to the United States (if they are foreign-born). Children can identify songs that they connect to and that are also part of their family history and traditions. For example, a 12-year-old who recently immigrated from Honduras created a list of songs she would listen to during holidays, and that she associated with different people or situations in her life. During this activity, she chose a song that her family used to listen to during Christmas, and as we talked about it, she was able to identify safe people in her family, which we used as resources, and at the same time identify target memories as she discussed some of the conflicts her family had with each other. When using a similar intervention, a 15-year-old born in the United States created two playlists—one was called "up," in which he listed all the songs that he could identify with in a positive way, and the other one was called "down," in which he listed all the songs that he associated with negative experiences or people. After he identified the songs, he assigned a feeling and a body sensation. For the positive associations, we installed them as resources with BLS. For those songs that had negative associations, we created an imaginary "cloud storage" that served as a container. Both of these examples can allow the therapist to gather information about the child's worldview and family dynamics in a gentle, playful way and at the same time can open doors to identify resources and potential memory targets.

Another example is a teenager who wanted to discuss issues of relationships and possibly dating violence. Since both the teen and her mother reported they liked Mexican music, we looked up popular Mexican songs and analyzed together the lyrics during the preparation phase of EMDR therapy to help grow our therapeutic relationship and build resources. Later, we danced together during desensitization going back and forth with our feet while we targeted an incident with her boyfriend. She reported at the end of treatment that she appreciated the use of her cultural background and music during therapy.

In the case of working with children who would rather write as we follow their interests when gathering history, therapists can guide children or parents in creating a booklet about the child's life and family. The child will start with the table of contents by writing the name of the chapters of his life including good things and not-so-good things.

Maria's Story—10 Years Old

> Chapter 1: My grandpa and grandma got divorced
> Chapter 2: My mom stayed with my grandpa and my uncle
> Chapter 3: My mom and dad got together
> Chapter 4: We got a dog, and I won a prize in the school
> Chapter 5: We moved to the United States—began living with uncle's family
> Chapter 6: Bad thing happened with uncle
> Chapter 7: My siblings were born
> Chapter 8: I told my teacher about what was happening with uncle
> Chapter 9: Moved out of uncle's house
> Chapter 10: What is next?

In this example, Maria, aged 10, chose the first chapter of her booklet to be the divorce of her grandpa and grandma that took place before she was born. The second chapter was when her mother and father began their relationship, and the third chapter was when she was born. This might be surprising for us, as therapists, because her story, according to Maria, began long before she was born with the actions of her grandparents. This provides an example of the importance of relatives and extended family for Latinx children. Also, Maria's story helps us to remember the strong role that the elderly/grandparents have in the life of Latinx children. The elders are highly respected and play a dominant role in the family. They have authority over younger members, and are considered a very important part of one's history (Samovar et al., 2017). Chapter four was when she got a dog and she won a prize in school. Chapter five was when the family moved to the United States and they began living with their uncle. Chapter six was when "bad things happened with uncle," which later she described as sexual assault. Chapter seven was when her siblings were born. Chapter eight was when she disclosed the abuse by uncle to her math teacher. Chapter nine was when they moved out of the uncle's house. Chapter ten was for the future that is coming for her and her family. It is important to clarify that the child or the parent of a young child does not write the *content* of the chapters of this booklet in the first meetings, but only discusses the title of each chapter as a table of contents in a book. The contents of the book might be further developed as resources or target memories for reprocessing later in treatment. In Maria's case, we began working with the book talking/drawing about her dog and when she won a prize in the school and utilized BLS with patty cakes (Tinker & Wilson, 1999) to install those as resources. In further sessions, Maria utilized the figures in the sand tray to describe her family members and play out some chapters of her booklet.

One way that we have found helpful in discussing treatment planning and the importance of processing one thing at a time with EMDR therapy is to use a pizza analogy. First, the therapist draws a pizza (like a pie chart) and asks the child to identify what are the things that the client worries the most, such as home, school, friends, or being with family in their home country or relatives in the United States. Each slice then becomes an issue to be treated. The therapist can ask a subjective units of distress (SUDs) scale reading on each of the issues and start working with the issue that has the lowest or highest SUDs score depending on what seems most appropriate for the client's treatment. Marta was a 10-year-old who was very guarded and did not want to talk about anything. When we started to talk about pizza, her eyes got bigger, and she was happily surprised to be able to talk about her favorite food and how she is able to enjoy it more when she eats only one bite at the time instead of trying to eat a whole slice in one bite.

Therapist: *Do you like pizza?*

Marta: *Yes. I love it.*

Therapist: *Which one is your favorite?*

Marta: *Pepperoni. Umm… delicious!*

Therapist: *Have you ever tried to eat a WHOLE extra-large pizza in only one bite?*

Marta: *Nope. That is impossible because my mouth is not that big.*

Therapist: *You are right! So, in order to decide what we are going to be talking when you come to see me, we are going to divide our work. In that way, we focus on only one bite at a time. Can we work together to do this?*

Marta: *Okay.*

Therapist: *Let's draw a pizza together and let's write in each piece the things that worry you the most now. It could be bad things that happened in the past, or recently, or worries that you have about the future.*

Marta: *Okay. Let's see. I am worried that my mom will not have enough money for food this month. I have bad dreams. I am worried about my uncle because he went to Mexico to visit grandma and we have not heard from him in some time…*

Therapist: *Thank you for sharing. Now, what if you tell me how much each one of these things bothers you? On a scale of 0 to 10, where 0 is neutral and 10 is the most bothersome, you can imagine how much each one of these things that you mentioned bothers you. This can help us to know which of those things is the one that we need to talk about first.*

After this short conversation about pizza and the things she likes, she was willing to talk more about her worries. Through the pizza drawing, we were able to partialize and identify the concerns that she brought to therapy, and we were able to identify targets for reprocessing. This strategy also served as containment in the sense of emphasizing the concept of working with one slice at a time and putting the rest in the freezer in order to be able to make things more digestible. If the therapist finds out that the child does not like pizza or enjoys another fruit/vegetable, we can modify the project. We have used watermelon, papaya, cookies, quesadillas, and other foods as a replacement for pizza in order to make it appropriate for specific clients.

Another playful way to engage Latinx clients when doing history taking and treatment planning is to make origami with child clients. A very creative 10-year-old boy, who liked origami, created an origami fortune-teller in session, and we used his origami fortune-teller figure as a way of gathering history and identifying resources. Each number under the fortune-teller's tab was linked to a question for history taking and preparation such as favorite place, name of his pets, favorite subject in the school, a time when he felt angry, a time when he felt happy, and places in his body where he felt his feelings; he was excited about playing and talking at the same time.

During the preparation phase of EMDR therapy, in order to teach BLS to children, the therapist can use toys or happy faces at the end of a wand or finger puppets in order to hold the child's attention. Drumming and the "butterfly hugs" can also be used (Jarero & Artigas, 2009). One way that we have taught BLS to children is the "horsey," since the tapping on their own knees sounded like a horse galloping. For example, an 8-year-old child who loves horses was more open to BLS once he heard the name horsey. As we moved through the reprocessing phases of EMDR therapy, we used the horsey taps as a form of BLS to keep him engaged in the process. In addition, the horsey taps also helped this client be more grounded, since the client was using his own hands to do the taps on his knees and had a more embodied experience.

During the assessment phase, the goal is to identify the parts of the target (traumatic memory that we are going to reprocess) and to establish baseline measures before we began the reprocessing phases of EMDR therapy (Shapiro, 2018). We are also trying to turn on a memory network so that it can be reprocessed by asking information about an image that represents this memory, a negative belief, a desired positive belief, emotions, and body sensations and location of those. One important aspect to consider with children is that the developmental level of the child impacts the procedural steps in this phase and the language to be used. During this phase, the therapist can ask the aspects of the target while playing a game. Also, drawings or sand tray can be used to show the worst part of the incident and discuss the other aspects of the target. It is important to consider that often the targets with children might be related with current events, not past ones (Adler-Tapia & Settle, 2017).

When engaging in the assessment phase with children, a therapist would need to accommodate to meet client's language and developmental stage. It is important to make the scaling questions easier to grasp, when in addition there might be a linguistical barrier. For example, we have asked clients to draw lines during the assessment phase when asking about a Validity of Cognition (VoC) or SUD scale. For instance, a child could draw three consecutive lines, as if she was doing tally marks, to represent a VoC of 3. During the installation phase, when measuring the VoC, the child could add or take lines away to depict where she is at in the process.

The goal of the desensitization phase is to introduce BLS and begin the reprocessing of the traumatic event. Those who have engaged in desensitization with children and teens know that shifts can happen in the blink of an eye. We have seen the need for the reprocessing phase to be very culturally sensitive with Latinx children and teens. Oftentimes, due to shame or even stigma, some children might not want to talk in depth about their traumatic experience and would be prompted to avoid talking about their trauma. We know that with EMDR reprocessing, clients don't need to give an extensive recount of their trauma in order to heal, and this can make trauma processing more doable for clients and therapists.

We have found a magic eraser board to be a great tool for young and school-age kids during desensitization. This board allows the child to create a drawing and erase it after each set very quickly by just pulling the handle of the board. The use of a board during this phase allows for a more concrete way of expression of images, thoughts, and feelings. Additionally, it also serves as a form of containment as the child can put the disturbing image in the board to process it or "digest it" and let it go away (Jarero & Artigas, 2009). Jorge, a 4-year-old, came to therapy due to having adjustment difficulties because of the recent birth of his youngest sister. Jorge's parents were very distressed because culturally, older male siblings are supposed to protect younger sisters or siblings. Jorge had been physically aggressive multiple times to his baby sister and had caused some minor injuries. When processing the last incident in which he pushed his sister while she was crawling, Jorge drew feeling faces in the magic eraser board after each set of BLS and pulled down the handle of the board to have a "clean slate" to work from. The concept of a clean slate helped Jorge transition to feel he could have a "redo" with his sister after he was able to process all of his anger for needing to make room in his life for a new little person.

During the EMDR installation phase, the goal is to continue reprocessing the target while integrating the positive desire belief for the client. Installation can be seen metaphorically as the light at the end of tunnel. For young children, using a crawl tunnel can provide a concrete way to exemplify how true and how far away the child feels they are from the positive cognition. This is a playful intervention that is providing proprioceptive input to make the installation process a more embodied experience. Sophie is a 6-year-old who liked to be very active in session. She was processing a target memory related to the removal from their home of her sister and herself after she had disclosed an incident of sexual abuse by her stepdad. During installation, we used the crawl tunnel to help her see how far she felt she was from her positive belief "It is not my fault." We wrote down her positive cognition in a piece of paper and placed it at the end of the tunnel. When asked how far away from the end of the tunnel she felt in regard to believing it was not her fault, she crawled inside and sat in the middle of the tunnel. Sophie did butterfly hugs as a way of BLS and after each set she began to move closer to the end of the tunnel that had the sign with her positive cognition. Once she got to the end, we celebrated her accomplishment with more butterfly hugs.

During the body scan phase, the goal is to reprocess any somatic residual disturbance from the targeted event. Research suggests that weighted blankets can promote calm and ease anxiety. Using a weighted blanket is like getting a big, warm hug for some children. A 5-year-old with sensory-processing issues came with her blanket to session most times. We used a dog-shaped weighted lap pad (that she called "Brownie") during body scan to help her feel more in touch with her body. She used a stethoscope to examine Brownie and see what and where Brownie was feeling things in its body. This intervention provided a sense of body awareness in a secure and playful manner for her.

BE CURIOUS, ASK QUESTIONS, AND MAINTAIN AN OPEN ATTITUDE

When working with children, teens, and their parents, it is helpful to have a curious approach in treatment rather than be a "know it all." This principle is important whether the therapist is from the same cultural background as the child or not. Even though Spanish is our first language, we have encountered families that use the same words but with different meanings because some words change their use from one country to another. For example, an expression that means "just kidding" in Colombia has a completely different meaning in different parts of Mexico that could be perceived as offensive. So an open attitude to asking questions allows the therapist to clarify any possible misunderstandings. In this part of the chapter, we discuss ideas to follow the principle of being curious, asking questions, and maintaining an open attitude in the context of EMDR therapy.

During the history taking and treatment-planning phase, it is important to include questions about culture, strengths, and challenges in a respectful and open way. From the suggestion of a colleague (R. Levis, personal communication, September 4, 2018), one of the questions that we began to ask during intakes, for both parents and children, is "What would you like me to know about you or your family including race, culture, religion, lifestyle, socio-economics, immigration, sexual preference, gender identity, or any other diversity topics?" Through this question, children, teenagers, and parents from the Latinx background could talk about their ethnicity and their country of origin (if other than the United States). The idea of asking an open-ended question allows clients to share what they think is appropriate. In addition, as a way to follow the child's lead and interest usually, we ask the intake questions while playing a game that the child has chosen; so we play and talk at the same time.

Siniego and Levi proposed some questions to use when conducting history taking with immigrants (in Nickerson, 2017), which we have adapted and added to for use with children.

1. *If your teacher asked you about your coming to the United States, what might you say? If your cousin asked you about your coming to the United States, what might you say?*
2. *What is your first memory of being in this country? What have you heard from your relatives about their first memories in this country?*
3. *If you friend from back home asked you what you like the most or the least about living in the United States, what would you say?*
4. *If I have a magic wand, what would you like to change about your experience of living in the United States right now?*

It is important to remember that Latinx immigrant children might change their response or story according to who asks about it, not because they are lying, but because they want to protect their family and themselves (Nickerson, 2017). So, the therapist needs to work on cultivating a genuine and positive therapeutic relationship so the child and his family might feel more comfortable to provide information. It might be important for therapists who work with the Latinx population to be willing to self-disclose some minor details about themselves in order to help with rapport building. Minor self-disclosure is considered in Latinx cultures as a way to show the self as caring, genuine, and real (Aviera, 2015). For example, when working with a child who loves playing soccer, a therapist can pass the soccer ball back and forth while taking turns asking and answering questions such as the child's and the therapist's favorite color, food, and games. As the therapist follows the principle of being curious and asking questions, the information gathered during playful engagement can be used later as potential targets or resources. Also, a therapist can create a bingo game and assign questions to different combinations of letters and numbers or use a Jenga where each one of the blocks has a number that is connected with a question. Also, the therapist must include questions to assess the level of acculturation such as: What language do you speak at home? And what are some of your family traditions?

For younger children as a way to gather information during history taking and treatment planning, the therapist can ask the child to draw a picture of her different settings, such as house, school, and neighborhood. When working on the drawing of the client's house, the therapist can ask clients to identify the following: favorite room, least favorite room, good and not-so-good things that have

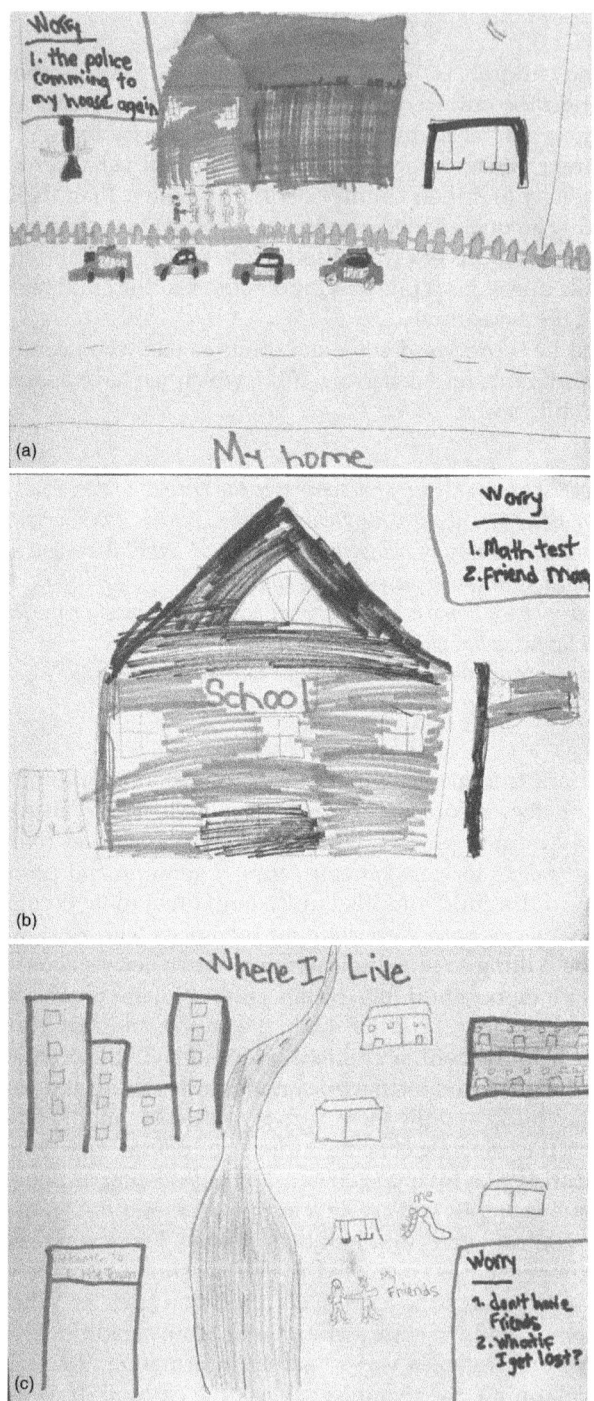

Figure 7.1 *Home, School, Neighborhood Settings Drawings. (a) Home Drawing During History Phase. (b) School Drawing for History Taking Phase. (c) Community Drawing for History Taking Phase*

happened in their house, things they would like to change about their home, people who live in the house, or whom they would like to live with. Therapist can do the same with the school picture and identify favorite and least favorite class, teachers, classmates, difficult events (Figure 7.1)

During the preparation phase, following the principle of being curious, asking questions, and maintaining an open attitude provides a framework to help children find resources, provide psychoeducation about EMDR therapy, and engage children with different types of BLS. The main goal of this principle of openness as a therapist is to see what interests the child and utilize them in the context of EMDR therapy. The therapist can think about the goal of the phase of EMDR therapy that they are working on and what tools will accomplish that goal keeping the child's interests in mind. If a client likes music, then the therapist should use music to gather information, find resources, and reprocess. If a client likes animals, then the therapist should use animals. If a client likes painting, then the therapist needs to use painting. We must be creative in the work with children in order to provide therapy from a strengths perspective and in an empowerment model.

It is also vital to pace the work when engaging children in trauma processing. As child therapists, we often play the role of a detective who reads the verbal and nonverbal cues our clients give us during the therapeutic process. Thus, we need to be skillful in the task of fragmenting the work or breaking down the processing into manageable parts to make sure children are maintaining stability inside and outside of session. The child needs to feel supported and in control.

During the reprocessing phases of EMDR, following the principle of being curious and asking questions allows the therapist to empower the client to lead the process and keep the work in manageable fragments. Ana Gomez (2012) uses the terms "titration and pendulation" as "in and out" strategies that help children layer the amount of trauma exposure and make trauma processing easier to digest. We have adapted some of her strategies when working with Latinx children and teens.

Katia, a 16-year-old teen, was processing her experience of ongoing sexual abuse by her stepfather. While processing, it was very important that Katia would stay within her window of tolerance. The *window of tolerance* is a term used to describe the zone of arousal in which a person is able to function most effectively. If a person is able to stay within the optimal zone of arousal, a person is able to think and feel at the same time, and in turn be able to manage trauma processing more effectively as typically they can receive, process, and integrate information easier. During Katia's treatment, we created a plan for what helps her be "in" and what pushes her to be "out" of her window. One of the things that helped her to be "in" was to listen to her "safe song," which was a hymn in Spanish from church that her grandmother used to sing for her when she was little. We were able to find this song on YouTube. During session, we agreed that we will stay "in" the memory for a few minutes and "out" of the memory by listening to her "safe song."

A 5-year-old boy was processing an incident in which he witnessed his dad being arrested due to an incident of domestic violence against his mother. We set up the target and played the game "two hats" using two hats from the pretend play area in the playroom. He wore one hat while thinking about the incident and the other hat while playing the *Veo, Veo* game, which is the equivalent of I Spy, beginning with a simple traditional rhyme that has a question/answer exchange.

Veo, veo / I see, I see
¿Qué ves? / What do you see?
Una cosita / A thing
¿Qué cosita es? / What thing is it?

This game served as a way of grounding and pendulating. At the beginning of the reprocessing of this memory, we would play it a couple of times each session while processing. After a few sessions, we just played it once as he was able to wear his "super hero hat" longer and keep reprocessing his traumatic memory.

Latinx children and teens might find themselves in an ongoing traumatic stress situation due to their or their family's immigration status or catastrophizing about their future. We must keep an open attitude to the fact that it is not uncommon for children to struggle with the uncertainty of not having the proper documentation to live and work in the United States. Therefore, providing a safe environment for children and families to process their feelings about a potential deportation is vital. One intervention that we have found useful to address this situation is to set up a target using the flashforward procedure, which helps clients to process an anticipated fear (Logie & De Jongh, 2014). Marcos, an 11-year-old from Venezuela, recently arrived in the United States with his family fleeing the political crisis in their country. Marcos and his family came to a community program seeking support. During individual therapy, after building rapport by asking him to talk more about his upbringing and what it was like to have been born and raised in Venezuela, we explored the present concern. He reported having ongoing nightmares of his family not being able to stay in the United States and having to go back to his country. When asked about the worst thing he imagined could happen, he stated that all of his family could be killed. We used the concept of a time machine to help Marcos imagine what he and his family would

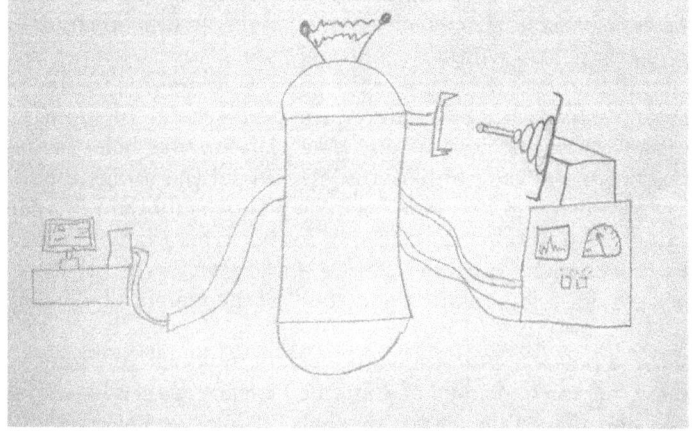

Figure 7.2 *Time Machine Drawing Sets the Stage for Processing Anticipated Troubles*

do if they have to go back to provide some distance when identifying the target to be processed during the flashforward. See Figure 7.2 for a "time machine" drawing example. After processing this target memory about the future, Marcos was able to realize that they were already safe in the United States, and that they were getting help. Also, he was able to recognize that no matter what, he can take advantage of the current time and enjoy their family relationships.

During closure and reevaluation, it is important that the counselor keeps an open attitude to recognize the child's needs because some children might need additional games and activities to regulate after reprocessing.

UTILIZE AND EMPHASIZE CULTURAL AND INDIVIDUAL STRENGTHS

When performing EMDR therapy with Latinx clients, it is important to consider that "the reason the client originally enters therapy may only be a minor portion of the trauma narrative, and, like an iceberg, much of it may be hidden from the view" (Nickerson, 2017, p. 81). Some clients and their families might have misconceptions around mental health and might feel uncomfortable about disclosing all their information, while others think that counseling is for "crazy people" and mistrust mental health providers. When working with Latinx children and their families, it is especially important to work on building a genuine therapeutic relationship, provide information to the child and parent about the purpose of gathering information, and clarify confidentiality. The child might have been taught that *la ropa sucia se lava en casa* ("don't air your dirty laundry in public"). Cultural norms may discourage disclosing family information to strangers because bad things might happen, they might take a child away and separate him from the family. For the Latinx culture, the concept of *Familismo* is very important. With *Familismo,* one has to protect the family unity because they are an extended part of the self. The sacredness and importance of the family can be seen in the Mexican proverb, "The only rock I know that stands steady, the only institution that I know that works, is the family." The family is the place where the individual finds security and emotional support (Samovar et al., 2017). Because of the concept of *Familismo,* when working with first-generation/foreign-born children, an attuned therapist should consider asking questions in a creative and culturally sensitive way so the child and family can feel safe to share information. The therapy playroom should include darker skinned dolls and typical objects and toys from the Latinx culture, such as tortillas, a *comal* (tortilla griddle), and a *balero* toy (cup and ball toy) to help children and families feel comfortable in a familiar environment. By introducing culturally relevant materials in the playroom, clients are able to share their story in a culturally sensitive way (Pradilla, 2007).

When working with Latinx children and families, we must recognize their cultural values as assets and resources during treatment. For instance, when doing history taking and preparation with Latinx children, it is vital to ask about the inclusion of religious beliefs and figures. Many Latinx have strong religious beliefs, which might impact how they see trauma and therapy. For example, it is culturally accepted that things will happen *"si Dios quiere"* (if God is willing). This belief is related to the concept of *Fatalismo* (Fatalism), which refers to the idea that divine providence governs the world (Aviera, 2015). This belief might influence how people see themselves in the aftermath of a difficult situation and might change their feelings and cognitions around guilt and responsibility in a traumatic situation. During preparation phase, an 8-year-old created a team of friends/helpers (as suggested in Gomez, 2012) where she included her mom, dad, her aunt Sonia (who was a close friend of the family and not blood-related), her cousin Antonia (Sonia's daughter), and the priest Jose (since her family were devout Catholics and the priest came to their house very often).

Preparation is very important in order to establish the foundation and prevent emotional blockages during reprocessing (Adler-Tapia & Settle, 2017; Shapiro, 2018); therefore, we want to look for ways throughout this phase to connect with the child emotionally and culturally. Preparation also includes assessing the client's resources and skills, assessing the client's home environment, determining what the child needs in order to begin reprocessing phases of EMDR therapy, and teaching the mechanics of EMDR (Adler-Tapia & Settle, 2017). When working with Latinx clients, this phase also involves assessing the level of acculturation and utilizing specific strategies to connect with the child emotionally and culturally.

One such way to establish a therapeutic alliance with Latinx children might be to engage in traditional games such as *loteria* (Mexican bingo, a game that uses images on a deck of cards instead of numbered ping-pong balls. Every image has a name, usually of traditional objects). The therapist and child should meet in a play therapy room that contains culturally sensitive toys, pretend foods that are representative of the Latinx culture, diverse art supplies such as multicultural crayons and paint that offer an opportunity for children to accurately depict their skin color when doing self-portraits or making family pictures, or musical instruments such as *maracas* or *matracas o raspas*. The therapist should be aware of the child's language preference; it would be important to include bilingual books and maps or globes that encourage conversation about where the family comes from (Pradilla, 2007). Another important factor might be to learn how to pronounce the name of the child as close as possible to their preferred pronunciation since a lot of names have been Americanized, meaning they have been changed to be easily pronounced by English native speakers without the consent of the owner of the name, such as "Maria" becoming "Mary;" "Viviana" becoming "Vivian;" and "Cristobal" becoming "Christopher." This idea of pronouncing the name as desired by the child will communicate *respeto* (respect) and will support the establishment of a genuine therapeutic relationship.

We have found the use of metaphors or analogies very useful when trying to explain the mechanics of EMDR during the preparation phase. Providing some context in which clients can easily relate to the process can greatly facilitate client's engagement during the course of treatment. One of our adult Latinx clients gave us a wonderful analogy to explain EMDR therapy that we have used successfully with children. She said that EMDR therapy is like cleaning your refrigerator. Sometimes, you have leftovers from past experiences that are just there, stuck in your refrigerator (your brain and body), and they smell, and they are not useful anymore; so, what we do with EMDR therapy is to take those leftovers out so we can have space for new, good food (experiences) to feed us. While using this analogy with a young girl, we can discuss how she would like to do some "cleaning of her refrigerator" because the bullying that she experienced at school left her sad and angry, and she wants those feelings to go so she can have space for other things.

Since the goal of EMDR therapy is to achieve the most profound and comprehensive effects possible in the shortest period of time while maintaining client stability (Shapiro, 2018), it is very important to teach children self-regulation skills including containment so they know how to handle their responses and fears outside of sessions. One way that we have used bilingualism as an asset and resource when working with children is to use their experience of knowing two languages to help them understand the concept of containment by explaining the idea of a "trauma language." If the child is bilingual, it is easy to understand that when you are using one language, you are not forgetting the other language. You are simply choosing which language to use in which context. The language that you are not using is still present, but you are consciously deciding not to access it. In the same way, when clients are outside of the therapist office/playroom, we do not want the use of the "trauma language," the one that contains the information about the hard things that they have experienced. We want them to restrict the use of this "trauma language" only to the processing time in the healing environment.

Therapist: *I know you speak both English and Spanish. Is that right?*

Client: *Yes. I do.*

Therapist: *How do you know which language to use?*

Client: *If I am at home, I speak Spanish. If I am at school, I speak English.*

Therapist: *How did you figure that out?*

Client: *Because my parents do not speak English and my friends think that it is more "cool" to speak English.*

Therapist: *One question, when you are speaking English, do you forget your Spanish? Or when you are speaking Spanish, do you forget your English?*

Client: *No. Of course not.*

Therapist: *Okay. So here in this space, we are going to use a special language, called "trauma language or the language of the bad things that happened" but we want to use it only here. Whenever you are outside of this room, you don't have to use it. You don't have to talk about the bad things that happened in the past. Okay?*

Client: *Okay.*

Therapist: *So, it is like speaking English and Spanish. You don't forget the other language, but you decide not to use it. Makes sense?*

Client: *Okay. I can do that.*

Another cultural resource we have used with Latinx children as a way of establishing a containment strategy is the use of worry dolls. Several authors and therapists have used worry dolls as a way to teach children and families to alleviate their anxieties. The indigenous tribes from Guatemala believe that if you are worrying about something, you can give it to a *quitapena* (a worry doll), and she will take your worry away. The worry doll becomes a symbol for clients with which they can separate from their worries and their "sad" memories and continue enjoying other things. For example, an 8-year-old was so excited when she received a worry doll. She took her home and named her Fanny. She carried Fanny in her backpack and pockets and every time that she felt sad/worry/overwhelmed, she would talk with Fanny. She told the therapist in the next session, "It is so good to have Fanny. I feel free and good. She carries everything that I do not want to think about. Thank you." During sessions, when we were reprocessing, she would hold Fanny in her hand as a way to get support.

One of our teen Latinx clients said, "Of course the worry dolls are silly, they do not work. It is only a doll." The therapist replied, "You are right they might not be magic. But what if they are a symbol for us? A symbol that represents that you do not have to carry your worries with you. A symbol that you can enjoy other things and not be so preoccupied. What do you think? Can we use it as our symbol?" and she said "Okay." In later sessions, she referred to the doll as our symbol, and used it very often as a way to separate herself from her worries. She did not carry the doll with her at all, but she remembered that she could contain her worries and give herself a break (Figure 7.3).

One consideration when working with Latinx children is the use of the *Realismo Magico* (Magical Realism) approach that might be helpful in setting up a target and help the child separate from the event. *Realismo Magico* is a literary movement from Latin America that uses the mixture of reality and fantasy as in the novel of Gabriel Garcia Marquez, *One Hundred Years of Solitude*. Comas-Diaz (2006) describes a study with traumatized Latinx children where the therapist encouraged the use of magical realism to attribute causality and cure to cultural heroes and villains and encourage clients to create images of symbolic figures to facilitate integration and processing of the traumatic event. Through magical realism, a child can have some distancing from the traumatic memory in an effort to facilitate the processing of painful life experiences as the child might be doing it in a third person narrative. Oscar, a 10-year-old, who had witnessed an incident of domestic violence at home between his mom and dad used a frog as the main character of his story. Oscar drew a time in which this frog saw his father hitting his mother. Oscar reported that the worst thing for him was that this happened in a house that he thought was safe because it was in a magical mountain protected by magical figures. The negative cognition of the frog was: "I am not safe" and the positive cognition was "I am okay now." Oscar continued to externalize his experiences using the frog, which allow him to distance himself from the trauma and effectively process this event. During assessment and reprocessing phases, Oscar included many magical things as part of the story, which were not discouraged by the therapist. The role of the therapist during this intervention is not to question or investigate the factual details of the event but facilitate the processing of this incident by allowing the client to engage in the memory in a way that feels safe and manageable, since the client is externalizing his internal pain through symbolic figures.

It is important to conceptualize our treatment when working with Latinx children from the perspective of a person in an environment. We emphasize the importance of understanding a client and their behavior in light of their environmental context. When facilitating trauma processing, especially during the reprocessing phases of EMDR therapy, it is important to note that there might be some issues that could be blocking the processing, and some of those could be related to cultural, political, or family beliefs.

7. PLAYFUL AND CREATIVE APPROACHES FOR EMDR THERAPY 243

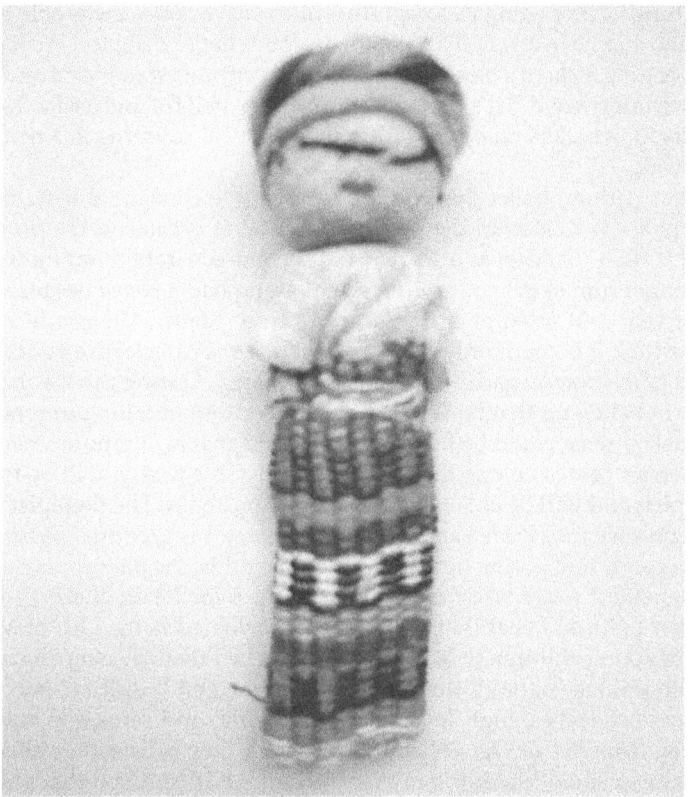

Figure 7.3 *Worry Doll as a Container*

Also, we would like to expand on different cultural beliefs that are important to consider when working with Latinx children and their families, as they could be key resources during the reprocessing phases of EMDR, and at the same time could provide understanding for why processing might be stuck. Jessica, a teen mom who was processing the intimate partner violence she has been experiencing in her relationship, was looping due to the fact that she believed that the abuse was "her cross to carry." Jessica came from a very traditional family with very strict religious values. She was living in a maternity house for teen moms while raising her baby. In the past, her family had communicated that as soon as she turned 18, she should plan to go and live with her boyfriend as it was her "duty" to be a good wife and mother although her boyfriend was abusive. Therefore, Jessica believed it was her job to be a good role model and stay in the relationship for her child and because that was her cross to carry. As we processed this memory, we had to give attention to this cultural value and perhaps blocking belief that was amplifying a maladaptive memory network for Jessica. We used a cognitive interweave to help Jessica process her shame and guilt and invited Jessica to see her experience from her baby's perspective. "Let's pretend that your daughter was going through a similar experience and she felt guilty because her boyfriend was calling her names and being controlling, would you expect her to stay with him?" After using this cognitive interweave, Jessica was able to process her guilt and shame in a way that did not discount her experience. We have found that approaching a client's blocking belief from a curious standpoint and using an imaginative interweave "let's pretend" can be very helpful and assist the client to process blocking beliefs related to cultural or political concerns in a nonintrusive unbiased way.

Another cultural belief that could be relevant to consider during the desensitization phase is related to the perception of what is causing the problem and what could "fix it." Andres is a 13-year-old second-generation immigrant, whose family brought him to get counseling after having had a *limpia* because he failed his school year and attempted to run away from home. A *limpia* is a spiritual cleansing ritual. It is commonly believed that a *limpia* can cleanse your emotions, mind, and body from negative thoughts and energy. During processing, Andres was stuck in believing that he is a bad person because of failing in school so the therapist asked what could be helpful and he said that his grandmother believed that if a person passes an egg through their body, this person will be freed from any bad spirit and will be able to be a good person again. The therapist used this as an imaginative interweave and Andres imagined his grandma passing an egg through his body and giving him a blessing. After this, the disturbance decreased and he felt neutral so we were able to move to the installation phase.

Another cultural belief that needs to be considered is the idea of *Mal de Ojo* (evil eye) in young children. It is commonly believed that when a person stares at a child with jealousy or envy, this causes the young child's spirit to become weak and triggers headaches, high fever, anxiety, crying, and refusal to eat or sleep, all suffering from *Mal de Ojo*. When this happens, they believe the child needs to be taken to a spiritual leader to pray for the child. It is common that parents will protect their children with a special bracelet that has been prayed over by the spiritual leader, and must be worn by the child at all times. A 4-year-old client wears this kind of bracelet and uses it as a resource to remind her about feeling safe from evil spirits and people. Esperanza, a teen mom with a 10-month-old baby girl, described how the baby has experienced fever recently and does not want to eat or sleep well. Esperanza says that she thinks it is her fault because she took the baby to see a friend that has a "very strong look" who might have given the *Mal de Ojo* to her daughter. Esperanza stated that she will take her daughter to the traditional healer and to the doctor after her session. The therapist focused on processing Esperanza's feelings of guilt and respectfully used a cognitive interweave such as "I am confused, how were you going to know that your daughter was going to be sick after visiting your friend?" Esperanza was able to decrease disturbance and feel calm and empowered to help her daughter heal physically. To complicate matters, the solution for *Mal de Ojo* changes from one country to another. In Colombia, we think that the child has to receive a prayer from a traditional healer. However, in other places like in Mexico, passing an egg around the child's body (like Andres) is the solution for an evil eye. For that reason, a therapist should be curious and ask respectfully about the client's beliefs instead of making assumptions.

A teen client named Carolina was stuck while reprocessing the sexual assault that she experienced by a classmate. She reported that she felt "damaged" and cannot be "valuable" again. When exploring this blocking belief, Carolina reported that when she lost her virginity due to the sexual assault, she lost her value as a woman. Carolina grew up in a traditional Catholic Latinx family where virginity and chastity are highly prized. Due to the influence of *Marianismo* (a belief that women should have attributes of the Virgin Mary and be pure and saintly), Carolina felt devastated to lose her "woman value" because of the assault. When processing with EMDR therapy, we utilized a cognitive interweave, "Let's pretend that you can recreate what virginity means and feels for you." She was able to decrease disturbance and was able to have self-compassion to process the fact that it was not her fault that she was assaulted. Also, she was able to remember that her aunt has told her multiple times that her value as a person is not conditioned by anything, and that she is valuable because of who she is and not because of what she has.

Research has found that Latinx clients tend to be more prone to somatization (Angel & Guarnaccia, 1989). Therefore, as mental health professionals we need to be more aware of differences in the way that Latinx report physical symptoms, especially during the assessment and body scan phases of EMDR therapy. Seven-year-old Mercedes came to therapy because her family believed that her medically unexplained fever, lethargy, and lack of appetite and sleep were due to *el Espanto* and that she had developed an *ataque de nervios*. *El Espanto* is an illness that can affect anyone at any age. It usually originates when someone is suddenly scared and terrified. It is commonly believed that after a person goes through a very frightening experience, a person becomes depressed, does not want to talk, does not want to eat, can't sleep, is feverish, feels chest pressure, and wants to remain in bed (Lizardi, Oquendo, & Graver, 2009). During history taking, Mercedes's family reported having taken her to multiple doctors and that they referred her to a mental health professional for her symptoms. No "major" trauma was reported by the family, and they reported that her symptoms began after she stayed the weekend with her cousins. The family reported that Mercedes's older cousins liked to do pranks and that while she was in their house, they were hiding under her bed at night and waited patiently until she went to sleep to pull her feet and scared her. Mercedes's reprocessing was very somatic in nature. Knowing that Mercedes was able to connect with her body very easily, we developed a game to help her identify her "comfy" and "not so comfy" body sensations. Mercedes loved pretend play and in the dramatic play she identified herself as a magical fairy. She had developed a special wand that could help get access to the "boss fairy," a resource she had identified earlier in treatment. When Mercedes was confused about what she was feeling or did not know what she was experiencing, the wand had a special button she could press and it would dial the number to the "boss fairy" and she could ask her any question. When we got to the body scan, Mercedes reported she still felt disturbance in her chest and was afraid that the *ataque de nervios* will not go away because the doctor could not find a medicine for it. We used our special wand to dial the "boss fairy" for help and used a modification of Ana Gomez's (2012) "interviewing a body part" technique to understand what was happening. Mercedes interviewed the fairy and asked her to help her find a medicine for her chest pain. Mercedes processed her *ataque de nervios* with EMDR therapy, and felt neutral after treatment. The therapist did not question her definition of her illness, and with this flexibility, offered a culturally sensitive intervention in a client-centered way.

During the reevaluation phase with children, it is important to assess how treatment is going from the perspective of both the child and the parent and continue resource-building and processing as needed. Culturally for some Latinx clients, going back and thinking about the past experiences can be seen as being ungrateful about the present or as not appropriate. Often you will hear a phrase that speaks to this belief *para atras ni para cojer impulso*, which translates as—never take a step back, not even to gain momentum. This phrase highlights the importance of cultural sensitivity if there is some resistance to going back and checking on a memory from the past session in the reevaluation.

ADDITIONAL IDEAS: GROUP PROTOCOL

We have used the EMDR integrative group treatment protocol (EMDR-IGTP) very effectively with Latinx children and teens, as during the group they don't have to talk about their trauma experience since they are drawing. The EMDR-IGTP allows for the administration of individual EMDR treatment in a group setting, which can be highly valuable in a setting where resources are limited (Jarero & Artigas, 2009). The literature on providing culturally competent mental health services to Latinx populations suggests that a key variable is access to treatment (Miranda, Azocar, Organista, Muñoz, & Lieberman, 1996). Being able to provide effective treatment to a group helps minimize the barrier of access to treatment. This protocol was designed to be used with children starting at age 7, but with permission from Dr. Jarero (the developer of the protocol), we have modified it to be used with ages 4 to 6. We organized "healing camps" and provided intensive EMDR group therapy for Spanish-speaking child victims of domestic violence from a waiting list at a community agency. In 1 week, we were able to treat 35 children using the standard EMDR-IGTP and the modified version for ages 4 to 6. This model was very effective and culturally appropriate as it created the experience of being "in the same boat" and at the same time provided reinforcement to the communal aspect of the Latinx culture. Between the sessions of reprocessing, we invited children to play traditional games from Latin America and do arts and crafts.

When conducting the group protocol, children identify the worst fragment of the event they would like to process and draw a picture of it, identifying the level of disturbance and doing self-administered BLS via butterfly hugs. At the end, they also draw a vision of the future that serves as the installation phase.

Since while doing the EMDR-IGTP, clients don't have to talk at all, we have found that using this protocol individually or with a family is very effective for those clients who are not comfortable talking about their trauma. Indeed, this protocol has been very culturally relevant to Latinx children and teens as it provides a protective layer of privacy and protection, especially when dealing with taboo issues or sensitive topics like a client's immigration status in the United States. Furthermore, this protocol was developed in the context of Latin America by members of the Mexican Association for Mental Health Support in Crisis (AMAMECRISIS) to deal with the need for mental health services after Hurricane Pauline in Mexico in 1997 (Jarero & Artigas, 2009). The origins of the protocol help it to be an excellent fit to work with Latinx clients.

ADDITIONAL IDEAS: USING A STORY TEMPLATE AND *CUENTO*

Joan Lovett (2007) created an EMDR processing intervention for children called the story template. It utilizes stories and BLS to process traumatic events. We have taken her work and adapted it to the work with Latinx children and teens. Stories are a way to relate to children in a nonthreatening way by bringing concepts to life and bridging gaps in making big concepts more accessible. Within a lot of cultures, including Latinx, folk stories and storytelling have been a way to engage with the younger generation and leave behind a legacy of information and beliefs. Latin American people commonly answer questions by telling a story, allowing the answer to come from the narrative (Comas-Diaz, 2006), so this is a model that fits very well with this culture.

Some of the ways we have incorporated Lovett's story template is by using familiar characters of the same ethnicity as the child, or animals they can relate to. This is similar to *Cuento* therapy, which is a model that uses Puerto Rican stories to promote adaptation and growth among children. However, *Cuento* therapy has a strong psychoeducation component (Comas-Diaz, 2006), and the story template's main goal is to process trauma. Estela is a 3-year-old who came from Central America when she was 2 years old with her mother to escape the violence there. When meeting with mom for the initial intake, Estela's mother reported that her daughter had been having extreme separation anxiety symptoms since mom began to work a few hours per day out of the home. As we embarked into exploring creating a story template for Estela to help her process her trauma, we created a timeline with mom as far as prenatal, birth, and life before and after arrival to the United States. Mom recalled having suffered domestic violence since she was pregnant with Estela until she was able to leave her country. She also recounted different experiences in which their lives were in danger while they traveled across different countries until they were able to arrive to the United States. We also went over present recent triggers, including mom leaving the house to go to work, and finally discussed mom's dreams for Estela's future including coping adaptively while mom was out knowing that mom will come back to be with Estela. Once all the information was gathered, we composed a story with relevant clip art pictures to resemble Estela's story.

We had mom read the story while tapping on Estela's shoulders as Estela was in mom's lap coloring the figures in the story. In this case, we took four sessions to go through the whole story with mom and Estela. Every session, we did a fragment in which mom read while tapping continuously on Estela's shoulders. By the end of the fourth session, Estela's mother began to report a decrease in Estela's disturbance when she left for work and being more cooperative during sleeping and eating times.

CONCLUSION

This chapter serves as a call to include interventions that acknowledge, value, and celebrate the culture of children and their families. It emphasized the importance of increasing our cultural awareness and sensitivity by following three principles to work with the Latinx population: (1) Follow the child's lead and interest; (2) be curious, ask questions, and maintain an open attitude; and (3) utilize and emphasize cultural and individual strengths. Playful and creative interventions throughout the eight phases of EMDR are essential to success, as well as becoming familiar with some common cultural values among Latinx people, with the understanding that Latinx are a diverse group with many different characteristics. We emphasize a strengths-perspective approach and the importance of seeing clients as people within an environmental context that sometimes invites them to grow and thrive and at other times is the cause of oppression and prejudice.

REFERENCES

Adler-Tapia, R., & Settle, C. (2017). *EMDR and the art of psychotherapy with children: Infants to adolescent's treatment manual*. New York, NY: Springer Publishing Company.

Angel, R., & Guarnaccia, P. J. (1989). Mind, body, and culture: Somatization among hispanics. *Social Science and Medicine, 28*(12), 1229–1238. doi:10.1016/0277-9536(89)90341-9

Aviera, A. (2015). Culturally sensitive and creative therapy with Latino clients. *American Psychological Association*, 1–2. Retrieved from https://www.apadivisions.org/division-31/publications/articles/california/aviera.pdf

Comas-Díaz, L. (2006). Latino healing: The integration of ethnic psychology into psychotherapy. *Psychotherapy: Theory, Research, Practice, Training, 43*(4), 436–453. doi:10.1037/0033-3204.43.4.436

Dingfelder, S. (2005). Closing the gap for Latino clients. *America Psychological Association, 36*(1), 58.

Fry, R., & Passel, J. S. (2019). *Latino children: A majority are U.S.-born offspring of immigrants*. Pew Research Center. Retrieved from http://assets.pewresearch.org/wp-content/uploads/sites/7/reports/110.pdf

Gil, E., & Drewes, A. A. (2006). *Cultural issues in play therapy*. New York, NY: Guilford Press.

Gomez, A. M. (2012). *EMDR therapy and adjunct approaches with children: Complex trauma, attachment, and dissociation*. New York, NY: Springer Publishing Company.

Hovey, J. D., & King, C. A. (1996). Acculturative stress, depression, and suicidal ideation among immigrant and second-generation Latino adolescents. *Journal of the American Academy of Child and Adolescent Psychiatry, 35*(9), 1183–1192. doi:10.1097/00004583-199609000-00016

Jarero, I., & Artigas, L. (2009). EMDR integrative group treatment protocol. *Journal of EMDR Practice and Research, 3*(4), 287–288.

Lizardi, D., Oquendo, M. A., & Graver, R. (2009). Clinical pitfalls in the diagnosis of *ataque de nervios*: A case study. *Transcultural Psychiatry, 46*(3), 463–486. doi:10.1177/1363461509343090

Logie, R., & de Jongh, A. (2014). The "flashforward procedure": Confronting the catastrophe. *Journal of EMDR Practice and Research, 8*(1), 25–32.

Lovett, J. (2007). *Small wonders: Healing childhood trauma with EMDR*. Riverside, CA: Free Press.

Markus, H. R., & Conner, A. (2014). *Clash: How to thrive in a multicultural world*. New York, NY: Plume.

Miranda, J., Azocar, F., Organista, K. C., Muñoz, R. F., & Lieberman, A. (1996). Recruiting and retaining low-income Latinos in psychotherapy research. *Journal of Consulting and Clinical Psychology, 64*(5), 868–874.

Nickerson, M. I. (2017). *Cultural competence and healing culturally based trauma with EMDR therapy: Innovative strategies and protocols.* New York, NY: Springer Publishing Company.

Pradilla, D. N. (2007). *Identification of play therapy strategies that are used with Latino children* (Doctoral Dissertation). Retrieved from https://commons.lib.niu.edu/bitstream/handle/10843/17255/Pradilla%2c%20Daphne%20N.pdf?sequence=1&isAllowed=y

Samovar, L. A., Porter, R. E., McDaniel, E. R., & Roy, C. S. (2017). *Communication between cultures* (9th ed.). Boston, MA: Cengage Learning.

Shapiro, F. (2018). *Eye movement desensitization and reprocessing (EMDR): Basic principles, protocols and procedures* (3rd ed.). New York, NY: Guilford Press.

Tinker, R. H., & Wilson, S. A. (1999). *Through the eyes of a child: EMDR with children.* New York, NY: W. W. Norton.

U.S. Census Bureau. (2018). *Hispanic Heritage Month 2018: Facts for features.* Retrieved from https://www.census.gov/newsroom/facts-for-features/2018/hispanic-heritage-month.html

8

Understanding and Responding to Dissociation in Children With Play-Based Approaches

ANNIE MONACO

INTRODUCTION

A journey into learning about dissociation usually begins with a therapist being unsuccessful in the treatment of traumatized children. An eye movement and desensitization and reprocessing (EMDR) clinician starts to seek information on how to help their clients by attending training, reading books, or engaging in "What am I missing?" discussions while in supervision. Therapists have an "aha moment" when they look through the lens of dissociation at the child's symptoms and behaviors. The gift of dissociation brings relief to many children in harmful situations. The transformation of therapists occurs when we truly understand the depth of this gift and work to find play-based approaches for children to be able to safely identify and discuss their *self-states*, the dissociated or fragmented parts of the self formed by trauma. This chapter provides an understanding of the internal world of self-states and what that might look like in the child's external world and in the playroom. Recognizing and knowing the guiding principles of how to access self-states provide therapists the tools for effective treatment for the child and all of their caregivers.

USING THE LENS OF DISSOCIATION

Many therapists feel discouraged with complex trauma cases due to the overwhelming behavioral problems, the family dynamics, and the challenge of managing other systems and providers. Also discouraging is the lack of proper dissociation training for therapists, which results in children's lives filled with extensive suffering and multiple failed episodes of inpatient and outpatient treatment. These children may end up with multiple diagnoses or living in residential or psychiatric centers for years instead of at home with a loving caregiver.

Dissociation defenses used regularly in childhood become a fixed behavioral pattern that continues into adulthood with further development of psychiatric disorders and repression of trauma. The lack of disclosure or awareness of the trauma, for both the client and therapist, can then lead to further problems in adulthood, including relationship issues, addiction, eating disorders, and violent behaviors. One of the most disheartening consequences of ineffective treatment of children with dissociative symptoms is the path that leads to the criminal justice system, resulting in spending years, if not a lifetime, in prison.

THE "AHA MOMENT" FOR THERAPISTS

Working with the complex layers of trauma-based symptoms and external concerns is daunting to therapists. This chapter offers a framework for understanding the serious behavioral problems evident when a child is utilizing pathological dissociation to escape painful thoughts, feelings, and overwhelming bodily sensations of a horrific trauma. Therapists will get a sense of the internal world and the struggles between self-states and how this internal world is clashing with the external world of family, schools, and friends (Waters, 2016). The hope is that the therapist has their "aha moment" about their own cases when reading about similar challenging and mysterious behaviors and recognizing that their client is also exhibiting dissociative symptoms.

Understanding levels of dissociation for both adults and children is a new phenomenon in many mental health agencies (Weiland, 2015). Many therapists want to refer these cases to experts, but it is the therapists themselves who are often the best possible solution for the child, and looking elsewhere will lead to another treatment failure for the child. Having a dissociative lens when conceptualizing a case is like putting on the right pair of glasses and realizing what you have been missing as a key piece in treating children with complex trauma. Learning about the dissociative parts of self is often a new language for therapists, and it can be frightening to learn about and witness hostile parts of the self. The information is foreign as it is not like any other treatment the therapist has learned before. After the "aha moment" of understanding that this client is utilizing dissociative strategies, there follows the apparent realization that they do not have the training, skills, or tools to treat the child. *Okay, this is dissociation symptoms, but now what do I do?*

Whenever working with children having complex trauma histories and problematic coping strategies, therapists are challenged to find play-based effective treatment that provides relief to children and their families. The work begins with curiosity in the playroom as the therapist and child explore what is hidden internally and find ways to work toward a future of being whole. Learning and treating in the play-based "language" of the child is an important skill, as working with children is not like working with little adults. The intervention discussed later in the chapter on how to access self-states in the preparation phase of EMDR embodies the principles of play therapy.

Properly educating parents on dissociation and teaching them how to communicate with the self-states is key in healing the child. Engaging caregivers to do this work is crucial as most parents are on the defense and feeling defeated.

They are traumatized themselves by the behaviors they have witnessed, and/or they are enduring physical attacks from the child. Many caregivers hang in there with their children and continue to seek knowledgeable treatment providers who can help, going through many treatment options before finding a therapist who has the knowledge and ability to treat dissociation. These parents are desperate for answers or treatment options that will allow them to live as a family that has some joy and for their home to feel safe for all members.

A motivated therapist can take advantage of a number of resources on dissociation. In the late 1990s, the Child and Adolescent Committee was formed under the auspices of the International Society for the Study of Trauma and Dissociation (ISSTD). Over the next decade, this group developed the guidelines for the evaluation and treatment of childhood dissociation, including frequently asked questions and information for parents and teachers on the ISSTD website. The Child and Adolescent Committee also offers a yearly course for therapists to gain advanced knowledge in the topic. Reading the great works of the leaders of childhood dissociation is a must: Richard Kluft (1985), Frank Putnam (1997), Joyanna Silberg (2013), Fran Waters (2016), Lynda Shirar (1996), Sandra Weiland (2015), and Renee Potgieter Marks (2018). Their research and books were part of my "aha moments" of how to treat children in foster care, in preparation for adoption, in residential treatment settings, or in out-of-country adoptions. Often, I was asked to work with a family who had numerous providers before me. In my early years of EMDR, I attempted to avoid dissociative children but that did not last long. I would ask the single question of *"Do you ever feel like you have different parts of you?"* or ask a parent *"Does your child act like different children?"* Even just these questions brought significant relief to families and children who realized I understood the internal world that was in conflict and in pain. Clinicians can work effectively with dissociation. Understanding the unusual symptoms, following a few basic principles, and staying curious are often the key elements in effective treatment. If the EMDR therapist can also be the play therapist utilizing the language of play to explore parts of the dissociated self in a way that helps children feel comfortable and safe, treatment can ultimately be successful.

Why therapists need to know about dissociation in children

> *I can't put my finger on what is going on with this child. He has an odd presentation of symptoms. He takes so long to answer my questions. He has blank stares and seems to be somewhere else. I tried EMDR, and it went nowhere. He just sat there blank and said he didn't remember anything about what happened to him even though we talked about that memory many times.*
>
> *This child has unusual behaviors at home and school and changes in personality. I don't understand his presentation of symptoms. In school, teachers say he doesn't seem connected to the other kids and does his own thing. He can't pay attention well. At times, he can do the school work, and other times he can't and turns into almost like a baby and starts sucking his thumb. Do you think he is on the spectrum? Or maybe I am dealing with ADHD* [attention deficit hyperactivity disorder]?

> His parents hear him talk to himself at home and he shouts out angrily sometimes. He seems to be in imagination a lot and may be hearing voices. When his parents ask him why he did something wrong, he says it wasn't him even though they are right there when he does it. I referred him to the psychiatrist as I think he is developing schizophrenia.

As an EMDR trainer and consultant, I have seen how therapists struggle with treating young children who are survivors of early attachment wounds, ranging from mild to severe, and who have problematic symptoms and limited coping skills that interfere with healing their traumas. The cases are often complex and overwhelming to the therapist, and the presenting behaviors mimic other psychiatric disorders. The therapist is confused about the presenting symptoms and often thinks they are the result of another disorder. Dissociation, being one of the most common defense mechanisms utilized to survive a traumatic event (Putnam, 1997), often is displayed with an unusual and confusing range of symptoms. Children exhibit behaviors that are strange, odd, and perplexing in the playroom as well as at home, at school, or in the community (Waters, 2016). The therapist may try a wide variety of treatments, such as child-centered play therapy (CCPT), directive play therapy approaches, behavioral plans with parents, cognitive behavioral therapy (CBT), and EMDR. Often, the use of these interventions is missing the key information that the child's internal world has conflicting self-states that are not working together or even being co-conscious, which prevents healing and growth through these various therapeutic approaches.

Growing awareness of the impact of dissociation is inextricably linked with EMDR. Screening clients for dissociation has long been a part of the basic training for EMDR, largely because dissociation makes memory networks less available for adaptive information processing, making EMDR with these clients more complicated. Activating the target memory can trigger extreme responses in these clients, so extensive preparation is needed (Shapiro, 2001).

Therapists face many challenges and obstacles in working with traumatized children with dissociative features. The following list is a series of problems that commonly occurs when working with this population.

Problem 1: Many clinicians have not received training in diagnosing and treating dissociative disorders (ISSTD, 2003). Other therapies have failed to recognize trauma and dissociation as being the core of the symptomology in children. In addition, most trainings address managing dissociation for adult clients, and therapists find it difficult to translate how to make the information "fit" with children.

Problem 2: Many therapists have high caseloads that are filled with children exhibiting severe and destructive dissociative symptoms that are disabling and disrupting daily life at home, daycare, and in the classroom. Children who use dissociative defenses regularly are not learning, participating in play, or practicing socialization skills with peers (Putnam, 1997).

Problem 3: The therapist working in a clinic is assigned a child with conflicting diagnoses and medication from medical providers. The therapist observes dissociation and does not agree with the provider but does not want to speak up to cause confusion with the caregivers. If the therapist does speak up, possibly the caregiver prefers the doctor's diagnosis and recommendations. In many professional circles, dissociation conversations among therapists and medical providers do not proceed well. There is still a notion that the dissociative symptoms are related to other disorders, and many therapists shy away from discussing dissociation with medical and psychiatric staff. In EMDR trainings and in consultation, this problem is reported as a frequent dilemma in working with complex cases.

Problem 4: The child's behaviors are harmful, and symptom management becomes the focus of treatment. The clinician does not recognize the dissociative strategies being used, and the therapies utilized may not be effective. This could result in an increase in mood fluctuation, behaviors, performance, and somatic concerns causing hospitalizations, residential placements, and unnecessary medication (Waters, 2016).

Problem 5: Therapists struggle to manage the magnitude of the dissociative symptoms and self-states that appear in the playroom. Therapist not recognizing multiple self-states, and therefore not welcoming all parts of the self or making them feel comfortable, could lead to a lack of trust and safety (Waters, 2016).

Problem 6: Therapists' role is multipurpose, and they often have to work with caregivers and systems such as schools to manage children's behaviors. Therapists have to provide treatment to the caregivers, many of whom have inherited this child through circumstances of foster care, adoption, or as part of an extended family network. Educating caregivers about dissociation is a must, but caregivers may not buy-in and are instead remaining stuck on the symptoms exhibited and a rigid understanding of the child as manipulative, lying, and defiant.

Problem 7: Children endure the termination of relationships and movement between multiple foster homes. This is in addition to visiting with the biological parents who may have harmed them, been in and out of jail, not shown up for visits, and so forth. Often visits are increased against the treatment provider's recommendations. These visits dysregulate the child as they are exposed to constant reminders of the abuse. This is all occurring while the therapist is stabilizing the child and working toward trauma therapy.

Problem 8: Children are hijacked by slight changes and triggers in the environment. Children's dysregulated and destructive behavior alienates potential new caretakers, such as foster parents and adoptive parents. Instead of the child receiving compassion and empathy, they again receive rejection and alienation, which is the original source of pain.

These layers of tasks and problems are often overwhelming to the therapist and take up a large amount of treatment time, making it a struggle to maintain the focus on working with the parts of self in the playroom.

WHAT IS DISSOCIATION, WHY DOES IT OCCUR, AND WHAT ARE THE THEORIES?

Dissociation is categorized along a continuum from mild to moderate to extreme (ISSTD, 2020), and these distinctions can assist a therapist in deciding appropriate interventions for treatment. Children and teens can experience normal dissociation due to a frightening event, such as an automobile accident, house fire, animal bite, or bullying episode. If the child has appropriate support, the situation is not recurring, and did not have devastating effects, the child can talk about the incident with a support person and most likely be able to continue functioning without any fragmentation of self. Further, in disasters or emergencies, dissociation is adaptive as it enables the person to function without being flooded by emotion until reaching safety.

We know from the polyvagal theory (Porges, 2011) that in traumatic events, it is instinctive that a person enters into a fight, flight, or freeze state. For a child, immobilization or freezing and surrender are often the only option due to their inability to escape or protect themselves from the terrifying reality. Children do not have the ability to physically escape but psychologically they can leave the situation and be somewhere else that feels safer (Weiland, 2015). Dissociation is one of the earliest available defenses for children, allowing them to escape the unwanted feelings, thoughts, sensations, and beliefs (Water, 2016). The child is mentally separating from the terrifying experience. The amazing gift of dissociation is that the child can deny and forget the painful reality both during and after the traumatic event (Weiland, 2015). Jonathan with glazed eyes walks into my playroom with his foster mom of 2 years.

> *My mom doesn't know where I am at. They took me away from her today, and I didn't get to say goodbye. I have to go home. She is worried about me.*

For Jonathan and many other children, this gift becomes problematic. As dissociation continues, the child's perception, feelings, physical sensation, or the knowledge of the world become stored outside active awareness. These parts of the experience continue to exist but are separate in the individual's internal world. The child's internal self becomes fragmented, and self-states are formed (Weiland, 2015). In an attempt to cope with the distressing feelings, the child's memories "pile up behind the wall" as a way to avoid all the pain from the beliefs, emotions, and body sensations. While this reaction appears effective at the time of the terrifying event, eventually a trigger hits this "sore spot" and the memory comes spilling back over the wall (Greenwald, 2005). These "spills" are typically the presenting problems that bring the child into therapy.

The avoidance of experiencing the event eventually takes its toll, and then more often than not, this very effective avoidance strategy is utilized regularly and causes the child to lose connection with feelings and physical sensations. The memories then only exist in a dissociated part of the self, and the child's internal working model of self is fragmented (Liotti, as cited in Weiland, 2015). This dissociated part may not share *co-consciousness* with the self and may cause erratic and disruptive behaviors for the child.

If a child is experiencing chronic, repetitive events with no ability to talk about the frightening and difficult events with anyone, the child will continue to utilize the protective response of dissociation instead of developing healthy coping responses (Weiland, 2015). Moderate dissociation occurs on a continuum, and children can experience depersonalization and derealization. In *depersonalization*, a child may experience a change in themselves like being outside of their body watching the event happening—in an almost dreamlike state (Shirar, 1996). In *derealization*, things do not seem real in the external world, such as for a child who experiences sexual abuse by his father in the middle of the night, wakes up in distress wondering if it was a bad dream, and goes into the kitchen to find his father cooking breakfast and his mother sitting at the table. Though having uncomfortable feelings, he tells himself it did not happen. Sometimes, the child can go as far as experiencing full amnesia for traumatic events (Weiland, 2015).

In extreme dissociation, self-states are formed to carry the traumatic experience or act as possible helpers to assist the child during the experience (a soothing part) or are hostile introjected parts that bear similarities to the perpetrator. Often, the child is unaware of what they have done, while in another self-state it becomes problematic for the child and the caregivers (Weiland, 2015). "I didn't do it," "It wasn't me," and "I don't remember" become common phrases for the child, which is frustrating to the caregivers and often becomes the topic of many therapy sessions between therapist and caregivers.

When children are switching self-states, parents will share the experience of having a nice and calm child one minute and seconds later a child who is angry, hostile, aggressive, and catches the parents off guard. Many times, caregivers are unaware of the trigger and of the self-state emerging. This part surfaces, and it may be an earlier traumatized infant state that is stuck in trauma time, and the present life of living in a new and safe supportive home may not have generalized across self-states (Weiland, 2015).

THEORIES OF DISSOCIATION

We can consider a number of conceptual models for the formation of dissociation as well as Silberg's (2013), Waters's (2016), and Weiland's (2015) suggestions for the treatment of self-states in children.

Putnam (1997) describes discrete behavioral states in infancy as the changing states of the baby when they go from waking, feeding, being fussy, crying, being tired, and sleeping. If the caregiver system responds calmly and appropriately to the infant's needs, the transition between states goes smoothly and the child can become an integrated self. Without experiencing positive mirroring from the caregiver system, the healthy states do not develop and the child's trauma-related states are formed. These states compartmentalize all or some of the memory and its components. This separating of the self is helpful at the time of the trauma, but this "estrangement from self" is the formation of the dissociative parts of self. These states are separated off and may hold the physical and emotional experiences and need to be bridged together through art and play as necessary interventions.

The affect avoidance theory (Silberg, 2013) refers to the avoidance scripts that children use when the affect is too much to handle whether related to a frightening event, such as terror, or to the lack of comfort or care on a regular basis. The child blocks the emotions, sensations, and beliefs with acting out behaviors like physical aggression, destruction, and self-harm. In this model, dissociation is seen as avoidance of the extreme pain of the event, which then activates the avoidance scripts: "Automatic activation of patterns of actions, thought, perception, identity, or relating, which are overlearned and serve as conditioned avoidance responses to affective arousal associated with traumatic cues" (Silberg, 2013, p. 22). Silberg developed the *EDUCATE* model to guide clinicians in discovering self-states:

*E*ducate about dissociation.
*D*issociative motivation; why is a child using this coping strategy.
*U*nderstand what is hidden/avoided.
*C*laim the aspects of the self that have been hidden.
*A*rousal modulation/affect regulation/attachment.
*T*riggers and trauma to be processed.
*E*nding with learning new ways to cope.

Waters (2016) uses the Star Theoretical Model for assessment and treatment of childhood dissociation. It includes attachment theory, developmental theory, family systems theory, neurobiology, and dissociation theory. Waters sees the attachment theory as the most prominent of the Star Model theories as the parent–child bond can be an underlying cause of dissociative strategies, and a strong attachment bond is beneficial to a child's healing from trauma. Waters considers all aspects of the theory when analyzing a child with dissociative features. When working with a case, Waters (2016) recommends considering the attachment history, developmental status, any neurobiological factors in play, and what family circumstances are contributing to the child's use of dissociation.

Van der Hart, Ninjenhaus, and Steele (2005) introduced the concept of structural dissociation, which is the concept that many EMDR therapists utilize in their approach with adults. The *apparently normal personality* appears normal and is the face that interacts with the world. The *emotional personalities* are most likely the child's parts that contain all the unprocessed traumatic experiences. These networks contain the emotional, cognitive, and the physical pain. Once the networks of dissociated self-states form, the traumatic material is removed partially or completely from consciousness and contained in the disconnected neural networks (Forgash, 2008). The traumatic experience is not integrated, and it is unprocessed and stored in a separate compartment or separate existences (Paulsen, 2009). The child may develop multiple self-states, including harmful introjects.

What Early Life Experiences Lead to Dissociation?

Overwhelming experiences such as violence, disasters, accidents, maltreatment, bullying, medical illness, and deaths of caregivers can cause posttraumatic stress disorder (PTSD) with possible dissociative symptoms. If there are supportive caregivers assisting the child through this type of event, then dissociation strategies are unlikely to continue (Weiland, 2015). In this chapter, we focus on the dissociation used as an ongoing strategy when consistent support from caregivers is lacking or absent. Research has shown that chronic dissociation can be linked to relational trauma in which there are exposure traumas in the early years that are repeated, chronic, and typically occur with caregivers (Spinazzola et al., 2005). These caregivers are frightening and unpredictable, and this is damaging to the development of healthy attachment between child and parent. One of the most profound adversities in childhood is betrayal by a caregiver. Freyd (1996) theorizes that betrayal trauma is why children use dissociate defenses and have amnesic episodes. Trauma in infancy is the underlying cause of many behavioral problems later in life. If treatment providers are unaware of early attachment history, the child's symptoms are often confusing to providers.

> As an infant in a bassinet, Jacob witnessed his father attacking his mother on almost a daily basis. He was also left in his father's care during the day, and when Jacob's mother called to check in while she was at work, she would hear her husband screaming at Jacob. One day when Jacob's mother returned home after work, Jacob was unable to use his legs and was unresponsive for days.

> Three-year-old Amber was found dazed and wandering at midnight in the streets calling for her mother who left earlier that night to go to a bar. There was history of neglect since Amber's birth as cited by the frequent visits from social services. This time, Amber was removed from her mother's home. She remained in a catatonic state and did not move or speak. She was diagnosed with autism and placed in a psychiatric center despite the daycare stating she was adequately functioning prior to the incident.

Jacob and Amber are examples of infants who are holding traumatic memories in implicit memory systems and exhibiting their traumas through sensory experiences. Bowlby (1980) and Frailberg (1982), as cited in Waters (2016), observed infants who experienced maternal separation and deprivation and found that they demonstrated freezing behaviors, trance states, and memory problems. As Waters (2016), citing Bruce Perry, states, "The younger the child when experiencing trauma, the more likely they are to suffer enduring and pervasive problems" (p. 7).

Significant neglect histories throughout infancy and the toddler years that are repetitive, chronic, and frightening have a profound impact on the child's coping abilities and increase their use of dissociative strategies as they increase in age.

> Do you see the blood on my arm! It's all over!! Do you see what that boy (from birth mother's house) did to me when he raped me? My mother is in the other room! Why isn't she helping me?

Tasha is in the tub bathing, screaming in the background as her bewildered foster mom is trying to explain to me on the phone that there is no blood on her

4-year-old foster child. Tasha and her sister suffered from a lack of food, regular bathing, and stable housing. Her older sister remembers Tasha being left in a crib overnight while her mother went out for the evening. Tasha had many disturbing memories, including, at the age of two and a half the rape, which her biological mother later confirmed when she stated she had sold her daughter for drugs. With profound attachment disruption, Tasha and other children like her live their lives in dissociative states. Even children who are placed in the home of loving caregivers continue to dissociate until they receive treatment.

The traumas that are often missed or overlooked while gathering trauma history are the covert traumas where children endure caregivers who respond to their traumatic experiences with rejection, ignorance, chaos, or instability, leaving the child vulnerable and relying on dissociation as the adaptive response (Forgash, 2008). Some examples of covert traumas might be rigid expectations of perfection, harsh criticism, showing the child love and affection only after the child meets the needs of the parent, or inadequate parenting leading to parentified children. All these instances can all lead to attachment disorders and dissociative disorders if not addressed early in life. Dissociation can become persistent and intense, making it difficult for the child to form relationships, have friends, learn in school, or manage emotions.

Diagnosis

Dissociative children present a challenge to treatment providers, as their fluctuating odd and unusual symptoms do not fit neatly in any diagnostic categories and often these children do not respond to traditional treatment. They have quickly changing moods, memory problems, voices in their head, destructive behaviors, and then other days are calm, relaxed, or normal. In the initial assessment of children, a therapist must employ a number of different ways of diagnosing a dissociative disorder. Dissociation is on a continuum and has four diagnostic subcategories: depersonalization/derealization, dissociative amnesia, dissociative disorder not otherwise specified, and dissociative identity disorder. Another possibility is the diagnosis of PTSD with dissociative symptoms (American Psychiatric Association [APA], 2013). Pathological dissociation is difficult to diagnose in children as similar symptoms are mimicked in other disorders. Similar features can be seen in anxious and depressed children, or disorders of oppositional defiant disorder, attention deficit disorder, obsessive compulsive disorder, or bipolar disorder (Waters, 2016). Children may be using dissociative defenses and may not have memory of doing certain behaviors such as lying, stealing, or aggression (Putnam, 1994). Self-destructive behaviors such as cutting and suicide attempts may be efforts to regulate overwhelming posttraumatic emotional states (van der Kolk as cited in Putnam & Peterson 1994).

Screening measures should be utilized that are appropriate to the age group, such as the Child Dissociation Checklist (Peterson, 1991; Putnam & Peterson, 1994), which is completed by caregivers, the Child Dissociative Experience Scale and Traumatic Stress Inventory (Stolbach, 1997), and for older children, the Adolescent

Dissociative Experience Scale (Armstrong et al., 1997). Also, we must rely heavily on interviews with children and their caregivers and can also include other providers such as school teachers. Joyanna Silberg (2013) and Fran Waters (2016) provide a list of comprehensive questions to utilize during interviews with caregivers and children.

The task force for children and adolescents has guidelines for the Assessment and Treatment of Dissociative Symptoms in Children and Adolescents (ISSTD, 2003). These guidelines along with a thorough description of children's symptomology are formatted into frequently asked questions of parents and children on the ISSTD website and are discussed later (ISSTD, 2003).

Symptoms of Dissociation

A study done on children with complex trauma by Cook, Blaustein, Spinazzola, and van der Kolk (2003) determined that half the children in the study had chronic problems across seven domains of impairment: attachment, biology, affect regulation, dissociation, behavioral control, cognition, and self-concept. When a child is utilizing dissociative strategies, these can be perceived as a being an odd avoidance reaction. These impairments are symptoms that are displayed through behavioral, emotional, cognitive, and somatic symptoms and witnessed by caregivers (Cloitre et al., 2009). On the ISSTD website, the Child and Adolescent Committee has outlined a thorough explanation of common symptoms to help parents, educational systems, and therapists identify if the child is displaying dissociative symptoms by paying attention to shifts across various domains.

Dissociation Interferes With New Attachments

Early on, children with complex trauma figured out that their own caregivers cannot be trusted and are weary to trust any other seemingly helpful adult. They are on guard and cautious to share any emotions or thoughts. This causes problems when placed in foster homes or with adopted parents, as these are children who are slow to warm up and reject nurturance and connection. As this rejection continues, they are not bonding to potentially good caregivers, thus causing the creation of more traumatic memories (Silberg, 2013).

Biological Symptoms

Children can have problems with coordination and balance and increased medical problems. Often, these are children that are going to the nurse's office in school for headaches or stomachaches. Children can have somatic experiences when their sore spot is triggered, and it is their body's way of expressing the past memory, such as pains in the arm that was grabbed and broken during the trauma.

Examples of Biological Shifts to Discuss With Parents

These physical problems may be a result of the tension or anxiety from a trauma that is being "held" (remembered unconsciously) in the body.

- Your child may wet or soil without knowing it is happening. She may not feel or smell it.
- Your child may get hurt (e.g., get a cut or break a bone) or may harm herself (e.g., cutting or burning) and not feel the pain or be aware that she has been hurt.
- Your child may have stomachaches, headaches, seizure-like motions, or other physical problems (for example, difficulty breathing, walking, genital pain) that cannot be physically explained.

Note: These symptoms may occur only a few times a year or may be much more frequent and occur several times a day.

Source: International Society for the Study of Trauma and Dissociation. Retrieved from www.isst-d.org

Affect Dysregulation

The failure to attach to the caregiver impairs the child's ability to learn to regulate affect (Schore, 2012; Siegel, 1999). These are children who have limited language for emotional states. They react often and powerfully with disruptive behaviors and have strong fluctuation of moods. Calming down these children requires numerous creative interventions and a skillful caregiver in their external world. An additional struggle that will arise for the EMDR therapist in the desensitization phase is that the client may struggle to close down emotional disturbances (Forgash, 2008).

Emotional Shifts to Discuss With Parents

Emotionally, a child may experience sudden shifts and move from one extreme feeling to a completely different or opposite feeling without showing any of the in-between emotions.

- Your child may be calm one moment and then in the next moment become explosive, aggressive, frightened, tearful, or panicky.
- Your child may show emotions that do not fit what is happening, such as laughing during a sad and upsetting situation or becoming sad or angry in a joyful situation.
- Your child may not show any feelings at all. They may not be aware of any feelings.

Source: International Society for the Study of Trauma and Dissociation. Retrieved from www.isst-d.org

Behavioral Control Symptoms

We know from state-dependent learning that people re-experience a memory more vividly if in a similar environment to where they learned it (Putnam, 1997). When children are experiencing intrusion, it is typically accompanied by fear and confusion as their conscious awareness is being invaded by fragments of unresolved memory material, experienced as nightmares, auditory hallucinations, or visual flashbacks. Greenwald (2005) uses the *sore spot* analogy of the multiple traumas piled up behind a *wall* and the present-day reminder of the past trauma hitting that sore spot with a powerful reaction. As the trigger can be a minor stressor, such as teacher's redirection or arguing about a toy with a sibling, the reaction may be stronger than others might expect. The reminders of the traumas can cause intrusion of the traumatic memory and can easily dysregulate a child. Children are overreacting, shutting down, or being destructive in their behaviors. When children are experiencing these behaviors in the classroom, home, or community, it causes relationship issues for the child.

Examples of Behavioral Shifts to Discuss With Parents

Behavior shifts that are most commonly seen by parents or teachers:

- Your child may act very grown up one moment and then behave like a much younger child (even a baby) at another moment.
- Your child may be aggressive and mean at one point and then become passive, loving, or caretaking at another time.
- Your child may talk about themselves with different names or may use "we" when referring to themselves.
- Your child may use different voices or specific mannerisms (e.g., picking at her skin) at one time and not other times.
- Your child may want to wear a favorite outfit or eat a favorite food, but then later on, or perhaps the next day, they will say they hate the outfit or food. They may not be able to explain this change and may say yhey never liked the outfit or food.
- Your child may have certain skills or be able to do certain activities easily and well (handwriting, sports, math, reading), but then, the next day, may have trouble with them or no longer know how to do them.
- Your child may seem to "space out" at home, school, or social events, and not know what is going on around them. Time may pass and they don't know what happened during that time.
- Your child's facial expression may change dramatically and suddenly from smiling to angry without any apparent reason.
- Your child's eyes may appear to be in a dead stare when you are talking to tjem (like they are miles away) or they may have a glazed look, particularly when they are aggressive or raging.
- Your child may find themselves in a place and not know how they got there. For example, they may be sent to the principal's office for

(continued)

Examples of Behavioral Shifts to Discuss With Parents (continued)

> misbehaving and not remember leaving the classroom, walking to the office, or even why they are there. Emotionally your child may experience sudden shifts and move from one extreme feeling to a completely different or opposite feeling without showing any of the in-between emotions. The reason for this change in emotion may not be clear or make sense to you.
>
> *Source:* International Society for the Study of Trauma and Dissociation; www.isst-d.org

Cognitive (Information Processing) Symptoms

Toxic stress in a child's environment impairs the development of the brain, and children with severe traumatic histories can manifest severely impaired school performance. These are children who have problems with language development, solving problems, completing details of a task, or even thinking clearly (Cook et al., 2005). They struggle to acquire a new skill or sustain it properly. Their attention may be lacking due to flashbacks of or being hyperresponsive to all stimuli in their environment as well as impaired memory making it difficult for them to progress in treatment. While in dissociative states, the child might not be learning educational material across all self-states (Waters, 2016).

When Tasha, the child described earlier, was 6 years old and through EMDR processed the rape she experienced at two and a half years of age, she had a shift in cognitive processing. Her adoptive mother called me the day after the session to say that Tasha (who had been labeled with severe learning disabilities) was reading her older sister's books! When Tasha came back to see me, I opened the waiting room door and she said *"I read all the kids' books you have here."* In 2 months, she was placed in a regular classroom with no accommodations.

Children may also experience memory problems as self-states may have emerged and acted out violence. The child may state, *"I didn't do it."* A foster mother in a private meeting with me stated in frustration about her 7-year-old, *"She lies all the time about everything saying it wasn't her. I was right there when she did it."* Meeting with the child separately, she tells me with tears in her eyes, *"I don't remember anything she is talking about . . . I feel like I have a bad memory."*

Examples of Cognitive Shifts to Discuss With Parents

> These are sudden changes and sometimes contradictory ways of thinking.
>
> - Your child may be able to do an assignment quite well on one day, but then not know how to do the same or similar assignment the next day. Without any additional teaching, they may be able to do the assignment again later.

(continued)

Examples of Cognitive Shifts to Discuss With Parents (continued)

- Your child may make a good choice when faced with a problem, but when faced with the same problem later on, they may make a poor choice and not recall the earlier situation and the earlier decision.
- Your child may think that a completely safe situation is extremely unsafe and be very fearful. Or they may interpret an unsafe situation as safe.
- Your child may not be able to recall important events, such as birthdays, holidays, family vacations, or camping trips.
- Your child may have no memory of having done something even when someone saw them do it.
- Your child may "hear" voices inside their head. (Children seldom talk about this unless directly asked.)
- Your child may report having "inside people" that say mean things and boss them around. These are different from the pretend or imaginary friends that young children commonly have and outgrow.
- Your child may think badly about themselves (perhaps even feel suicidal) and see the world as a frightening, threatening place. Then suddenly they may feel good about themselves and the world, and hopeful about the future.

Your child may have flashbacks (reliving a traumatic event) and be unaware of present surroundings.

Source: International Society for the Study of Trauma and Dissociation. Retrieved from www.isst-d.org

Determining if there is the presence of a dissociative disorder is crucial to the treatment plan of the child. It does not always manifest right away with children. It is important to note that the internal system does not want to be exposed (at first) and does an excellent job of hiding and being secretive. Children and adults go to great lengths to hide the internal voices and do not offer the information willingly without a therapist asking the right questions (Shirar, 1996).

What Do Self-States Look Like In and Out of the Therapy Room?

Fantasy play in the early years of childhood is considered normal dissociation. Children have mastered living in fantasy worlds, being a princess, having imaginary playmates, and having full conversations with their dolls. Imaginary playmates can help with expanding an experience, alleviating loneliness and boredom, and working out internal worries (Baum, 1978; Trujillo et al., 1996 as cited by Weiland, 2015). All children explore how they can "get away" inside their heads. When things become scary or overwhelming to children, dissociation is one of the earliest coping tools that they can use to reduce anxiety and fear. As imagination is a familiar experience in the early years, chronically traumatized children turn to it again and again (Putnam, 1997).

> Questions about imaginary friends (from Silberg, 2013):
>
> Have you ever had or have imaginary friends? Do they seem real to you? If so, in what way?
>
> Does your imaginary friend bug you, and you wish it would go away?
>
> Does your imaginary friend try to boss you around?
>
> Does your imaginary friend tell you to keep secrets?
>
> Does your imaginary friend take over and make you do things you don't want to do?
>
> (Older kids) Some children had invisible friends. Do you have this now or did you have it when you were younger? Do you feel like the friends are still there? Can you see them or hear them?
>
> Do you feel like there is a fight going on in your brain? Like there are several parts fighting with each other? Do you hear the fight?

If danger continues, the child utilizes dissociation on a regular basis, and this patterned response becomes automatic. The overwhelming feelings, thoughts, and body sensations associated with the traumatic memory are still present but are stored in a separate self-state of the child. The self-state who holds the memory may regularly intrude into conscious awareness especially when the child is experiencing a similar situation where the emotions, beliefs, and body sensations arise (Putnam, 1997).

I give this narrative to explain what is happening:

> *When you went through that event and you decided that it was too much for you to handle, a part of you stepped out of you and said: I will take this awful memory, and you go on and live a good life like going to school and having friends. But when you are older, don't forget me. Come back and take care of this "little me" who is holding this yukky memory for you.*
>
> *So, this "little you" is reminding you that it is still here inside of you and still holding that yukky memory. And there might be a few parts of you that want help with these memories and feeling better about it. This is why you keep hearing voices or seeing the images of that yukky time. We can use puppets or sand tray figurines to show all the parts of you.*

As learning may not generalize across self-states, the child may be unaware of all the other positive learning and experiences such as coping skills taught by the therapist or the presence of loving supportive adults in their life (Weiland, 2015). The self-state can reject the caregivers' help and love. This is challenging and confusing to providers and caregivers who are providing safety and nurturing environments. I explain to parents in the following way:

> *When your child went through that difficult time in their life, it was too much, too many big thoughts and feelings for them to handle. They escaped into an*

> imaginary world where another part of them emerged and holds that difficult time in their life and the strong feelings that go with it. So, when your child is nice, kind and themselves, that is who you like to have around . . . but when something happens and it reminds your child of that past event and triggers their sore spot, they get nervous and upset. This other part of your child is trying to figure out a way to protect themselves and make sure they don't get hurt again. And then what happens is you have a child in front of you who is difficult to manage and you don't feel like you know who they are and they seem like a different kid.

In extreme dissociation, children may not remember their behaviors or see the other part of themselves committing the behaviors. The scariest situation for most caregivers and therapists is when the extreme form of dissociation occurs, and these dissociated states or parts take over the child's functioning, as opposed to functioning *through* the child. The child appears as though they are separate people (Weiland, 2015). It can appear as if the child has a demon in them as their voice, facial presentation, and demeanor change right in front of the adult. This the moment when most therapists are frightened and unsure of what to do.

- A 5-year-old child says *"My (preadoptive) mom says I stole at the store, but that wasn't me. I can see who did it but it wasn't me."*
- A 6-year-old boy was unable to protect himself when his older cousin was sexually abusing him. A sweet and calm boy would change into what parents described as "an evil monster," and he would viciously attack anyone he thought was trying to harm him.

Children use their adaptive strategies to maintain safety, to avoid being harmed again, or if potential for harm arises, to escape in their mind. Valuing and recognizing the resourcefulness of these creative strategies is the first step in understanding the meanings of their behaviors. The self-states must be recognized as having been formed by and holding the specific memory, related feelings, body sensations, irrational beliefs, and details of the experience (Forgash, 2008). The self-states can present as a different age and gender and have different mannerisms, body language, and voices than the child. The child may also have parts that are animals. A 5-year-old girl would get on all fours (only at home) and bark like a dog in hopes that her mother would love her the way she perceived her mother loved the three family dogs.

These self-states can also be an imitator of the perpetrator and be hostile or aggressive (Van der Hart et al., 2005). Children may take on a part of their abusive parent and mimic their manner and actions. We know that this ability to imitate caregivers is due to mirror neurons in the brain (Weiland, 2015). An example of this hostile imitator is in the following case:

> A father recently got custody of the 9-year-old daughter he never knew he had after he was contacted by social services in another state. In our third session together, he stated in front of his daughter: *"She is like three different people. At school, they say she is perfect, a teacher's helper, and she gets all these outstanding reports and privileges. After school, at home, she*

cries for 3 hours in a temper tantrum. Then other times, she tries to hurt her stepbrother and stepmom!" After the father leaves the room, I asked, "Do you ever feel like there are other parts of you?"

Susan hesitated for a brief moment and then said, "Yes, there are three of us, do you want to know our names, ages, and what happened to us that we were formed? 'Violet' is older and goes to school and is the 'good' girl and wants a better life. The 'crying baby' is mad as she was left in a crib overnight so her mom can go out with her boyfriend. The 'killer' wants her stepmother dead as she finally has been reunited with her dad and wants him to herself."

Switching

The therapist may notice switching of the child between self-states with either obvious or covert behaviors, such as blinking, eye flutter, a gesture such as flipping their hair, or using either regressed speech or mature speech as if they are older (Shirar, 1996). They might "become small" and slump or go in a fetal position. Some children go from calm to rage in seconds. Showing caregivers "switching" can be useful in treatment. I had a father watch me and his son behind a one-way mirror with a predetermined signal from me when his son was switching. This intervention was helpful to the dad as then he was able to position himself to implement strategies at home when he noticed "switching" occurring. To get his son's "9-year-old self" back in the room, the father showed him funny videos of a neighbors' dog. Within minutes, the child would start laughing and became oriented in the present.

TREATMENT

Children, identifying and working with their inner world, must have certain components to be successful in treatment. Adequate safety will allow for the awareness of self-states to emerge, along with communication among these parts of the self, and the eventual processing of traumas (Weiland, 2015). Children will need safety in the play therapy room and within the therapeutic relationship, as well as in their environment, including home and school. Addressing attachment concerns with caregivers wherever the child resides is vital. The child should be having new experiences of emotional regulation that work within the family.

At the beginning of the chapter, we identified the challenges therapists face when working with dissociation. Children with complex trauma should be seen by a therapist trained in the developmental stages of children, play therapy, EMDR training approved by the Eye Movement Desensitization and Reprocessing International Association (EMDRIA), and additional training in attachment and dissociation. A play therapy environment is key, as is it allows self-states to surface naturally in the playroom. Both nondirective and directive play therapy approaches allow the dissociative parts of self to be projected through metaphors, and for memories to be processed in the playroom. Play is the best "language" of the child, and it allows the child to remain more comfortable and to tolerate and approach strong beliefs, feelings, and body sensations in small doses. Gradual exposure through sand and miniatures, art, puppets, and a dollhouse allows children to symbolically and unconsciously express their self-states for therapists to observe. Play allows children to "touch" and move closer to their emotional pain and trauma (Goodyear-Brown, 2010; Shirar, 1996).

I encourage all newly trained EMDR therapists to receive consultation from an EMDRIA-approved consultant, who has training and experience with attachment and dissociation in children. Many newly trained EMDR therapists are hesitant to work with parts of the self, and it becomes especially frightening when hostile introjects take over a child and enter the playroom. Sometimes, this sharing is in the form of extreme posttraumatic reenactive play in the playroom. If a child is able to show a therapist the different parts of self and share their traumatic experiences, this speaks to the safety of the therapeutic relationship. There are a number of principles the therapist can follow to guide them in their work throughout the phases of treatment.

EMDR PHASES 1 AND 2 TREATMENT OF A DISSOCIATIVE CHILD

Many of the items given subsequently are occurring in EMDR Phases 1 and 2 and focused on stabilization of the child to move toward the safety of self-states being disclosed.

Meaning of Behavior

Often in consultation, I talk about the importance of being a detective and finding out the meaning of the behavior that is occurring within the problematic symptoms (Greenwald, 2009). Understanding transition moments is an important part of this work, such as when the child switches from "being okay" to avoidance patterns and a different self-state (Silberg, 2013). Parents say *"It came out of nowhere,"* but careful questioning always leads to further clues and details about as to what triggered the child into a dissociative state. The therapist, family, and child must work together to detect what the child is attempting to voice through their behaviors.

Evaluation

Attachment assessments, dissociation scales, trauma history, and interviews of the caregivers including extended family, babysitters, schools, and other providers help to develop the clinical picture of the child in many different contexts. Our understanding of the child's inner world develops by observation in the playroom and careful questions utilized from Silberg (2013), Waters (2016), and ISSTD on understanding the different parts of the child.

Building the Future

Utilizing the concept of Future Movies (Greenwald, 2009), I work with children to see the potential in the next few years of growth. Seven-year-old Tommy, often hopeless about life and verbalizing wanting to die, was able to draw all of his problems with parents, harming his younger brother and having no friends as well as having flashbacks of a severe car accident with his whole family. I asked him to draw what his life could be like in 1 year. Seeing his future in a drawing of harmony with his family, new friends, playing video games with his brother, and using this as a positive image to install allowed him to talk about the steps along the way that could get him to his goals.

Improving Attachments Between Child and Caregivers

Effective psychotherapy with children is only as good as the relationship between the caregivers and the child. Children feeling safe and supported is key in the work of dissociation. When the environment is chaotic and unsafe, when the exposure to trauma is ongoing, or if there are other external stressors such as school and peers, increasing safety must first be the focus of care. The child will continue to use dissociative strategies if they feel in danger (Shirar, 1996; Silberg, 2013; Waters, 2016). There are never easy solutions in managing these situations, and when only the therapist is intervening with the family, it is difficult to meet the expectation of making significant changes within the structure of the home. The child in this situation may begin to explore their self-states in the playroom, but processing of the trauma cannot occur until stabilization is in place. Consultation is helpful in determining if a "good enough" level of stabilization is present to move ahead with reprocessing. If children are living in alternate placements such as residential centers or group homes, the agency staff must be included in the treatment. Requesting a favorite staff to be a support after a session is key in the closure phase of EMDR, as is informing the therapist of concerns in the reevaluation phase. School staff can be educated on noticeable symptoms and offer the child an outlet to deescalate.

As Normal as Possible

Waters (2016) emphasizes working closely with parents on identifying appropriate resources. When it became apparent that play dates for Tommy were problematic, I suggested he attend a center-based program where karate and yoga were offered. Because these were solo activities with other kids in the classroom, it became a successful peer experience until he was able to have more self-control.

Reducing Triggers to Create Safety

Creative and relentless problem-solving to reduce triggers is a therapeutic skill that can result in successful movement toward stabilization. An 8-year-old processing early memories from his country of origin was gaining great relief of his symptoms. However, the 24 hours following the EMDR session would result in him feeling emotional and sensitive, and this would lead to him physically fighting with peers and/or seriously harming himself. His specialized school for emotional disturbances of youth, his parents, the therapist, and the child all agreed he would stay home from school the day after an EMDR session and mom would be the support for the day. This safety intervention created success for him and allowed the therapist to provide trauma resolution without fear of serious problematic incidents.

When a 5-year-old foster child had stabilized in her relationship with foster parents and showed increased emotional regulation, she was ready for trauma work. The courts implemented the start of visitations with the biological parents the week that desensitization sessions were scheduled to occur. I contacted the law guardian, wrote a letter to the judge, and requested 4 weeks of intensive therapy three times a week prior to the beginning of the visitations. I also contacted the biological parents and explained my rationale that the child doing the trauma work could potentially offer a calmer and more engaging child. All parties agreed, and this allowed the trauma processing to occur without regular triggers and decreased the behavioral problems.

Psychoeducation and Working With Parents to Understand Dissociation

After several meetings with caregivers who have completed assessments and scales and answered questions, I provide information about the role and use of dissociative strategies. Many therapists have great ideas on how to explain trauma and how and why dissociation is utilized as a coping strategy. I use several different resources including reviewing the ISSTD website with caregivers. I share Waters's (2016) analogy of a child's dissociation being similar to a power outage and the lights going out when circuits become overloaded. It is important to explain to parents that when a child's circuitry or nervous system is overloaded, the mind goes blank or the brain turns off, and the lights keep going out if the child thinks they are in danger or feeling overwhelmed. I also share Ana Gomez and Sandra Paulsen's book: *All the Colors of Me: My First Book about Dissociation* (2016). *Polly and Her Parts* (Biggs, 2013) is another resource, which comes from the Internal Family Systems literature, written by Alison Biggs and illustrated by Danielle Mulcahy. *Rob the Robin and the Bald Eagle* (2015) by Madge Bray is another valuable resource for children and parents.

Caregivers are often overwhelmed by the symptoms of their child's behavior and the effects on the child's development and daily functioning. Caregivers need extensive support on how to handle dissociation as well as their own outlets to discuss sadness and frustration. If the caregiver is the nonabusive parent, they have to do a lot of reparenting and working with the child's self-states (Shirar, 1996). It is good practice to have separate sessions with caregivers or refer caregivers to a therapist who is trained in dissociation with children to practice techniques and effective soothing and grounding tools to use when the child dissociates. Especially important is teaching caregivers to accept all parts of the child, to expect switches, and to respond appropriately to the self-states that are all vital to keeping children safe and out of the hospital. With this information, parents' experiences of seeing their child being calm and loving one moment and hostile and attacking seconds later are less scary and overwhelming. I role-play with parents on what to say to a child when the child is switching, especially, if a hostile part emerges. I teach caregivers that switching is a moment of the child's self-states wanting to communicate a message. These "messages" can be around fear of abandonment, feelings of not being heard, or of being misunderstood. Some switches are a flashback of a past trauma or "big" emotions of pain or sadness from the past. Having parents react with curiosity, calmness, and soothing can reduce the possible outburst of anger or the child going blank (Shirar, 1996). These are responses that are not intuitive and may take many practices and role-plays to instill.

Kluft (1985) recommends that children of dissociative identity disorder (DID) parents be evaluated for dissociation. The caregiver may not be able to provide effective parenting until they have progressed in their own treatment (Shirar, 1996). Mary was living with her grandmother who exhibited different self-states and was not in treatment. "Your grandma acts like different people at times, can you show me in the sand what that might look like?" This allowed Mary to express what she has known all along and to work with me on how to manage her grandmother's switching of states.

PREPARATION ACTIVITIES IN EMDR (PHASE 2)

The *Playroom Parts of Self* process described later will occur within the preparation phase, but several important steps need to occur prior to accessing self-states. Affect regulation skills have to be in place prior to and during the accessing of dissociative parts of self. With children who have experienced early traumas, Gaskill and Perry (2014) recommend calming the brainstem with somatosensory activities such as breathing, music, and movement in a repetitive pattern. Schore (2012) emphasizes right hemisphere art and play activities to be used during the preparation phase, and these can be directed toward developing a repertoire of calming activities such as drawing a Safe Place and using clay for emotional containers and other affect tolerance-related activities.

> *Tommy, an active young boy of 7, used hyperactivity, aggression (including hitting the therapist), and dissociation to push away all the sad and angry feelings he had about his life. I introduced yoga and guided meditation with the use of HeartMath™ to him and his mom. At first, he resisted any of these interventions and would watch as me and his mom did yoga and meditation. The HeartMath became an opportunity to be oppositional to us when I told him I wasn't sure if he was capable of getting the blue and green level. His mother started crying when she saw him sit calmly for 20 minutes and be able to gain coherence in his body. She bought the mobile version of HeartMath, and he began doing meditations prior to school and in the evening (HeartMath, n.d.).*
>
> *Five-year-old Jonathon was raised in a violent neighborhood and was eventually removed from his home due to neglect and abuse. He was*

triggered multiple times a day by noises, touch, and interactions with adults and children. I had taught him the container exercise several weeks in a row. He was moved to a new therapeutic preschool and daily would run out of the front doors into busy traffic with staff chasing him. One day the counselor asked, "Why do you do that?" He said, "Because every day my head fills with bad things (memories) and you don't do 'container' like Miss Annie does with me."

For very young children, traumatic memories will be stored in body sensations, movements, feelings, images, or sounds; the ability to encode and recall experiences verbally does not develop until 28 to 36 months. The child retains a behavioral memory that usually comes out in nightmares and posttraumatic reenactment with others (Terr, in Lynda Shirar, 1996, p. 17). By using a neurobiological clinical approach, EMDR and play therapists can select developmentally appropriate play therapy activities that will help regulate these children, which will then improve relationships and enhance cognitive functions (Gaskill & Perry, 2014).

When Children Do Not Remember Harmful and Destructive Behaviors

At the beginning of treatment, it is important not to uncover amnesia of early events as children must be stabilized. Working with children who destroy property, are aggressive, and *"can't remember"* is often a delicate balance between getting parents to understand the amnesia that has been used for traumatic events and a child's current need for generalizing their dissociative strategies to serious incidents in the present. Silberg (2013) recognizes the importance of children remembering their present-day destructive behaviors and working to increase memory detail. We can work with parents to eliminate the barriers to children remembering their behavior by lowering the threat of severe consequences that are typically implemented for harmful behaviors.

I work with the parents and child on remembering the trigger right before the event. Often, if we can figure out the upsetting emotional memory that may have triggered the problematic behavior, the child starts to have some details come back into consciousness. The child may not want to share coconsciousness with the part that took over and committed the harm. Once children remember the details, they are filled with shame and hatred toward themselves.

Samantha, a sweet and caring 10-year-old child who was a protective older sister to her young siblings in the biological family's home, became so upset at her behaviors toward her young sister. She told me repeatedly she did not remember, until I tuned into her shame and how hard it was for her to remember the violent act the self-state committed. Her tears helped her father see the pain that comes with having parts of self as well as her remorse.

I do not focus on whether a child is telling the truth; I focus on reducing the learned behavior of forgetting actions and encouraging all parts of the team to work together (Waters, 2016). I often handle this by having parents reverse their parenting and offer a reward for "remembering," having the behavioral consequence focus more on reparation. The reparation includes the child repairing the harm with good deeds such as doing something for the harmed victim, as in washing the parent's car, cleaning, or baking a treat, which allows a parent to see that the child is receiving a consequence but in a more therapeutic and less punitive way.

> *Kevin had stolen a computer at school and police were called (not his first incident). Kevin's parents agreed to give him his video games back if he could remember. He would have to agree to admitting guilt and write an apology letter to school staff and the police officers as well. He was highly motivated to get his games back, and I included a special prize as well. We talked about his feeling really angry that he didn't get to go on the school trip to the zoo due to previous acting-out behavior.*

It took two sessions with Kevin to help him to remember and admit guilt. One of the sessions was playing out the scenario in the sand of what triggered him. Role-playing what it might feel like to have one's own property taken is important as it encourages insight and empathy (Silberg, 2013).

> Therapist: *I would be really angry if I didn't get to go to the zoo. In fact, I feel angry you didn't get to go. Your principal should know you didn't mean to hit that kid. So, I know when I feel angry, I might do something I know I shouldn't. Then later, I might feel like stupid I acted that way.*
>
> Kevin: *I didn't mean to hit that kid, and I said I was sorry. I wrote him a note. And they don't care about me at school and just think I am a bad kid.*
>
> Therapist: *How did you feel after you hit him?*
>
> Kevin: *I get so mad at myself about doing that.*
>
> Therapist: *I got a big word for you . . . can you handle it?* (He nods) *Shame . . . it's when you feel so awful inside.* (I starting wriggling my body and showing how awful I feel by covering my face and head and putting it down to my lap.)
>
> Kevin: *Yeah* (he puts his head down low), *and then you know what I want to do when I get so angry at someone—and the school doesn't care about me at all. I want to get them back!*
>
> Therapist: *Yeah, I get it. I wonder if that is when you did something else and you pushed it out of your mind.*
>
> Kevin: *I remember—it was like it wasn't me though . . . I can see myself going there. . . and taking the computer. . .* (his face changed to shame).
>
> Therapist: *And this is when you feel that "shame" . . . Come on wriggle with me and let's fall to the ground as it feels so awful and make noises so I know how awful it feels.*

THE PLAYROOM PARTS-OF-SELF PROCESS

PREPARATION OF THE THERAPIST IN ACCESSING SELF-STATES

A therapist's role with complex trauma can be understood as the "loving eyes" (Knipe, 2015) of a caring adult who guides the client to leave their survival symptoms behind. These children will repeat patterns of helplessness and lack of control throughout their lifetimes without intervention. The therapist who is conveying resonance and attunement can help the child to feel safe to reveal the parts of self so that all parts can be seen, heard, and otherwise have a witness to their story. This following list is guiding the therapist as they work over time to access and work with self-states. Many of these concepts come from Gonzalez and Mosquera (2012), Martin (2015), Waters (2016), and Silberg (2013).

The effective therapist:

- Stays in curiosity and increases the chances of learning about the parts of self.
- Allows gradual exposure to the self-states. If the child says "I don't know," it is okay to allow the child to tolerate in small doses.
- Welcomes and engages all self-states in treatment *through* the child.
- Respects all parts of the child and understands the internal hierarchy if one exists.
- Helps the child to understand that no parts are eliminated.
- Sees the internal world as a family or as part of the child.
- Helps caregivers respect and love all parts of the child.
- Recognizes the role of being a witness to the pain and suffering of these parts.
- Works to engage hostile parts instead of reacting with fear.

Inspired by Waters (2016), I use a dissociation doll (see Figures 8.1 and 8.2) to help "see" and acknowledge all parts of the child. The doll also normalizes for the child what is going on in their internal world. The doll contains mini figures inside the head and heart openings with expressions of various feeling states.

The Conference Room Technique (Fraser, 1993) is an intervention to help adult clients to gain access to the parts of self. This technique is used to create an opportunity for the client to see all parts of themselves in one room and start to learn about each other and build cooperation and empathy. In my work, I have adapted the concept of Fraser's table in the Playroom Parts-of-Self Process in order to introduce children to parts of themselves in the language of play.

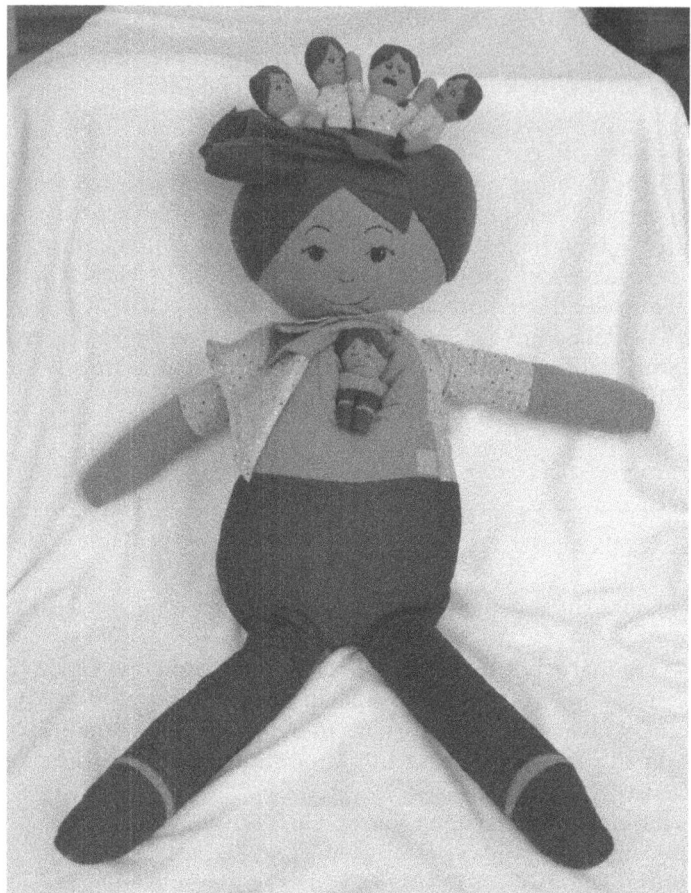

Figure 8.1 *The Dissociation Doll*

WHAT IS THE USE OF THE PLAYROOM PARTS-OF-SELF PROCESS?

- Chance to explore the internal world. *Do we know each other?*
- Chance to allow all parts to have a voice. *Do we hear each other, respect each other, care about each other, help each other, and do we appreciate each other's role in holding the painful memory?*
- Chance to reduce the phobia of the child to the dissociated and disowned parts of self.
- Chance to obtain resources like Safe Place, containers, or resources: superpowers, superhero strength, or guiding angels.
- Chance to be open and share the deepest sadness that exists in each part of self.
- Chance for parts to be healed from past traumas and protector parts to have a new role.
- Chance to increase conversation between the parts.

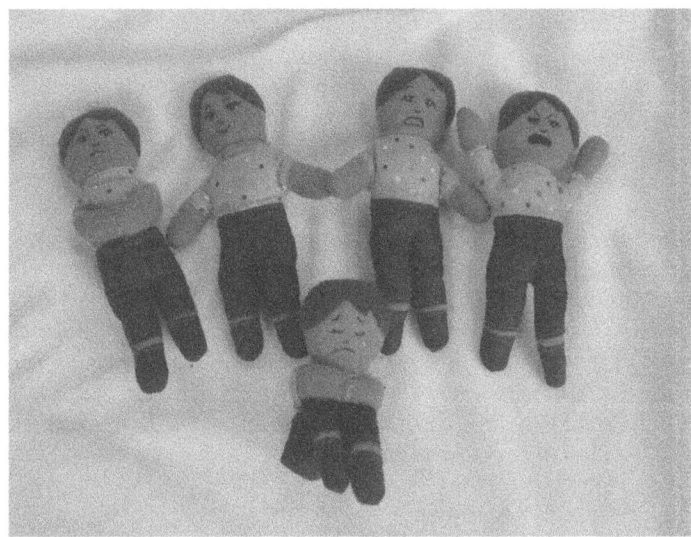

Figure 8.2 *The Dissociation Doll's Parts of Self*

- Chance to increase acceptance and understanding of the parts.
- Chance to reframe the parts especially hostile parts that scare the child and "takeover."
- Chance to increase compassion among the parts.
- Chance to increase internal awareness of switching parts.

Throughout these interactions, we are working to increase internal awareness and allow dialogue to occur within the child to access the parts in a safe and supportive way, which is allowing co-consciousness to occur.

PHOBIA OF THE DISSOCIATED PARTS OF SELF

Why would I want to know what happened? I do so many things to pretend it isn't true. I tried so many times to tell family members what was happening. Sometimes, I am not sure I was that girl in the bedroom. —7-year-old Samantha

Children are phobic to talk about their traumas due to the intense painful emotions, and the child will go to great lengths to avoid talking about the trauma or that feeling. This becomes habitual and automatic for the child (Silberg, 2013). What follows is severe acting-out behavior in the home, school, and playroom: self-harm, lying, stealing, including aggression, defiant behaviors, and so forth. In the play therapy room, the child does not "hear" the therapist, ignores the therapist, or has concerning behaviors. At home, children will do anything to avoid the feeling of the trauma memory.

THE PLAYROOM PARTS-OF-SELF SCRIPT: THE SETUP

It is important that the following questions be paced slowly and interspersed with play so that the child does not feel overwhelmed with the exploration. Accepting the child's limit on how much they can respond provides safety (Shirar, 1996).

> *Explanation*: Everyone has different moods or feelings that seem strong and powerful. We may feel like these feelings are so strong that they can even take us over. You might feel so mad and do things that you can't believe you did! Or maybe someone said you did something, and you don't remember doing it. Or maybe you hear a voice inside that tells you to do things, and it doesn't seem like you. Getting to know these different parts of ourselves can help us feel better. We all have different parts like from the movie Inside Out, when that little girl had different parts inside of her.

Imagining/Creating the Space

The child is invited to make a special place for the parts to come together, which can be done by drawing, sand, puppets, or utilizing some or all of the playroom as the special place or playroom.

> *We are going to make a playroom with everything that you and your parts want or need. This playroom is a nice place where nothing bad can come to you. It's a chance for all parts of you to come in and tell their story. They can show themselves, maybe talk about what they need, or if they are upset or maybe talk about why they act the way they do.*
>
> *Can you think about this playroom, let me know what it looks like, what is in it? What colors are the walls, what toys are in it, what furniture, what color is the play table, any stickers or drawings on it?*
>
> Or if in the sand tray:
>
> *Set up in the sand a comfortable and safe place for all parts of you can come to and meet each other.*

Give the client/child time to decorate and imagine the playroom or special place and create a play table or a circle. Have them describe what they would most like in the room—colors, door placement, windows, and so forth. Also, they should consider where the playroom might be—a large building, house, the forest, and so forth. Suggest that the room might also have an adjoining room or space outside.

> *Playroom—entering the room:*
>
> *Now I want you to imagine **you** entering this space. Now I want you to pick a figure or symbol to represent this part of yourself at the play table* (child chooses a figurine, image, or draws).

Playroom—inviting other parts to the play table:
Now I want you to go inside and just listen . . . and see who is there. Invite the other parts of yourself into the playroom. What part of yourself do you notice first?

Here is where most clients will first begin to struggle. Give a short menu of possible parts. Remember there are no wrong answers, and whatever the client comes up with is okay and useful. It is important that they are the ones who provide the answers, but of course assistance might be necessary.

Feelings: Happy, sad, mad, afraid, guilty, shameful, tired, hyper, shy, and so forth.
Roles/ages: Baby, little me, little girl/boy, wise me, mature me, me in-charge, me being bullied by others, bad part, bad me, angry part, mean part, devil, monster, superhero part, and so forth.
Other descriptive parts: Creative, wise, strong, productive, musical, worried, scared, yelling, crying part, and so forth.
Animals/object parts: Cat part, dog part, cloud part, slime part, black hole, and so forth.

What Should the Therapist Be Thinking While Using the Playroom Parts-of-Self Process?

Why was this self-state created? What is the function?

What life development stage (Erickson, 1994) was interrupted? Are they developmentally stuck at a certain age?

What age does the child seem as they talk about the parts?

Are there hidden self-states that are influencing the child's mood and behavior?

If a hostile part, did the child witness this behavior, and is this a person that the child imitated?

Is that imitator part holding the anger of the child?

Considering the words the child is saying, how are these related to the traumatic incidents: Do the words have similarities? Could the child have heard this, witnessed this?

Is the child phobic to having parts of self and denying them (telling them to "go away" or "not real")?

GRADUAL EXPOSURE

Allowing for gradual exposure to the parts of self is key, as these parts may feel vulnerable to exposure and be untrusting and worried that the therapist might not accept them or their stories and pain. The child may have mixed emotions in exposing such strong feelings of helplessness and powerlessness. Having children reconnect to their emotion pain must be done with play-based opportunities and at the child's pace. Reconnection to emotional pain can allow healthy expression of anger and deep wounds, but it can also flood a child. The safest way to start might be allowing the child to just expose the self-states without much conversation with the therapist. Reflective listening and commenting on what you are possibly noticing could help with the gradual exposure. Asking "light" questions in the beginning and allowing the child to distract or end when they want is an important process in allowing the self-states to feel safe enough to show.

PLAYROOM PARTS-OF-SELF PROCESS: INVESTIGATING PARTS

After each part enters the room, gently explore with the child. (Make sure to make your own notes and sketches as you go along to carry over between sessions.) Explore until the client no longer is able to identify another part. Investigating parts is a process that occurs over time. Working with a child in identifying the dissociated parts of self can take months of exploration. As this process can be overwhelming to a child and they may be phobic and confused about the different emotions, exploring has to be gradual and at the pace that is bringing awareness to the child in a titrated fashion.

Types of Parts of Self

Most of the self-states that therapists witness are the parts of self that hold the memories of the past such as baby or young parts of self. But, there are additional self-states that may have been created such as helpers, recordkeepers, and introjects. Helper parts can assist the child in school to do well, make friends, or can be a helper part that mimics a nurturing caregiver for when they were lonely.

DID children may have observers who record their trauma and who have all the details of their experience (Hilgard as cited in Shirar, 1996). Perpetrator–imitator parts can be the imitation of the one who harmed the child or witnessing domestic violence (Van der Hart et al., 2005). It is not uncommon for the child to take on the powerful stance of the harmful person. This imitator part can also be the sexualized part of self that is harming other children. "The child may not consciously remember context and details, he may still play it out or reenact it in therapy quiet accurately" (Hollingsworth, 1986; Terr, 1990 as cited in Shirar, 1996, pp. 189; concepts come from Martin, 2015; Potgieter Marks, 2018; Shirar, 1996).

When Exploring the Parts of Self, Consider Asking These Questions

- Where would that part go at the play table, playroom, and sand tray? Can you mark it with a symbol? What are they playing with?
- Does that part have a name? How old do they feel?

- *What do they want us to know about them? If you look inside, what are they trying to say?*
- *What do they like doing or not doing?*
- *Does that part like any other parts at the play table? Who is it friends with or who doesn't it like? Is there any part they stay away from or they are afraid of?*
- *What do the parts want them to know about each other?*
- *Who is the protective part? How do they protect? For example, by getting angry, screaming so that others leave them alone, never answering adults' questions about the past.*
- *What do they want to accomplish? Or do for other parts? For example, do they take care of the younger parts, be the good child in school, or criticize?*
- *Why were they formed? Do they hold bad memories? How did they help you survive? Which part was there at the time of the [trauma]? How did this part help you when "that" happened to you or when you lived with your birth parents?*
- *What worries them most? Are they worried about other parts and how they act?*
- *Who knows what about whom?* (e.g., does *Angry* know *Shy* is under the table?)
- *What is a good way to symbolize or show them (drawing, puppets, sand)?*

CHECK FOR *HOSTILE OR PERPETRATOR–IMITATOR* PARTS

Go inside and see who it is that is doing the things you don't like or getting you into trouble.
Is there any part of yourself that did not want to come into the room?
Is there a part that the other parts are afraid of?
If the child names the perpetrator as being inside of them, clarify that it is "Dad part of you."
If the answer is yes, would it be okay for that part to be in a different part of the playroom or adjoining room?
Is there a part that doesn't like counseling or like me being your counselor? Maybe they are afraid I will hurt them or ask too many questions?
Which parts do not want to listen or obey your caregiver?

Things to Remember Once Parts Have Been Established

Checking In

It can be helpful to check in with parts of the self at the beginning and end of the session. *"I am just checking in with all parts of you and seeing if there is anything any part wants me to know or show me in the sand."* This check-in can guide you to hear information that may not have been stated outright by the child. It is important to remember that parts may be listening and are scared and not trusting the therapist. If they have had previous experience with therapists, especially from being hospitalized after sharing parts of self, then it is possible the child is hearing messages of distrust.

Talking to the Parts Through the Child

Utilizing the child to engage in the communication and conversation with the parts of self is important. The therapist should refrain from having direct conversation with the parts of self so as not to encourage the brain habit of avoiding affect by creating more neural networks that support the coping of dissociation (Silberg, 2013). Here are common statements: I might say to a child, *"What is that part of you trying to tell us about that yukky time?" "Can you close your ideas and check inside what the parts think of this idea. What are they telling you?" "Can you see who inside had some big feelings over the weekend and got really upset?"*

Who Does the Therapist Need to Befriend?

Sandra Paulsen (2009) describes the necessary intervention of engaging the "head honcho" who may be operating the whole system of parts or who is capable of causing harm to other parts if they perform behaviors (like disclose trauma) that it deems detrimental to the system. This part may not like the therapist or therapy, and my common questions are: *Is there a part who doesn't like me? Or is there any part of you that doesn't like what I am saying?*

Hostile Parts/Perpetrator Parts

The most important concept in working with angry or perpetrator parts of self is that the therapist accepts the part without judgment and works to align with this part of self (Paulsen, 2009; Waters, 2016). These angry, rageful, self-destructive parts are likely to be baby parts or very young parts of the child and serve as a protection to the child so they will not be hurt again. (Waters, 2016). Talking to these parts through the child is important, as is engaging them in conversations about their functions, their roles, and what they can do to relieve stress. Being curious and accepting with these parts is important, which can be difficult if this part is threatening to kill the child, hurt another person, or saying things that promote hatred, violence, and pain. The part may be attempting to create safety for the system by pushing away any adult who comes near the child. Or the part may be expressing hatred, disgust, and rage for what it witnessed or had to experience. The child may feel that they *are* the perpetrator or this person lives inside of the child. The therapist must frame that it is "a part of you" and *it is* not you. It is important to reframe any negative part of self that the child dislikes and wants to disown. *That part might be trying to protect you so no one hurts you again* (Shirar, 1996; Silberg, 2013; Waters, 2016).

CREATING DIALOGUE AND COOPERATION AMONG PARTS

Once self-states are identified, having dialogue between the parts of self allows each part to state their needs and wants and fears. Encouraging the child to have internal dialogue takes patience and time for the therapist and the child. Much like families, habits are hard to break and many different ways have to be tried for healthy internal communication.

> *"Does that baby part want you to know their story?"*
> *"How do you feel when that (hostile part) hurts your sister?"*
> *"Can you ask that part what it needs to feel safe or feel better?"*
> *"Can this part and you work something out so you don't go to the hospital again?"*

PARENT INVOLVEMENT

After psychoeducation regarding self-states, I involve parents to work with me and the self-states. Having the parent as a co-therapist is valuable and allows the work I do in the playroom to be carried on in the home environment (Waters, 2016). An example might be asking the caregivers when saying goodnight to include the statement "I am saying goodnight to all parts of you." A good caregiver can help shift even the most hostile part. "I am walking on eggshells" is a common phrase from parents in dealing with their child's switching between self-states. I teach parents to acknowledge the switching at home and to acknowledge the parts of self. One parent I worked with who observed her son switching into a very young part say, "I see that the 4-year-old part of you is out, and I know that part is really mad at me for staying with (perpetrator) when you were so young. I let you get hurt by him." Her son started to cry and express anger, and mom was able to soothe that part of self.

After discussing possible interventions, a child who was struggling to stay co-conscious with their violent part was able to pass a note to her mom "get my sister out of the room" when she felt the part getting ready to take her over.

TREATMENT EXAMPLES

CHILD-CENTERED PLAY THERAPY

With young children, the parts will sometimes make themselves known initially through CCPT. This case involved a 5-year-old child called Sally with disorganized attachment who had experienced the death of her father at 18 months and been subsequently raised by her teen mother who would rage at her.
In the first session, Sally entered the play therapy room and was invited to play any way she wanted.

> Sally: *Sally is a baby. She is not allowed to be here. I'm the wolf.*
>
> Therapist: *Wolf, you are welcome to play here. You are not sure if it's safe for babies here.*
>
> Sally (growling and crawling, loud, eccentric voice): *Grrrr! Stay away, where is my cub?*
>
> Therapist: *You are looking for the baby wolf cub to protect. You want me to stay away until you are sure it is safe.*
>
> Sally (finding a puppy puppet): *Run away!* (To therapist) *You have to chase us.*
>
> Therapist: *You want to be chased, tell me how to play this story the way you want.*

Over a number of sessions, Sally reenacted a play involving threats to the baby and protection by the bad wolf (hostile to therapist); therapist consistently tried out reflections that recognized that the wolf, while scary, might have good intentions as a protector, which was intriguing to the child.

(This reflection fit because the therapist saw this as an introject and wanted to make space for that shift.)

In the next session, the child entered the playroom:

Sally: *Sally is here today . . .*

Therapist: *Sally, you are welcome here, I've been wanting to meet you . . . Should we find you a safe place in this room to play?*

Therapist helped client build a safe nook using the tent in the playroom, bean bag chair, blanket, and stuffed animals, and the client curled up in the bed with the blanket and pretended to sleep for several minutes.

Therapist: *You can rest while I make sure no one disturbs you. I might be able to help Wolf to protect you. What else does Wolf think we need?*

Sally: *Shhh . . . baby needs quiet . . . ..*(She spent nearly 10 minutes curled up in the fetal position in repose, therapist breathing deeply with her, playing soft music and "watching over her.")

In further child-centered play sessions, she played the same story with similar themes enacted in sand, puppets, other places in the room.

> *Gradually, a storyline emerged of a baby who lost her Daddy. (This is the baby part beginning to share how she was formed when Dad died suddenly.) There were many opportunities within the metaphor of the play to get key ideas about parts, safety, cooperation, and so forth across, in preparation for the more intentional and directive work of the conference table where the child could acknowledge her baby part and wolf part.*
>
> *During this period, she stopped referring to herself as a separate person and the presence of parts became more playful. Her adoptive mom was encouraged to welcome the baby play and stop any focus on correcting the "wolf-like" behavior. A sudden surge in affection toward adoptive mom, increased periods of calm, and a leap forward in her learning occurred during this period.*

DIRECTIVE PLAY WITH PARTS

In another case example, at the start of each session with 7-year-old Tommy, I would invite him to put his parts in the sand. It allowed me to see new self-states that may have been hidden and were now willing to emerge, any new shifts that occurred in the states, and conflicts among the states. Tommy and his parents had done significant attachment work, had talking openly about the past traumas, and he had done considerable internal exploration work. Tommy had worked hard on problem-solving for the parts of self that were destructive to reduce the chance of possible removal from the home. In one session, Tommy put a new figure for his most mature 7-year-old part and said, "This is the new leader." He talked differently about the parts, and this "new leader" was guiding everyone down a more cooperative path. One of the most significant changes was when he managed to include two parts that had been hated by the others.

WHAT NEEDS TO HAPPEN PRIOR TO EMDR

If a therapist is preparing to process a memory with EMDR, it means that the child's part of self that holds this memory agrees to allow this trauma back into consciousness (Shirar, 1996). At this point, all the parts are working together and have agreed that the system needs relief to feel better.

Communication

When communication is not happening among parts, safety concerns should be investigated. Usually a trigger within the environment is causing the child's parts to be highly activated and conflictual or there is a lack of internal safety and the child is not wanting to face the past traumas (Shirar, 1996). The parts may be naturally dialoguing and communicating, and this may be occurring through the visual representation that the child created with the Playroom Parts-of-Self process. The child can show how the various parts are communicating, and therapists can give ideas to encourage internal safety, such as meeting on the playground, meeting inside a certain part of the space they created, or "have a meeting with everyone's favorite snacks." Sometimes, the internal dialogue between the parts of self has brought significant relief to the system, and the child's symptoms have reduced considerably. The therapist is looking for the parts to be co-conscious with each other, become fairly acquainted with each other, and experience each other more or even play internally together. I noticed improvement in the cooperation of parts of self with a 6-year-old girl, when she told me two of her parts always played, then included another part to join the fun, and then all three invited the hostile part to come with them on a horseback ride. "We told that (perpetrator) part that it would be happier if it just played with us." When there is high-risk behavior such as violence and/or self-harm and hospitalization is imminent, I ask the parts to come together to hear the possible course of outside treatment that might need to become involved to keep all parts safe. With one boy, once all self-states understood they would have to go to the hospital, they agreed to find a different way to express anger and were able to stabilize those behaviors.

PROCESSING PHASE OF EMDR

Containing the Child Parts

The child and parts of self may decide that the small children parts should not be part of trauma processing (Paulsen, 2009). A separate Safe Place for the child part or "little children" can be created with blinds drawn or "window closed" to the outside world. I encourage the child to put in comfy furniture, animals, a grandmother/fairy godmother, food, TV, videogames, music, or an intercom that can talk to the child or a safe member. Containment is important in dealing with the child feeling flooded.

Phase 4: Playing While Processing Through EMDR

Phase 4 of EMDR can be implemented with children once all the parts of self are in good communication and willing to dialogue about trauma work. I introduce it as an option for a part to "feel less upset," "think less about it," "feel stronger about it," and how this can help everyone involved "if the baby is crying less." When allowing the child to metaphorically play out the traumatic event with acknowledgment of all aspects of the memory, including the dissociated emotions, body sensations, and beliefs, these dissociated aspects become closer and closer to the child's awareness (Shirar, 1996). It is in these moments that a therapist may capture in moments of processing the image, emotions, beliefs, and body sensations in the desensitization phase of EMDR (Adler-Tapia & Settle, 2012).

Sometimes, with children we may set up the actual processing session like we do with teens or adults. An 11-year-old adopted from her country at age 9 agreed to allow me to process one early memory that occurred at 2 years of age. Two older and helper type self-states agreed to stay to support the 2-year-old part, and she said about one of the parts, "It would be watching me to make sure I didn't mess up." Another part who was annoyed that everyone wanted to do this agreed to stay in their Safe Place while the processing was occurring. Once we were done and the self-states noticed that the 2-year-old was more at ease and less "fussy," they agreed to continue with other memories.

INTEGRATION

Integration is knowledge, feelings, sensations, and behaviors coming back into the child's consciousness, and fusion is when two parts have joined together (Shirar, 1996). As soon as the child starts to explore self-states, integration is occurring (Shirar, 1996; Waters, 2016). Throughout the gradual exploration of self-states, promoting awareness, acceptance, appreciation, dialogue, and cooperation, integration is naturally occurring. A self-state that held a traumatic memory and processed it in the desensitization phase may no longer need to be separate. Children are not invested in staying separate as much as adults might be (Kluft, 1985), and integration for a child may gradually and naturally occur especially if the child is very young, has good attachments, and has successfully processed their memories with EMDR. If the child's symptoms and behaviors have improved, the child may be less interested in talking about the parts of self (Waters, 2016). When asked to "go inside and check in," a child who had worked very hard on past trauma said, "It's very quiet . . . I think everyone is okay." Through sand, clay, or drawing, children may symbolize everyone getting along, working together, and start to use the word "I" instead of "we." A 5-year-old girl who had processed her past traumas and whose symptoms had disappeared chose one figurine for herself in the sand and proudly announced "Momma now has only *me* to love!"

If integration is not naturally occurring, we can encourage it by talking about the self-states joining their "special parts" of each of them and becoming one. Susan, a 9-year-old child, agreed to have two parts meet in her playroom to talk about her joining with an older self-state, "Violet," who had been going to school and getting good grades and was very well liked by teachers. While doing sand work, I did a visualization of her standing behind "Violet" and eventually stepping inside of her and "getting all her smarts about Math and English and feeling good about the grades they now got together." By the next session, instead of naming the other self-state who got the school achievements, Susan was stating, "*I* got an A on my Math test" and her father reported much less switching at him between school and home.

Integration can be observed by a number of different indicators. Typically, what is first noticed by caregivers is a reduction or elimination of problem behaviors and symptoms. The child is using less dissociative strategies and more verbal communication with caregivers in handling problems. The mother of 7-year-old Tommy, whose case was mentioned earlier, said that "I never knew he had such deep feelings" as he now talked about his sadness and pain of the past instead of his violent aggression. His most profound statement was "Can I *tell* you if I feel jealous when you are playing with my sister instead of *showing* you by being bad?"

In the playroom, what is typically noticeable to the therapist as healing and integration occur is the child talking in the singular, and affect being more regulated. Overall, children start to flourish at school and at home with caregivers. The child's physical appearance may even shift (Waters, 2016) as they walk taller and prouder, and our conversations are more about their daily accomplishments instead of talking about the conflict in their internal world.

This approach is challenging, but my presence as a therapist assisting a child and caregivers to leave their pain in my playroom and live in harmony is the greatest gift I can give to those who have chosen me to free them of their past.

CONCLUSION

The manifestation of dissociation in children is often a confusing presentation of symptoms and behaviors that are not easy to identify and are often missed among even seasoned therapists. Managing dissociative states and self-states feels overwhelming to many therapists, and this chapter's goal was to give some direction in following the guiding principles. I encourage all therapists to stay in the curious part of their own selves even when it feels difficult to know the next steps. The greatest gift you can give a child is bearing witness to the pain of their internal struggle and to the trauma's that are held deep within their heart.

REFERENCES

Adler-Tapia, R., & Settle, C. (2012). Specialty topics on using EMDR with children. *Journal of EMDR Practice and Research*, *6*(3), 145–153. doi:10.1891/1933-3196.6.3.145

American Psychiatric Association. (2013). *Diagnostic and statistical manual of mental disorder* (5th ed.). Washington, DC: Author.

Armstrong, J. G., Putnam, F. W., Carlson, E. B., Libero, D. Z., & Smith, S. R. (1997). Development and validation of a measure of adolescent dissociation: The Adolescent Dissociative Experiences Scale. *Journal of Nervous and Mental Disease*, *185*(8), 491–497. doi:10.1097/00005053-199708000-00003

Biggs, A. (2013). *Polly and her parts*. Waltham, MA: Front and Center Press.

Bray, M. (2015). *Rob the robin and the bald eagle*. Vincennes, IN: Artsake Publishing.

Cloitre, M., Stolbach, B. C., Herman, J. L., Kolk, B. V., Pynoos, R., Wang, J., & Petkova, E. (2009). A developmental approach to complex PTSD: Childhood and adult cumulative trauma as predictors of symptom complexity. *Journal of Traumatic Stress, 22*(5), 399–408. doi:10.1002/jts.20444

Cook, A., Blaustein, M., Spinazzola, J., & van der Kolk, B. (2003). *Complex trauma in children and adolescents white paper from the National Child Traumatic Stress Network Complex Trauma Task Force.* Retrieved from https://www.nctsn.org/resources/complex-trauma-children-and-adolescents

Cook, A., Spinazzola, J., Ford, J., Lanktree, C., Blaustein, M., Cloitre, M., . . . van der Kolk, B. (2005). Complex trauma in children and adolescents. *Psychiatric Annals, 35*(5), 361–373.

Erickson, E. (1994). *Identity and the life cycle* (rev. ed.). New York, NY: W. W. Norton.

Forgash, C. (2008). Applying EMDR in and ego state therapy in collaborative treatment. In C. Forgash & M. Copeley (Eds.), *Healing the heart of trauma and dissociation*. New York, NY: Springer Publishing Company.

Fraser, G. (1993). Special treatment techniques to access the inner personality system of multiple personality disorder. *Dissociation, 6*, 193–198.

Freyd, J. (1996). *Betrayal trauma: The logic of forgetting childhood abuse*. Cambridge, MA: Harvard University Press.

Gaskill, R., & Perry, B. (2014). The neurobiological power of play: Using the Neurosequential Model of Therapeutics to guide play in the healing process. In C. Machoidi & D. Crenshaw (Eds.), *Creative arts and play therapy for attachment trauma*. New York, NY: Guilford Press.

Gomez, A. (2013). *EMDR therapy and adjunct approaches with children*. New York: Springer Publishing Company.

Gomez, A., & Paulsen, S. (2016). *All the colors of me: My first book about dissociation*. Phoenix, AZ: Agate Books.

Gonzalez, A., & Mosquera, D. (2012). *EMDR and dissociation: The progressive approach*. Assam, India: A.I. Publishers.

Goodyear-Brown, P. (2010). *Play therapy with traumatized children: A prescriptive approach*. Hoboken, NJ: Wiley.

Greenwald, R. (2005). *Child trauma handbook*. Binghamton, NY: Hayworth Press.

Greenwald, R. (2009). *Treating problem behaviors*. New York, NY: Routledge.

HeartMath. (n.d.). *The HeartMath experience—New online program*. Retrieved from https://www.heartmath.com

International Society for the Study of Dissociation Task Force on Children and Adolescents. (2003). *Guidelines for the evaluation and treatment of dissociative symptoms in children and adolescents*. Retrieved from https://www.vkjp.nl/media/files/De%20praktijk/childguidelines-ISSTD-2003.pdf

International Society for the Study of Trauma and Dissociation. (2020). *Child and adolescent FAQs*. Retrieved from https://www.isst-d.org/resources/child-adolescent-faqs/

Kluft, R. P. (Ed.). (1985). *Childhood antecedents of multiple personality*. Washington, DC: American Psychiatric Press.

Knipe, J. (2015). *EMDR toolbox: Theory and treatment of complex PTSD and dissociation*. New York, NY: Springer Publishing Company.

Martin, K. (2015, November). *Mastering the treatment of complex trauma, transforming theory into practice*. Amherst, NY: Western New York Regional EMDR Network.

Paulsen, S. (2009). *Looking through the eyes of trauma and dissociation*. Charleston, SC: Book Surge Publishing.

Peterson, G. (1991). Children coping with trauma: Diagnosis of "Dissociation Identity Disorder." *Dissociation: Progress in the Dissociative Disorders, 4*(3), 152–164.

Porges, S. (2011). *The polyvagal theory*. New York, NY: Routledge.

Potgieter Marks, R. (2018). When the sleeping tiger roars: Perpetrator introjects in children. In R. Vogt (Ed.), *Perpetrator introjects: Psychotherapeutic diagnostics and treatment models* (pp. 87–110). Kroning, Germany: Asanger.

Putnam, F. (1997). *Dissociation in children and adolescents: A developmental perspective*. New York, NY: Guilford Press.

Putnam, F. W., & Peterson, G. (1994). Further validation of the Child Dissociative Checklist. *Dissociation: Progress in the Dissociative Disorders, 7*(4), 204–211.

Schore, A. (2012). Playing on the right side of the brain: An interview with Allan N. Schore. *American Journal of Play, 9*(2), 105–142.

Shapiro, F. (2001). *Eye movement desensitization and reprocessing: Basic principles, protocols and procedures*. New York, NY: Guilford Press.

Shirar, L. (1996). *Dissociative children: Bridging the inner and outer worlds*. New York, NY: W. W. Norton.

Siegel, D. J. (1999). *The developing mind: Toward a neurobiology of interpersonal experience*. New York, NY: Guilford Press.

Silberg, J. (2013). *The child survivor: Healing developmental trauma and dissociation*. New York, NY: Routledge.

Spinazzola, J., Ford, J., Zucker, M., Kolk, B., Silva, S., Smith, S., & Blaustein, M. (2005). National survey of complex trauma exposure, outcome, and intervention for children and adolescents. *Psychiatric Annals, 35*(8), 624–624.

Stolbach, B. C. (1997). The Children's Dissociative Experiences Scale and Traumatic Stress Inventory: Rationale, development and validation of a self-report measure. *Dissertation Abstracts International, 58*(3), 1548B.

Van der Hart, O., Nijenhuis, E., & Steele, K. (2005). Dissociation: An insufficiently recognized major feature of complex PTSD. *Journal of Traumatic Stress, 18*(5), 413–423. doi:10.1002/jts.20049

Waters, F. (2016). *Healing the fractured child: Diagnosis and treatment of youth with dissociation*. New York, NY: Springer Publishing Company.

Weiland, S. (2015). *Dissociation in traumatized children and adolescents: Theory and clinical interventions*. New York, NY: Routledge.

Section II

Play-Based Interventions for EMDR Phases

9

Taking a Play-Based Trauma History

ANN BECKLEY-FOREST AND MELISSA LAVIGNE

INTRODUCTION

Finding ways to complete Phase 1 of the EMDR protocol, history and treatment planning, presents unique challenges when working with children. The therapist often has many other sources of information about the child's trauma history; still, developing a shared understanding of the trauma and the impact of trauma is just as important in child therapy as it is in the adult protocol. In this chapter, we present an option for using storytelling, props, and metaphor to elicit trauma history from a child in a way that is sensitive to their age and their window of tolerance for distress.

PHASE OF EMDR

History and treatment planning (Phase 1)

MATERIALS

- Bowl or open container of some kind
- Stones of various sizes
- Sand tray (optional)

RATIONALE

When working with children who have experienced trauma, it is important that the therapeutic relationship is built around safety, security, and healing. Gathering trauma history from the child early on in treatment in a play-based and developmentally informed way creates an opportunity to obtain some of the painful information while keeping the child feeling emotionally grounded and safe. Developing a clear understanding of the history of adversity through a trauma-informed lens helps the therapist proceed at the child's pace and implement the most effective approach (Greenwald, 2005, 2007). Asking children about the bad things that have happened to them, within the context of a safe relationship, fosters a level of acceptance (Gomez, 2012; Greenwald, 2005, 2007). Not every child has the distress tolerance to complete even this basic approach to obtaining a trauma history (Phase 1 of the EMDR protocol) early in treatment. However, many are capable of doing so and feel relief in having this intervention serve as a kind of safe container for these experiences until they are ready to proceed with trauma digestion later on in therapy. For some highly reactive children with complex trauma, the therapist might delay this intervention until after safety and stabilization have been established.

A play-based, metaphorical story is a common tool in play therapy settings to help the child receive information in a more implicit way (Mills & Crowley, 2014). Therapists are looking for a way to convey a number of messages early in treatment, including the idea that other children have had bad things happen to them, too. Even though bad things have happened, others were able to learn how to overcome them and get better (Greenwald, 2005, 2007). Using props and items that the child can handle, such as stones and sand, is grounding and satisfying to the child and can help to "detoxify" the intensity of bringing up the traumas (Goodyear-Brown, 2019).

Joyce Mills and Richard Crowley (2014) describe an ancient Hawaiian story called *The Perfect Bowl of Light* that offers a metaphorical framework for gathering a trauma history in a developmentally appropriate way. Using this metaphor as the foundation and adding some of the straightforward language from the Greenwald (2007) approach to taking a trauma history from a child enable the therapist to elicit some information and put trauma work on the agenda without overwhelming the child. Keeping the story and corresponding intervention quick, play-based, and early on in treatment will not only meet the developmental and emotional needs of the child, but it will also set the precedent that the therapist can handle knowing whatever has happened to the child (Gaskill & Perry, 2013; Gomez, 2012; Greenwald, 2005, 2007).

DESCRIPTION OF INTERVENTION

In this intervention, the therapist tells the *Bowl of Light* story with some simple props as a set up for asking the child to list some of the bad things that have happened in the past and get a quick read on the child's current level of distress in bringing up these events. The intervention is designed to be accomplished quickly and kept within the child's ability to tolerate and is usually done at the beginning of a session, so there is ample time to re-regulate with child-centered play or fun activities.

STEP-BY-STEP DIRECTIONS

GETTING THE HISTORY (STEPS 1–3)

Step 1: Start off by letting the child know you are going to tell them a quick story. Place the bowl into the sand while you tell the tale (Figure 9.1):

> *"There was once a tribe in Hawaii who believed that every child was born with a bowl of purest light inside them. Sometimes, some bad things would happen, and these things were like stones in their bowl, blocking some of the light."*

Step 2: The therapist gives examples of bad things while moving stones into the bowl one by one. Giving a menu can normalize these experiences and help the child recall some of their history. *"Things like someone close getting really sick or hurt or dying, getting really hurt yourself, being taken away from family, being made to do sex things, being threatened, seeing parents having really bad arguments or fights or get divorced ... you know, the kinds of things that could really hit you hard"* (Greenwald, 2007, p. 67).

If the therapist is aware of a specific trauma from the child's past, it can be added to the menu. It is important to make sure that the list is broad enough to make room for possible disclosures or previously undisclosed events.

Step 3: Now, the therapist asks the child to very briefly list some of the past upsetting experiences. *"Some kids who come to work with me have some stones like this, and later on when they are ready and if they want to, we can help some of the stones to get smaller so they don't block so much light. So I just need to know what are the some of the stones in your bowl. Some things like that which have happened to you? ... I am just going to make a quick list, no details, just the thing and how old you were when it happened"* (Greenwald, 2007, p. 67). It is important that the therapist keeps this quick and not allow the child to start telling the story, as this might lead to overwhelming feelings we are not yet ready for at this point in therapy.

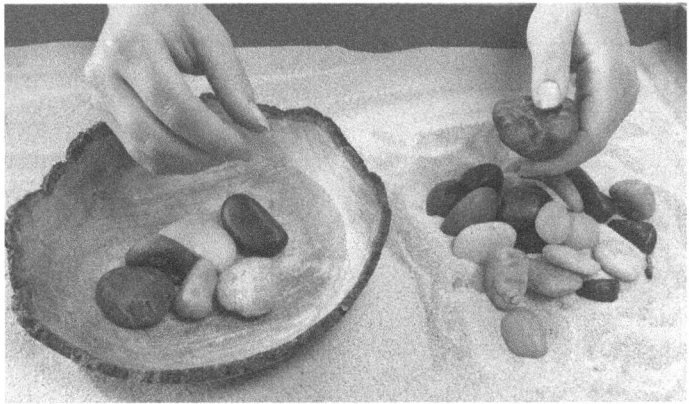

Figure 9.1 *The Bowl of Light* Story

RATING THE LEVEL OF DISTRESS (STEP 4)

1. After the child has placed their rocks into the bowl and identified the bad things, the therapist gathers a quick rating of the current level of distress. This is done by quickly listing the items back to the child one by one, and asking the child how much that item still bothers them on the 0 to 10 Subjective Units of Distress Scale (SUDS). With young children, we want to offer a visual, interactive SUDS, which keeps the activity play-based and developmentally appropriate. Hanging a large 0 to 10 "bothering scale" on the wall and asking the child to throw a ball at the number that represents the amount of bothering for each item would be one example of how to get the SUDS rating.

REESTABLISHING SAFETY (STEP 5)

2. After this activity, some kind of playful containment activity that helps reestablish a sense of safety is needed. We might make a "best things" list using the colors of the rainbow, invite child-centered play or do another fun activity along with deep breaths or a calming activity. Due to the time needed to reestablish safety, this intervention should not be started near the end of the session, but only when there is adequate time to contain any upsetting feelings.

MODIFICATIONS

When parents have knowledge of traumas that children "don't remember," a variation of this story can be used to introduce information about the event, setting the stage for later processing. Likewise, for children with complex early trauma, the therapist may do more of the naming and keep the description of the stone deliberately nonspecific and within the child's tolerance. For example: "I guess there should be a stone for you having to leave your bio family when they could not take care of you."

When engaging a child with complex trauma in this intervention, it is important to consider delaying its implementation until later on in treatment. When we want to proceed with a trauma history in those cases, we offer grounding and soothing strategies throughout. One way to do this is to offer the child a piece of chewing gum prior to the story. If the therapist notices that the child is becoming overwhelmed, they can ask them to try to blow a big bubble with the chewing gum. As the child becomes regulated through the use of the gum, the process can continue.

Additional modifications would be made for extremely young children, aged 4 and under. This can be done by only listing a few items, in an effort the keep the intervention short and more age appropriate.

CONSIDERATIONS

WHEN NOTHING IS SAID

If the child is struggling to identify events, offer a few more choices by rephrasing the question (Greenwald, 2007, p. 67):

> *"How old were you for the worst time you got into trouble at school?"*
> *"How old were you for the worst time you got into trouble at home?"*
> *"How old were you for the worst time you saw grownups get angry or fight with each other?"*

If you are aware of a traumatic experience the child has had from the parent's report, you can offer that as a suggestion, if the child does not offer it. *"Your mom told me about that bad thing that happened with your dad. That might be a rock..."* If the child agrees in some way, verbally or nonverbally, place a rock into the bowl to represent that event.

We know that we do not always get all the child's traumas on the list, and some items that the child lists might not be traumatic so much as they are descriptions of recent triggers. The therapist accepts each item calmly without expressing too much sympathy (as that might open the floodgates of emotion) or minimizing the events, which may not be as significant but are relevant to the child at the moment.

CASE EXAMPLE

This is an example of the dialogue with an 8-year-old child.

> Therapist: *Today I am going to tell you a quick story, after that we will get to play.*
>
> Child: *Okay.*
>
> Therapist (places bowl into sand along with container of rocks): *There was once a tribe in Hawaii who believed that every child was born with a bowl of purest light inside them. Sometimes, some bad things would happen, and these things were like stones in their bowl, blocking some of the light. Things like someone close getting really sick or hurt or dying, getting really hurt yourself, being taken away from family, being made to do sex things, being threatened, not seeing a parent for a long time, seeing parents having really bad arguments or fights or get divorced...you know, the kinds of things that could really hit you hard. Some kids who come to work with me have some stones like this, and later on when they are ready and if they want to, we can help some of the stones to get smaller so they don't block so much light. So, I just need to know what are the some of the stones in your bowl? Some things like that which have*

happened to you?... I am just going to make a quick list, no details, just the thing and how old you were when it happened.

Child: *Hmmm, maybe when I got into trouble at school.*

Therapist: *How old were you?*

Child: *It was last school year.*

Therapist: *So you were 7?*

Child: *Yeah.*

Therapist: *What else would be a rock in your bowl?*

Child: *When my dad moved away, and now I don't get to see him.*

Therapist: *How old were you when that happened?*

Child: *5.*

Therapist: *What else?*

Child: *Well, nothing really.*

Therapist: *Other kids have spoken of the worst times when they got into trouble at home or school, or a time they got really mad or scared.*

Child: *When I got mad at my brother for stealing my candy.*

Therapist: *How old were you?*

Child: *This was just the other day!*

Therapist: *So you were 8?*

Child: *Yeah.*

Therapist: *What else would be a rock in your bowl?*

Child: *I don't know.*

Therapist: *Your mom told me about that time you guys got in a car accident; would that be a rock in the bowl?*

Child: *Hmmm.*

Therapist: *How old were you when that happened?*

Child: *I think I was 5.*

Therapist: *What else?*

Child: *Hmm, nothing else.*

Therapist: *Okay, so now I am going to ask you tell me how much these rocks still bother you. Not when it happened but right now when you think about it, on a scale of 0 to 10. Zero is no bad feeling and 10 is the worst possible feeling. When you got into trouble at school, how much bothering did you have? Does it feel like a 10* (motions a ten with arms really far apart) *or does it feel like a 5* (hands a medium width apart) *or like a 0* (hands touching)*?*

Child: *It feels like a four* (places hands a medium distance apart).

Therapist: *What about your dad moving away and not getting to see him? How much does that bother you now? Does it feel like a 10 amount of bothering or more like a 5 or more like a 0?*

Child: *It feels like a 10!* (places hands really far apart)

Therapist: *What about when your brother stole your candy?*

Child: *Oh, that made me really mad; that bothers me like a lot!*

Therapist: *So would you say it bothers you still like a 10 or somewhere else on the scale?*

Child: *It bothers me like way more than 10, so off the scale!* (Motions arms as far apart as possible)

Therapist: *So what about when you guys were in the car accident, how much bothering do you have about that?*

Child: *Hmm. It bothers me like a 3.*

Therapist: *Later on when you are ready and we know each other better, there are some special things we can do to make those stones feel smaller. But today that is enough hard work. Let's do something to relax a bit.*

Rest of Session: After the child engaged in the *Bowl of Light* Intervention, the therapist and child practiced deep breathing. After a few rounds of deep breaths, the therapist invited him to play with the toys in the playroom. The therapist stated that he could play with the toys in "anyway you like" for the rest of the session. During this time, the therapist used a child-centered play therapy approach to stay connected to his play.

Using a story or metaphor in the context of play can help lower the intensity of the process of taking a trauma history.

REFERENCES

Gaskill, R., & Perry, B. D. (2013). The neurobiological power of play: Using the Neurosequential Model of Therapeutics to guide play in the healing process. In C. Malchiodi & D. A. Crenshaw (Eds.), *Play and creative arts therapy for attachment problems*. New York, NY: Guilford Press.

Gomez, A. (2012). *EMDR therapy and adjunct approaches with children: Complex trauma, attachment and dissociation*. New York, NY: Springer Publishing Company.

Goodyear-Brown, P. (2019). *Trauma and play therapy: Helping children heal*. New York, NY: Routledge.

Greenwald, R. (2005). *Child trauma handbook: A guide for helping trauma-exposed children and adolescents*. New York, NY: Haworth Press.

Greenwald, R. (2007). *EMDR within a phase model of trauma-informed treatment*. New York, NY: Haworth Press.

Mills, J., & Crowley, J. (2014). *Therapeutic metaphors for children and the child within* (2nd ed.). New York, NY: Routledge.

10

Building a Calm/Safe Place in the Play Therapy Room With the Fort Tent

ALICE STRICKLIN

INTRODUCTION

The Fort Tent Calm/Safe Place (Fort Tent) is an intervention designed to help create safety within the constructs of the therapy office. This creative intervention heightens present moment experience of safety in real time. The Fort Tent allows clients who need a more concrete, kinesthetic intervention to be involved in the development of the safe place, thus empowering them to have a level of control in their own sense of safety.

PHASE OF EMDR

Preparation (Phase 2)

MATERIALS

- Two king-size top sheets
- Small clamps
- Three or four chairs
- Stuffed animals (varying types and sizes)
- Various play therapy items from the play room

RATIONALE

When children are exposed to toxic environments for many years of their childhood, they may have a difficult time even imagining a calm or safe place. Neurologically, their brains have developed adaptively to stay on high alert, keeping a hypervigilant awareness of their surroundings. When children's brains are in this hypervigilant state, their behavior can appear fidgety, inattentive, and impulsive. It is hard for them to focus on schoolwork or even take in cognitive-based information and process it. Their brains are constantly scanning their surroundings, attempting to predict people's reactions and moods, to assess potential dangers (Levine, 2007; Schore, 2003; Siegel, 2012; van der Kolk, 2014). When these clients begin treatment, the play therapy room may feel overwhelming with too many choices. They may show inattention in session or may impulsively move from one area to another distracted by all that is around them. The opposite could also be true; they seem to hover in one area without looking or interacting with much else or may seem disinterested. Some children may display sweaty palms or feet, have short rapid breaths, or even show visible trembling. Others may outwardly look calm, have slow-to-almost nonapparent breathing, display slow deliberate movements, have rigid body posture with little movement, or show extreme compliance. All can be signs of high stress and an overwhelmed nervous system. Peter Levine (1997) focuses on the housing of trauma in the body and nervous system and the symptomatic somatic byproducts of this housing process. Levine's work aligns with Shapiro's adaptive information processing (AIP) model used in EMDR (Shapiro, 2001).

When children have experienced or witnessed repeated incidents of abuse, they can begin to internalize a belief that the world is not safe. They may also begin to internalize beliefs about themselves such as *"I am weak"* or *"I am powerless."* Such beliefs begin to set up the framework in which they view themselves and the world, which then becomes the construct with which they then respond to the world. These beliefs seem to be about the self or the world at the time of the trauma, and these beliefs get stuck in the maladaptive memory networks right along with the trauma response of fight, flight, freeze, or collapse and submit (Shapiro, 2001). Because of this, the development of a felt sense of safety and control is the foundation of all trauma-treatment models. Van der Kolk (2014) states, "Being able to feel safe with other people is probably the single most important aspect of mental health; safe connections are fundamental to meaningful and satisfying lives" (p. 79). This intervention begins to lay the foundation of safety with the therapist in the therapy room.

Fort Tent has been adapted from Francine Shapiro's (2001) Calm Place exercise. This adaptation is designed to better suit children's needs. Abused and neglected children have very few internal and external resources (adaptive networks) to enhance the original Calm Place. The initial goal of this intervention is to create a specific experience of a Calm Place. By doing so, we hope new neuropathways of a corrective experience can begin to develop in the brain, creating a corrective adaptive memory network. This new experience can be added and enhanced in subsequent sessions. A second goal of this intervention is to begin to offer empowering opportunities for the child who previously has not had choice. The child can then access this developed adaptive network and utilize it as a resource outside the office. Additionally, the resource will be available, if needed, in later phases of EMDR processing.

DESCRIPTION OF INTERVENTION

This intervention involves constructing a fort or tent in the therapy office using large bedsheets, furniture, and other office items such as pillows, stuffed animals, and figurines. The therapist assists the client and offers permission to the client to ask for help as needed. The therapist first describes what the client will get to do and then offers the sheets to them. The therapist and client then work together to arrange furniture in order to drape sheets and create a structure that the client can climb in and out of. After the Fort Tent is created, the therapist invites the client to bring in any items from the office that would help the client feel safe, peaceful, and relaxed in their fort. The client may grab figures to put outside of their fort as protectors, or comfy pillows and stuffed animals that act as comforters or nurturers. Once the Fort Tent is constructed, the therapist begins creating new neuropathways in the brain by enhancing the present moment's felt sense of safety using slow bilateral stimulation (BLS), such as the butterfly hug (Jarero, Artigas, Mauer, López Cano, & Alcalá, 1999; Jarero, Artigas, & Montero, 2008).

STEP-BY-STEP INSTRUCTIONS

Step 1: The therapist explains to the child that they get to create a space in the therapy office that is their very own, using as many sheets and items any way needed to make a special place. The therapist offers support by offering to move furniture, arranging the sheets to make the fort, and fetching items as needed. It helps to give examples of what support may look like, *"If you need help moving something, you could ask and I would move it"* or *"If you need help getting a 'wall' (sheet) to stay up, all you need to do is ask and I will help."*

Step 2: Building the Fort Tent is an opportunity for the therapist to offer help and always immediately respond when asked. This part of treatment is important in building up three resources for clients: (a) *I can ask for help and get it*, (b) *I can trust an adult*, and (c) *I have a say in what happens.*

The therapist's attunement to the client through the construction phase begins the process of building a therapeutic alliance and is also foundational to the client developing a new adaptive memory of safety and empowerment.

Step 3: Once the Fort Tent has been constructed, the therapist invites the client to choose items from the playroom that would help the space feel relaxing, fun, and peaceful. The child can arrange them in a way that promotes a sense of safety. The therapist may use language like, *"Put the items you have chosen in your Fort Tent exactly where you need them to be. Move them around until it feels just right inside."* See example in Figure 10.1.

Encouraging the child to have a safe space with personal boundaries is important to enhance the feelings of empowerment and choice. *"This is your space, and in this space, you get to have a choice. I will not come in unless invited."* If the child chooses not to invite the therapist in, they can notice what it feels like to not invite an adult in and have the adult be okay with that. The child can choose where the

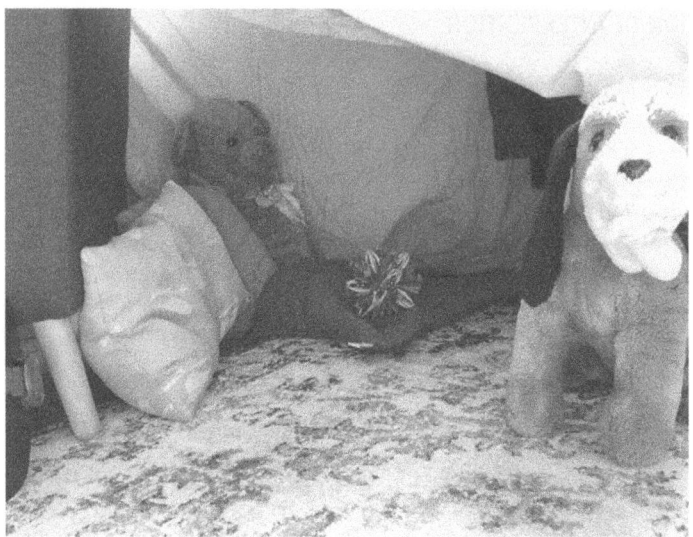

Figure 10.1 *The Inside of the Fort Tent Safe/Calm Place*

therapist should sit by offering, *"If at any time, you want me to leave, you can say, 'I need you to leave my special place, please.'"* This offer can be another way to empower a child to have choice.

Step 4: Once the child is inside the Fort Tent, the therapist teaches the butterfly hug. The butterfly hug helps establish safety through social engagement and rhythm, which is important for calming down the sympathetic nervous system (van der Kolk, 2014).

The child is invited to look around their Fort Tent and do four to six sets of slow BLS. If there is positive feedback between sets, add more sets of slow BLS with the butterfly hug. Once it is enhanced with contextually looking, feeling, and experiencing the present moment in the Fort Tent, the therapist recalls the building of the tent by saying, *"What was it like to ask for help and then have me help you?"* With positive responses or empowered responses, add four to six sets of slow BLS. *"What was it like to choose how big or little your fort is?"* Again, if positive, add four to six sets of slow BLS.

Other examples of questions: Add four to six slow sets with positive or empowering responses. (Note, the therapist does not need to do all of these statements but should choose two or three that most apply.)

"How do you think the stuffed animals feel in the Fort Tent?"
"What was it like to get to choose what goes in your Fort Tent?"
"What was it like to know you didn't have to let me in your Fort Tent?"
"How does it feel with me outside the Fort Tent and you inside the Fort Tent?"
"What is it like having both of us in the Fort Tent?"
"What was it like asking me to get out of your tent and me getting out?"

Possible follow-up responses to their answers to help with awareness and empowerment:

"What tells you that that was a good experience?"

"How do you know that felt good? Is something inside of you telling you it felt good?"

"I'm noticing your body isn't wiggling as much and seems more still, would you like to notice that too?" (For the child who presents as impulsive and fidgeting)

"I'm noticing your legs and arms want to move around a little more than they did before and even your eyes seem to want to look around more. Would you like to notice what that's like to want to move a little more?" (For the child who presents as very rigid and extremely compliant)

Step 5: Enhance the resource that has now been developed. It is advisable that the therapist proceed with caution as to not overstimulate, overwhelm, or cause the child to shut down. The therapist can certainly complete this portion of the intervention in subsequent sessions. Allowing the child to spend the first session developing and experiencing the Fort Tent is plentiful and begins the development of an adaptive memory network.

(The next steps can be done in subsequent sessions.)

Step 6: (Have the child reconstruct the Fort Tent.) Have the child get inside and find a comfortable place to sit or lie down, whichever is most comfortable. The child is invited to close their eyes or stare at one particular place in the Fort Tent. Using imagination, have the child picture themselves inside the Fort Tent. Invite them to imagine where everything is located in the Fort Tent without looking around.

"Imagine what it looks like on the outside, and on the inside, and even where you are lying down. Can you see it?" With positive replies, add four to six slow BLS or invite four to six taps with the butterfly hug. If the child says no, then invite the child to slowly look around, looking at each part of their Fort Tent slowly, almost studying it, while using the butterfly hug. Then go back to the beginning to try to remember all of it using only the imagination. With positive results, add four to six slow BLS.

Step 7: To access the inner experience, invite the child to check inside. If it feels good in the body, the child should notice how thinking about the Fort Tent feels good; add four to six slow BLS. If not, then invite the child to move around the tent and pick up each item and hold it until they find something in the tent that feels good. Wait patiently until the child finds something or a position that they indicates feels good. Add four to six sets of slow BLS.

Step 8: Finally, the child can create a challenge and imagine using the Fort Tent as a resource. This step may not happen until an even later session. First, have the client sit inside the Fort Tent and find a comfortable spot and position. The child should think of a time outside of therapy where they might feel a little nervous or worried. The therapist should wait for a response and may assist by asking questions like, *"I wonder if you feel a little worried when your tummy makes noises you are hungry,"* or *"I wonder if you feel a little nervous when you have a test at school."* Once you have the potential future moment in time where they might feel worried or nervous, the child can imagine the event happening and take a moment to look around and notice the Fort Tent, what the child likes about it, and how it feels to be in there. Ask the client to notice about the worry or nervousness now. If the distress is reduced, encourage the butterfly hug for 4 to 6 slow sets of BLS. If there is no reduction in disturbance, spend a little more time playing there and trying new positions until the positive effect is noticed.

Step 9: Next, invite the client to find another place in your office to sit other than the Fort Tent and then think of a time which might feel negative in the next few days. Considering this worry, the child might even *"feel it right now a little bit."* Then ask permission to try a little trick to see if it helps the negative feeling go away. Ask the child to close their eyes or stare at a place on the floor and imagine they are in their Fort Tent. The therapist may say *"Imagine you are looking around and seeing all the things in your Fort Tent, and that you can even imagine moving around inside the Fort Tent picking up toys and finding the right place to get comfortable."* Give them about 30 seconds to a minute and ask if they can imagine it. If they can, then ask them to check in on the worry and see if it feels different. If it has reduced again, add four to six sets of slow BLS.

MODIFICATIONS

For some clients who are younger or have lower verbal skills, staying with the first five steps of this intervention may be adequate. These particular clients will supply less verbal cues for safety or positive shifts. The therapist will need to watch for more nonverbal cues such as the client relaxing into the pillows, using slower breathing, or being curious about the space that indicates calm.

CONSIDERATIONS

With clients who have had few opportunities to develop adaptive networks of safety, the therapist may need to spend several sessions just developing these networks before beginning to enhance it or test it. For these clients, taking the extra time to ensure a truly felt sense of safety in the Fort Tent will be essential for the later phases of EMDR processing.

In subsequent phases of treatment, the Fort Tent can be used for regulation in a session if needed. It can also be used in Phases 3 to 7 if a client needs added resourcing when processing traumatic memories. The therapist can have the client sit in the Fort Tent to process the memories. This added resource can only be effective in these phases if adequate time has been spent to develop and enhance the resource in previous sessions.

CASE EXAMPLE

Billy* was a 6-year-old, biracial child. He came to treatment as required by family court. He was previously in his mother's custody, but at the time he presented for treatment, he was in his father's custody. His mother had a history of drug and alcohol abuse, a mental health diagnosis which included paranoia and psychotic episodes, and a history of becoming violent. The father had a history of alcohol abuse and depression. Part of the mother's episodes of paranoia included a narrative that the father was trying to kill her and Billy.

Billy presented in therapy as either extremely compliant, sitting rigidly in a seat with hands in his lap, or as fidgety, impulsive, and hyperactive, moving from

---

*In order to protect client confidentiality, the information in this case example has been modified.

one thing to the next in the play therapy room. I recognized early on that Billy had experienced very little sense of safety in his life. Billy was also now living in the custody of the person whom his mother told him was dangerous and out to kill them. I utilized the Fort Tent intervention to begin the process of developing a sense of safety for Billy.

In the fourth therapy session, Billy did not make eye contact, but he slid off his waiting room chair and started toward my office carrying a stuffed toy. He walked in and sat down on a chair, ignoring the toys, and sat rigidly with eyes downcast. I decided to create an opportunity for Billy to feel empowered by asking if it was okay if I introduced myself to his friend. Billy nodded, still not making eye contact. Introducing myself to the stuffed toy, I explained what the therapy room is all about and the simple rules (all the same things I had told Billy in previous sessions). I then asked Billy if he thought his friend might like to help us build something in my office. I explained to Billy that I thought it might be fun to build a fort in my office. I explained to him that it was actually a fort just for him, and that he got to choose where it went, how big it was, and how he wanted it to look. I asked if he would like to give it a try. Still not making eye contact, Billy shrugged but started to look around my office checking out the different corners and open spaces. This let me know he was interested and beginning to engage.

I showed him the big sheets and clamps I had and shared a few pictures of Fort Tents. I explained that we would use these supplies to build his Fort Tent. I said we would be co-leaders on this project but that he got to make all the final decisions. I started by asking him where in my office he would like the Fort Tent to be. Billy looked around the office and pointed to a corner of the office close to the window. I explained that he got to decide how big the fort got to be, how many sheets to use, and which furniture we might pull over to help make the fort, and that my job was to support him by helping move the furniture and putting it in place, or helping drape the sheet and clamp it, and then later by getting items he wanted in the office. Then I asked him if he was ready to start building. He looked at me for the first time in the session, looked away quickly, and reached for the sheet.

He walked away from me and started draping the sheet over a doll house that was nearby. He looked around and saw my office chair, looked away and around my office then back to the chair. I sensed he wanted to use my chair but was too scared to ask. I stated, *"I notice you keep looking at my chair. Remember you can use anything in my office to help build your fort. And you can even use me to help hold things or push things around."* He nodded his head and went over to the office chair and pushed it over to the corner. He lifted one end of the sheet to drape over the chair and it slid off the doll house. He stood back and looked at the sheet and chair and tried draping it again. It slid off the chair this time. I noticed his jaw clench and cheeks turn a little pink indicating that he might be getting agitated. I offered, *"Would you like it if I helped you get this first sheet attached somehow so it will stay up?"* Billy glanced at me and nodded. I walked over and asked, *"Would it be okay if I try to turn the chair around so the back is facing the wall?"* Billy nodded. I moved the chair around so the back was facing the inside of the fort. Then I asked Billy, *"Where should we put the sheet first you think?"* And Billy, talking for the first time said, *"Over the chair."* I draped the sheet over the chair first. I then said, *"It seems to be sliding on this chair. I have these clamps. Would you like me to see if*

I can find a way to clamp the sheet to the chair?" Billy nodded and I showed him how the clamp worked. We attached one on the back of the chair holding the sheet in place. He then picked up the other end of the sheet, draped it over the doll house and then reached for a clamp in my hand. He was able to maneuver it and get it to clamp onto the doll house. I made the observation, *"You catch on to things pretty quickly. Would you like to add another sheet? Or do you like the size we have?"* Billy stepped back and looked at the fort and went over and got the other sheet. He draped it over what we already had up, and asked me to pull over a cart I had in the corner of the room to make the third corner.

I then invited Billy to go into his Fort Tent and explore the inside. I remained on the outside. I noted, *"I will never come into your Fort Tent without your permission to come in. If you ever want me to come in you can say, 'Ms. Alice can you come in?' And you never have to let me in the fort if you do not want. It will not hurt my feelings. This is your Fort Tent and it's important that you know you can feel comfortable and safe inside of it. Also, if you ever do invite me in but you decide you want me to leave, all you have to do is say, 'Ms. Alice, I would like you to leave my Fort Tent,' and I will get out."*

I then invited Billy to choose items from my therapy room he thought might help his Fort Tent feel even more comfortable and safe. Billy crawled out of the tent and walked around the therapy room. He chose a bean bag chair and took it in; then he came out and grabbed a pillow off another seat and took it in. He then chose a large wolf puppet and sat him right outside the opening of the Fort Tent. Billy retrieved the stuffed toy he had brought to therapy. Billy then sat on the bean bag chair, looked around, and sat quietly. I remained on the outside of the Fort Tent. I offered, *"I noticed that you seem relaxed sitting in there and I'm wondering if it feels good to you in there?"* I didn't hear anything and simply said, *"You may have to say the words so I can hear you out here."* He then said, *"Good."* I asked him if he remembered the butterfly hug we had learned in another session, and he said yes. I asked him if he could do that right now while he sat in his fort and looked around, and notice how it feels good. I heard rustling and then slow tapping in the Fort Tent. I asked Billy how the Fort Tent was to him now. He stated *"I really like it."* I could hear a smile in his voice. I invited him to get as comfortable as he could in there and do the butterfly hug one more time. This time I invited him to notice if he smelled anything he liked or heard anything that was special in his Fort Tent. I heard more rustling and then the slow tapping again. After a few seconds, I asked, *"What's it like in there now?"* Billy responded with a yawn and said, *"I feel happy"* a short pause then, *"Can you sit in the door?"*

I moved to the doorway and peeked my head in. I looked around and exclaimed over his work, *"You are quite the handyman! This looks very well built and quite cozy inside."* Billy smiled. I asked Billy if he would like to name his Fort Tent. He thought a minute and said, *"Billy's Fort."* I asked if he would like to say that name out loud while he did the butterfly hug again. He agreed to do it and said his fort name while slowly tapping. He started giggling and picked up his stuffed toy and squeezed it really tight. I decided to do the next stages of the intervention in the next session and spend the remaining time of the session letting Billy just enjoy feeling safe and happy.

In the following session, I reconstructed the Fort Tent before my session with Billy and placed the bean bag chair inside with the pillow and wolf puppet. When I met Billy in the waiting room, he made brief eye contact, hopped off his seat, and led the way to my office. He paused in the door and when he saw his tent still up, he ran into the office and into the tent. I noticed he had brought his furry friend back. *"It seems like this place brings you happiness."* I heard a little giggle in the tent. I did my usual session introduction, only Billy sat in the tent and I sat outside of the tent. I invited Billy to see if he wanted to add anything else to the Fort Tent. He asked if I would sit in the opening again this time; so I did. I asked Billy if he would like to try a little experiment with Billy's Fort. With his agreement, I invited him to get comfy and this time close his eyes. He looked at me nervously and I realized I had introduced a stressor. I simply stated, *"Something I said, maybe it was lying down or closing your eyes seems to have made you nervous all of a sudden."* Billy looked away and nodded. I simply said, *"Remember the rules in here is that there is no hurting. If you would like to keep your eyes open for this to help you feel safer you can do that."* He nodded. I asked him if he would be willing to try our experiment outside of Billy's Fort for a few minutes. He hesitated, but agreed. I invited him to sit in another area of the therapy room and asked him to look at a place on the wall and see if he can imagine being in Billy's Fort. He looked at a place on my wall and focused for a few seconds; then he nodded his head. I asked him to do the butterfly hug while he was imagining being in the fort. As he tapped, I noticed his shoulders relax a little. I said, *"It might not seem as good as being in it, but I wonder if you can see if you can imagine it to where it almost feels like you are in it. And get that feeling as big as you can."* He focused on the spot on the wall. I noticed him tense again as if he was working hard, then I saw him smile and relax. I said, *"I'm noticing you seem happier all of a sudden."* He nodded and then without me saying anything he reached up and did the butterfly hug. I stated, *"How cool is it that you can imagine being in your fort and it can really feel like you are there!"* He smiled. I then asked what he would like to do next, and he crawled back into his Fort Tent. At the end of the session, I reminded him that he could imagine being in the Billy's Fort when he is at school or at home and he might be feeling nervous or scared about something. I asked if he'd like to imagine being in his fort at night before bed. He nodded his head.

By the eighth session, I had introduced EMDR therapy to Billy and his family. Billy and I had already chosen the targets to work on; we had identified the negative cognitions and he was more familiar with emotion words and body awareness. In this session, we had agreed together to start processing one of his target memories. In the session, Billy entered the office and went into his Fort Tent. He had been asking me to come in for the last two sessions. I still waited outside the tent until he asked. When he did, I sat in the entrance. I handed Billy my little stop sign (this was introduced in a previous session when introducing the mechanics of EMDR to Billy and the tools used. The small stop signal is a tangible stop signal my clients use to indicate they want to stop in processing.) I reminded Billy what we had discussed and agreed to work on with EMDR in this session. Billy got comfortable in his Fort Tent. I used the thera-tappers for BLS. We completed Phases 3 to 7 processing in the Fort Tent. The Fort Tent had been used for several sessions and continued to strengthen in the adaptive networks. Evidence of this resource was seen in the sessions where Billy was more interactive and relaxed. His father reported he was sleeping better at night and that he regularly reminded Billy to imagine his Fort Tent before bed. The father also reported that Billy seemed less agitated at home and more relaxed in his posture. By developing and strengthening this resource and then using the resource specifically in reprocessing phases, Billy was able to smoothly process the traumatic memories in a safe way.

REFERENCES

Jarero, I., Artigas, L., Mauer, M., López Cano, T., & Alcalá, N. (1999, November). *Children's post-traumatic stress after natural disasters: Integrative treatment protocol.* Poster presented at the annual meeting of the International Society for Traumatic Stress Studies, Miami, FL.

Jarero, I., Artigas, L., & Montero, M. (2008). The EMDR integrative group treatment protocol: Application with child victims of mass disaster. *Journal of EMDR Practice and Research, 2,* 97–105. doi:10.1891/1933-3196.2.2.97

Levine, P. A. (1997). *Waking the tiger: Healing trauma.* Berkeley, CA: North Atlantic Books.

Levine, P. A. (2007). *Trauma through a child's eyes: Awakening the ordinary miracle of healing.* Berkeley, CA: North Atlantic Books.

Schore, A. (2003). *Affective dysregulation and disorders of the self.* New York, NY: W. W. Norton.

Shapiro, F. (2001). *Eye movement desensitization and reprocessing: Basic principles, protocols, and procedures.* New York, NY: Guilford Press.

Siegel, D. (2012). *The developing mind: How relationships and the brain interact to shape who we are* (2nd ed.). New York, NY: Guilford Press.

Van Der Kolk, B. (2014). *The body keeps the score.* New York, NY: Penguin Group.

11

Using Trauma-Sensitive Yoga and Embodied Play Therapy for Stabilization and Resourcing

JENNIFER LEFEBRE

INTRODUCTION

Trauma-sensitive yoga and embodied play therapy blend well with eye movement desensitization and reprocessing (EMDR) therapy to address the preverbal and somatic challenges often associated with children who have experienced complex trauma. In order to demonstrate how to best integrate embodied play therapy and trauma-sensitive yoga techniques into the preparation phase of EMDR therapy, this chapter presents an overview of trauma and the brain–body connection, yoga, and play therapy. In addition, specific trauma-sensitive yoga and embodied play therapy exercises are presented that can be used with children during the preparation phase of EMDR.

PHASE OF EMDR

Preparation (Phase 2)

MATERIALS

- Sticky bubbles
- Pom-poms
- Yoga mat
- Animal pictures
- Toy ice-cream cone

RATIONALE

Trauma and the Brain–Body Connection

The term *complex trauma* has been coined to encompass both the nature of a survivor's exposure to multiple, prolonged traumatic events and its long-term developmental outcomes, with the consequences on development and overall functioning becoming more severe as the frequency and severity of traumatic events increases in a child's life (Cook, Blaustein, Spinazzola, & van der Kolk, 2003; Herman, 1992; National Child Traumatic Stress Network [NCTSN], 2014; Stolbach et al, 2013; van der Kolk, 2005). The human brain is organized in a hierarchical manner, with the lower brain (i.e., brainstem and diencephalon) developing first, mediating the simpler, more regulatory functions, which facilitates the development of more complex and executive functions within the limbic and cortical areas of the brain. When a child is exposed to traumatic stress prenatally or early in life (particularly stressors imposed by their primary attachment figures), there is a shift in the activation of the brain in regard to cognitive, social, emotional, and motor functioning, thus disrupting and dysregulating higher cortical functioning (Perry, 2001, 2006; van der Kolk, 2014). Traumatic experiences are primarily stored and processed in the body and the sensory networks of the brain, rather than the higher functions (i.e., hippocampus and verbal declarative memory), leading to a lack of narrative memory or rational thought (Ogden & Minton, 2000; van der Kolk, 2014). When the memories of trauma and adversity are activated by environmental stimuli, children will see their environment through the lenses of these memory networks and as a result will provide an inaccurate assessment of the situation in terms of danger and safety. This "faulty neuroception" (Porges, 2004) may activate the defense system in situations that may be in fact safe or, on the contrary, inhibit defense responses in environments that are actually risky.

The prefrontal cortex and Broca's area go *off-line*, with the amygdala and medial prefrontal cortex becoming reactive. The ability to reason and put thoughts and feelings into words fails; emotions, impulsivity, and hypervigilance take over, and everything becomes a threat. The amygdala, which is involved in the processing of emotions such as fear, anger, and pleasure, in part fuels the *fight-or-flight* responses (Gaskill & Perry, 2012; Ogden, Minton, & Pain, 2006; Perry, 2009) (Table 11.1).

The sympathetic nervous system engages during stress, with catecholamines, hormones, and neurotransmitters flooding our system. The parasympathetic nervous system, served by the vagus nerve, balances and calms the sympathetic active part. It also fuels the *freeze-or-faint* responses and at times moves us into immobility or dissociation (Porges, 2004; van der Kolk, 2005). The parasympathetic nervous system, according to the polyvagal theory, also employs the social engagement system, a mixture of activation and calming that may contribute to the *fawn-or-fool around/fidget* response (Porges, 2004; van der Kolk, 2005).

Keeping children within optimal arousal states where dual awareness can take place is pivotal to the assimilation of memory systems (Shapiro, 2001, 2018). The concept of the *window of tolerance* (optimal level of arousal) was conceptualized by Dan Siegel (1999) and highlights the capacity to tolerate various intensities of arousal or the ability to perceive, process, and react to sensory stimuli and

Table 11.1 *The 6Fs of Faulty Neuroception*

Fight	Flight	Freeze
• Sympathetic nervous system • Hands (clenched, fists, punch, rip) • Legs and feet (stomp, kick, smash) • Flexed/tight jaw, grinding teeth • Glaring eyes, snarl in voice • Feelings of anger/rage • Homicidal/suicidal feelings • Metaphors like bombs, volcanoes erupting	• Sympathetic nervous system • Hands (tapping, fluttering) • Legs and feet (restless, numbness, jumpy) • Shallow breathing • Big/darting eyes • Feeling trapped • Sense of running in life • Elopement or escape/avoidant behavior	• Parasympathetic nervous system • Dorsal vagal nerve • Sense of stiffness, heaviness • Feeling stuck in some part of body • Feeling cold/frozen, numb, pale skin • Holding breath/restricted breathing • Sense of dread, heart pounding • Decreased heart rate • Orientation to threat
Faint	**Fawn**	**Fool Around and Fidget**
• Parasympathetic nervous system • Dorsal vagal nerve • Child begins in freeze • Hypoarousal continues • Child emotionally or physically collapses • Dissociation occurs • Completely disconnected from reality • Other reactions may take place at this time given the dissociative response	• Parasympathetic nervous system • Social engagement system • Merge wishes and demands of others • Stockholm syndrome • Identification with the abuser • Codependency and compliance to increase safety	• Parasympathetic nervous system • Social engagement system • Playfulness • Use of humor • Physiological responses (farting, burping, hiccups) • Self-soothing or stimulation (head-banging, masturbation, hair pulling, scratching, self-biting)

Adapted from Gaskill, R. L., & Perry, B. D. (2012). Child sexual abuse, traumatic experiences, and their impact on the developing brain. In P. Goodyear-Brown (Ed.), *Handbook of child sexual abuse: Identification, assessment, and treatment* (pp. 30–47). Hoboken, NJ: Wiley; Ogden, P., Minton, K., & Pain, C. (2006). *Trauma and the body: A sensorimotor approach to psychotherapy*. New York, NY: W. W. Norton; Perry, B. D. (2009). Examining child maltreatment through a neurodevelopmental lens: Clinical application of the neurosequential model of therapeutics. *Journal of Loss and Trauma, 14*, 240–255. doi:10.1080/15325020903004350; Porges, S. W. (2004). Neuroception: A subconscious system for detecting threats and safety. *Zero to Three, 24*(5), 19–24. Retrieved from https://static1.squarespace.com/static/5c1d025fb27e390a78569537/t/5ccdff181905f41dbcb689e3/1557004058168/Neuroception.pdf; van der Kolk, B. A. (2005). Developmental trauma disorder: Toward a rational diagnosis for children with complex trauma histories. *Psychiatric Annals, 35*(5), 401–408

information in a timely manner (Ogden & Minton, 2000; van der Kolk, 2014). It is congruent with the notion of "dual awareness" brought up by Shapiro (1995), when the child can maintain present and mindful awareness while accessing the memories of trauma and adversity in order to reprocess. When a child is hyperresponsive (i.e., overresponsive or hypersensitive), a minimal amount of stimulation of the amygdala activates the cerebral cortex, and they are extremely sensitive to sensory input and can easily go into sensory overload. A child who is hyporesponsive (i.e., underresponsive or hyposensitive) has low amygdala activity, indicating they need a greater amount of sensory stimulation to trigger the cortex. Many times, these children misinterpret or misidentify bodily sensations, or how those sensations are associated with emotions. *Interoception* is the sense of knowing what is going on inside of the body, or the physiological condition of one's body, such as feeling hunger, thirst, tired, pain, temperature, using the bathroom, and other internal sensations (Moroz, 2005; Ogden & Gomez, 2013; Ogden & Minton, 2000).

PLAY THERAPY, YOGA, AND EMDR

Play therapy allows children to develop a rich variety of resources for complex trauma. Making a safe therapeutic space for the activation and the adaptive processing of traumatic memories has been a central theme in play therapy literature (Gil, 2016; Goodyear-Brown, 2019). Over the past two decades, integration of EMDR and play therapy has been a focus of many child trauma therapists (Adler-Tapia & Settle, 2008, 2017; Gomez, 2012; Greenwald, 1999; McGuinness, 2001). Embodied play therapy techniques, more specifically those that integrate trauma-sensitive yoga, allow children to develop a rich variety of resources for stabilization and affect regulation during the preparation phase of EMDR.

In the preparation phase of EMDR, children are establishing an appropriate therapeutic relationship, learning more about EMDR, and identifying and ensuring their readiness to move further through the phases. Children are learning additional grounding, stress reduction, and state change skills, which meld well with yoga and embodied play therapy. Bilateral stimulation (BLS), the back-and-forth eye movements, sounds, or tactile sensations that help the right and left hemispheres to process the traumatic material and activate the brain's adaptive information processing (AIP) system are explained during this phase, and children should be offered metaphors to understand trauma and encourage successful processing. They must learn self-regulation techniques in order to deal with the disturbing information that may arise during and between sessions (Gomez & Jernberg, 2013; Shapiro, 2018). Additionally, the child will learn about positive cognition (PC) and negative cognition (NC) as well as interoceptive cues to assist in the body scan in future sessions.

Of particular importance is the child's ability to feel contained, the creation of a calm/happy place, and the development of resources. Competency is compatible with resource development and installation (RDI) building and essential in the treatment of childhood trauma (Blaustein & Kinniburgh, 2007, 2010; Korn & Leeds, 2002), with goals to access and install a positive resource (e.g., bravery, confidence, assertiveness). Teaching emotional regulation, grounding, breathing, and mindfulness are all part of stabilization and resourcing, and trauma-sensitive yoga and embodied play therapy are ideal strategies to enhance EMDR in the preparation phase.

According to Perry (2006), if a child is provided with patterned, repetitive, rhythmic input via child-directed free play and somatosensory routes, they will feel safer and become more regulated, thereby assisting the child's availability for therapeutic change. The somatosensory experiences in many play activities have been viewed as the neurological foundations for later advanced mental skills, such as creativity, abstract thought, prosocial behavior, and expressive language. Accordingly, play therapists will often need to use bottom-up modulatory networks (somatosensory) to establish some moderate self-regulation prior to the implementation of insightful reflection, trauma experience integration, narrative development, social development, or affect enhancement. Doing so will require therapeutic methods to access and provide reorganizing input to the regulatory networks of the lower brain areas (Kleim & Jones, 2008; Perry, 2008, 2009).

Yoga has been increasingly studied as an adjunctive treatment modality for anxiety, chronic stress, and complex trauma reactions (e.g., Kirkwood, Rampes, Richardson, Pilkington, & Ramaratnam, 2005; Spinazzolla, Rhodes, Emerson, Earle, & Monroe, 2011; Telles, Singh, Joshi, & Balkrishna, 2010). The practice of yoga helps to calm the central nervous system, decreasing the physiological and biochemical byproducts of stress. Trauma-sensitive yoga (TSY) offers a platform for body-based interventions that emphasize integration of the mind and body when treating trauma-related disorders by utilizing somatically based bottom-up processing to build internal strengths and resources in a manner that cannot be accessed through talk therapy alone (Duros & Crowley, 2014; Emerson & Hopper, 2011; Emerson, Sharma, Chaudry, & Turner, 2009). TSY connects with the therapeutic powers of play of self-regulation, positive emotions, stress management, resiliency, and the therapeutic relationship (Schaefer & Drewes, 2013). Bringing embodied play into EMDR work, therefore, not only makes sense; it is often an essential element for therapeutic progress. TSY and embodied play therapy blend well with EMDR to address the preverbal and somatic challenges often associated with children who have experienced complex trauma.

INTERVENTIONS

TSY DEEP BREATHING FOR CO-REGULATION

Lion-Kitty

Step 1: Introduce intervention to client/family, explaining that deep breathing increases co--regulation, allowing for the development of self-regulation and the understanding of state change.

Step 2: Roll out a yoga mat and have the client kneel in front of the clinician or their caregiver.

Step 3: Using mirroring, the clinician/caregiver should take a deep breath and breathe out while growling like a lion. (See Figure 11.1; demonstration by a young friend, not a client.) Hands can be waved gently on either side of the face to mimic a lion's mane.

Step 4: After taking another deep breath, both client and caregiver/clinician would stretch forward into child's form (bottoms on heels, belly toward knees, chin toward floor, arms reaching out).

Step 5: Using mirroring, the clinician/caregiver should take a deep breath and breathe out while meowing/purring like a kitten.

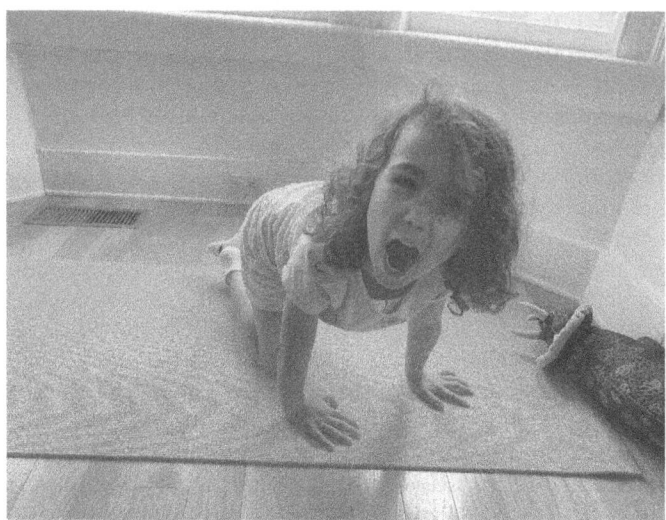

Figure 11.1 *Lion-Kitty Form in Yoga With Children*

Bubble Piles

Step 1: Introduce intervention to client/family, explaining that deep breathing increases co-regulation, allowing for the development of self-regulation.
Step 2: Hand sticky bubbles to client and caregiver.
Step 3: Bubbles should be blown back and forth to encourage diaphragmatic breathing.
Step 4: Bubbles can be "caught" with the goal of growing the largest pile possible, with the bubbles sticking together.

Pass a Breath

Step 1: Introduce intervention to client/family, explaining that deep breathing increases co-regulation, allowing for the development of attunement and connection while further developing regulatory capacities.
Step 2: Hand a large pom-pom to the client's caregiver.
Step 3: The caregiver should place the pom-pom in their hand and place their hands together and assist the client with placing their hands together.
Step 4: The pom-pom should be blown back and forth between client and caregiver in a slow, controlled manner.

Be Spaghetti

Step 1: Introduce intervention to client/family, explaining that a quick progression of tightening and loosening muscles in the body leads to the activation of the sympathetic and parasympathetic nervous systems, thus increasing regulation, grounding, and the ability to shift states.

Step 2: Have the client stand tall in mountain form, with feet shoulder width apart and arms raised above head.
Step 3: Clinician has client tighten each muscle from head to toe, squeezing tightly…like uncooked spaghetti.
Step 4: Client is instructed to loosely wiggle out all of their body (arms, legs, hips) like a cooked spaghetti noodle. Client is told to "shake out the worries."

Noodle Hug

Step 1: Introduce intervention to client/family, explaining that slow bilateral stimulation and midline crossing lead to an activation of the parasympathetic nervous system, increasing regulation, grounding, and the ability to shift states.
Step 2: Client is instructed to twist their arms around their body to give themselves a "noodle hug," providing their own slow BLS by tapping opposite hips as they slowly twist back and forth.

Fight-or-Flight Charades

Step 1: Introduce intervention to client/family, explaining 6Fs (fight, flight, freeze, faint, fawn, fool around/fidget) and the importance of understanding how our brain responds during a trauma or adverse event or stressor.
Step 2: Using Dan Siegel's (2010) hand model of the brain to assist in psychoeducation, the clinician should briefly explain how the brain responds during a stressor. This is an elementary explanation that can be used for all ages. The clinician should hold their hand in a fist, with thumb locked inside, and then flip up all fingers, revealing their thumb across their palm.
"This is the part of our brain…the prefrontal cortex… (point to fingers in closed fist) that helps us think and make decisions. It is the upstairs part of our brain. It helps us keep our bodies under control, and balances our emotions, and helps us understand the emotions of others. It is still growing until we are in our mid-20s! When we get stressed out, this upstairs part of our brain flips (clinician flips up fingers and points to thumb), *and we are in the downstairs part of our brain…the amygdala…the part of the brain that helps us breathe, where our emotions rule over everything!"*
Step 3: Using an integration of several neuroscience theories (Gaskill & Perry, 2012; Ogden et al., 2006; Perry, 2009; Porges, 2004; van der Kolk, 2005), the clinician will briefly discuss the 6Fs (fight, flight, freeze, faint, fawn, fool around/fidget) by employing animal metaphors with corresponding pictures, to assist in psychoeducation. This is an elementary explanation that can be used for all ages. If the client has shown a preference for certain animals, this should be adapted to those animals wherever possible.
"When we are in the downstairs part of our brain, we might respond in a lot of different ways. Some people are like a bunny rabbit and scurry away and hide (flight). Others are like opossums, and they seem disconnected…like they're not even there (faint). Have you heard of a deer in headlights? Some people aren't able to do anything…they are frozen (freeze). Others become a tiger, snarling and fighting their way to safety (fight). Some people become wiggle worms, and they may use playfulness or do things with their bodies

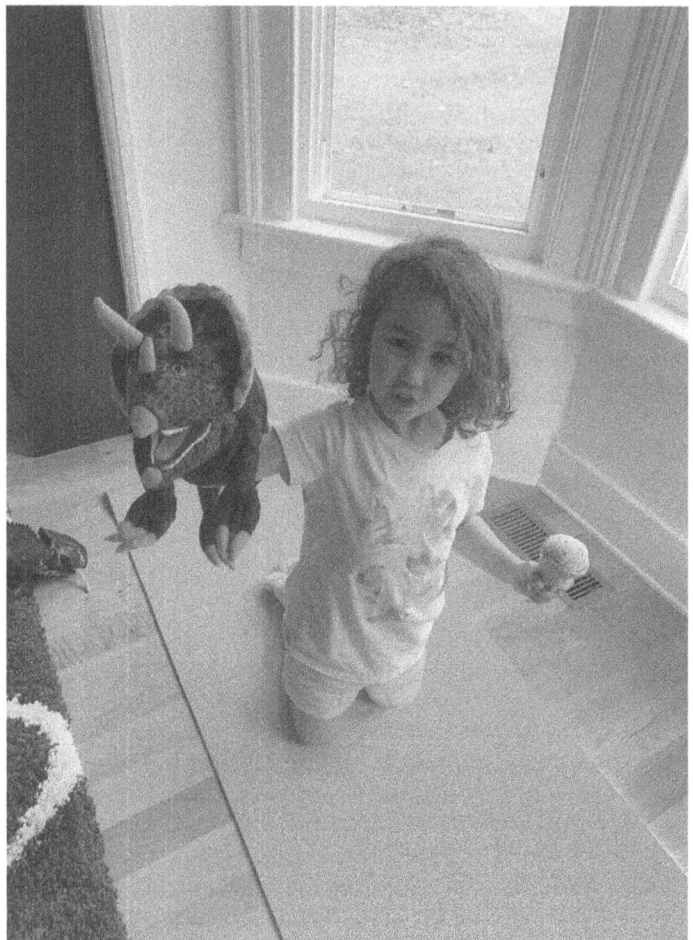

Figure 11.2 *Introduction of 6F Charades With Children*

to try to feel better (fool around and fidget). Lastly, do you know what a chameleon is? They change colors...to adapt to their surroundings. Some people change their behavior to match the stressful situation they are in (fawn). Many people can be different animals at different times, and sometimes we want to be two animals at once!"

Step 3: The clinician will demonstrate the 6Fs (fight, flight, freeze, faint, fawn, fool around/fidget) via an embodied play activity. The clinician will ask the caregiver to hand them an ice cream cone and then engage in a dramatic enactment of responding with one of the 6Fs. The client will verbalize or point to which of the Fs is being acted out. See Figure 11.2 (demonstration by a young friend, not a client).

Step 4: The client and caregiver will play a game of charades, acting out the 6Fs. Interoceptive cues, such as *"When you are a (animal), show me what your hands do?"* or *"Wow, your (body art) did ____ when you were a wiggle worm* (see Figure 11.3; demonstration by a young friend, not a client) *and ____ when you were a tiger,"* should be used to create mastery with these embodied play therapy activities.

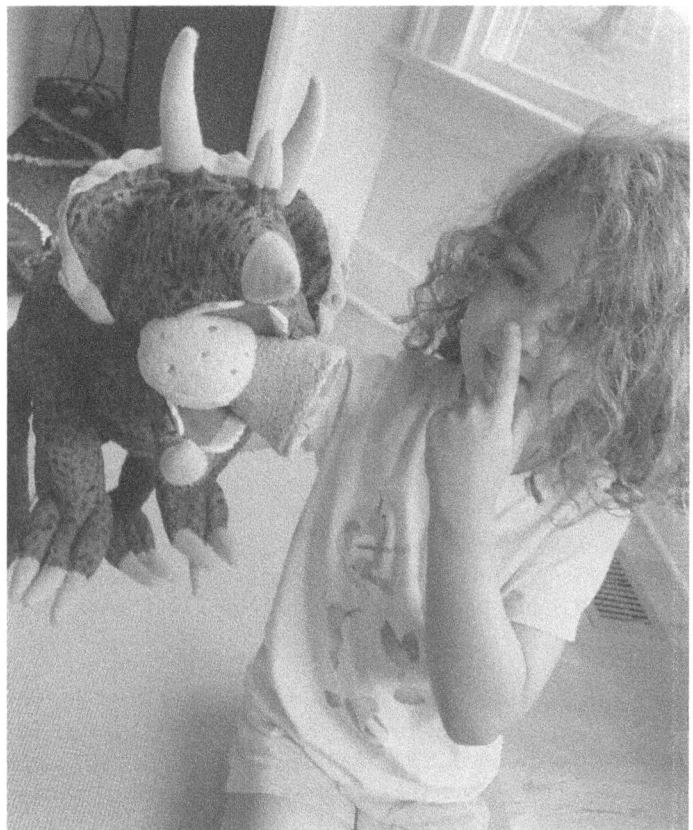

Figure 11.3 *Wiggle Worm (6Fs) Form in Yoga With Children*

Walk Like a...

Step 1: Introduce intervention to client/family, explaining how the 6Fs can be used to change how our brain and body respond during a stressor. The goal of this intervention is to access and install a positive resource or state (e.g., bravery, confidence, assertiveness), building competency.

Step 2: After the client has practiced all embodied responses, they can begin to shift responses to other triggers, gradually going up the scale.

"Now that you've shown me all of the animals, I'd like (caregiver) *to tell me about a time when you were a little bit scared/mad/sad. Great! So in that situation, your body was a* (tiger, fawn, etc.). *Let's think about that, and see what it would be like if we were an* (opossum, deer, etc.)." *See Figure 11.4 for the 'opossum' form* (demonstration by a young friend, not a client).

Step 3: After the client has engaged in embodied play therapy and shown they can shift their behavioral response, building resources can occur, and the client can pick an animal or figure that they can embody to handle one of their targets. This can be anything that would elicit feelings of bravery, assertiveness, strength, and so forth.

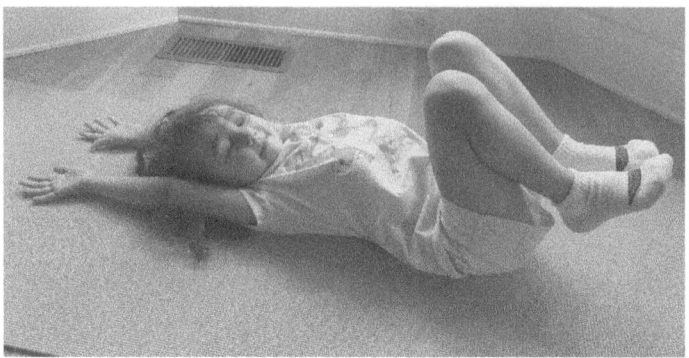

Figure 11.4 *Opossum Form (6Fs) in Yoga With Children*

"Now that you've shown me how all of the animals could respond in real situations, I'd like us to find an animal or figure that might be able to help you when you are scared/mad/sad. Great! So how would this (animal/figure) sound? Walk? Where might it live? Let's think about that, and practice what it would be like if we were an (animal/figure)."

Step 4: Once the client has demonstrated mastery over this embodied play experience, slow BLS can be utilized to strengthen and install this positive resource.

Modifications and Considerations: If a child/parent has breathing restrictions, deep breath work could cause lightheadedness. Embodied play could be modified to a seated position as needed for mobility purposes. Some activities have the potential for dysregulation given the activation of the nervous system.

CASE EXAMPLE

The following case example demonstrates TSY and embodied play therapy exercises that can be used with children during the preparation phase of EMDR, focusing on teaching children how to autoregulate and also on their ability to learn interoceptive cues in order to prepare them for the processing phase of EMDR.

Seamus* was a 3-1/2-year-old boy who had been sucked under the water and pulled down the hallway out of reach of caregivers after a water main exploded in his day care. He had previously been an outgoing, cheerful, secure little boy. Following the flooding incident, Seamus developed significant separation anxiety, fear of his day care, and an intense fear of water, to include sinks/toilets, bathing, drinking water, and the rain. He would freeze or run away and hide when having to leave his mother or the house. Seamus's mother wanted to alleviate his fear of water and assist him in eliminating his fear of his day care (it should be noted he needed to continue to attend there while the building was being fixed, as she was a single mother and there were no other options for childcare).

From an EMDR perspective, the goal for Seamus was to reprocess the memories of the flooding incident, and his memories of being sucked under the water and separated from his day-care worker were placed in his targeting sequence

---

*In order to protect client confidentiality, the information in this case example has been modified.

and treatment plan. Developing Seamus's ability to regulate affect and his capacity to reconnect to his secure base were primary goals. This writer decided to incorporate TSY and embodied play therapy activities to soothe Seamus's nervous system to increase regulatory capacities, and integrated his mother in all sessions to restore trust and connection with her.

Seamus and his mother were taught full-body deep breathing to increase co-regulation, allowing for the development of self-regulation and the understanding of state change. Lion's breath and child's form were used, and Seamus mirrored his mother by kneeling in front of her, taking a deep breath, and growling/breathing out like a lion. They then would stretch forward into child's form, keeping their bottoms on their heels, and reaching out their arms, meowing/purring like a kitten. Sticky bubbles were blown back and forth to encourage diaphragmatic breathing. They were then "caught" with the goal of growing the largest pile possible, with the bubbles sticking together. Additionally, Seamus and his mother would blow a pom-pom into each other's hands to increase attunement and connection while further developing regulatory capacities. These playful breathing games were used at the beginning and end of each session to help Seamus stay within his window of tolerance.

Seamus was drawn toward the sand tray and created worlds where storms, water, small animals, and a brontosaurus interacted. He was invited to create a calm/happy place and other resources in the sand tray. The small animals found safety within the sand tray worlds, and Seamus was able to express and bring into the external world the adaptive memory networks held by him. Although never verbalized, his NC was "I'm in danger" and his PC was "I'm safe now."

Given his age, verbalizations were limited while engaging in EMDR or play therapy. By following the metaphors observed in Seamus's play, it was evident that he saw the dinosaur as being strong and brave. This became the avenue for embodied play therapy and TSY to be integrated within EMDR. In the preparation phase, the therapist is trying to provide the child the resources and skills to proceed through the trauma and engage in healthy information processing. The dinosaur was used as a resource for Seamus through several embodied play exercises, and slow BLS was applied during sand tray play, and embodied play techniques when appropriate.

As previously stated, Seamus would not leave home or would run away (freeze and flee response) after the flooding incident. Seamus's mother described multiple situations where she was proud of Seamus for being brave and walking like a dinosaur, prior to the flooding. This writer used the hand model of the brain (Siegel, 2010) to briefly explain how the brain responds during a stressor, and then demonstrated the 6Fs (fight, flight, freeze, faint, fawn, fool around/fidget) via an embodied play activity. Seamus's mother offered this writer an ice cream cone, and this writer engaged in a dramatic response of responding with the 6Fs. Seamus was able to run away, pretend to be frozen or pass out and drop to the floor, and then walk like a dinosaur to get the ice cream. These embodied play therapy activities created mastery and interoception, as he was able to demonstrate an understanding of how his body was activated. Slow BLS was utilized to strengthen the positive state found by walking like a dinosaur and his mother's statements, increasing Seamus's connection with his mother and competency within himself. In order to address the targeting sequence, Seamus walked like a dinosaur with BLS, while his mom and this writer discussed the flooding incident and reminding him that he was safe now. When Seamus would become activated, he was taught to "be spaghetti" and shake his worries away. He learned to tighten his muscles and release them, shaking out his worries by twisting his arms around his body to give himself a "noodle hug," providing himself with his own BLS by tapping opposite hips as he slowly twisted back and forth.

Seamus began to add water to the sand tray, and the small animals found safety with the help of the brontosaurus. His fear of water began to subside, and he would breathe like a lion while taking baths, and walk like a dinosaur into the bathroom at his house. He began to walk like a dinosaur while leaving therapy sessions…progressing to being able to enter his school and separating from his mother without severe anxiety. His mother indicated that Seamus was back to his spirited self, and he was again the outgoing, cheerful, secure little boy he was prior to the flooding incident.

REFERENCES

Adler-Tapia, R. L., & Settle, C. S. (2008). *EMDR and the art of psychotherapy with children: Treatment manual and text*. New York, NY: Springer Publishing Company.

Adler-Tapia, R. L., & Settle, C. S. (2017). *EMDR and the art of psychotherapy with children: Infants to adolescents*. New York, NY: Springer Publishing Company.

Blaustein, M. E., & Kinniburgh, K. (2007). Intervention beyond the child: The intertwining nature of attachment and trauma. *British Psychological Society Briefing Paper, 26*, 48–53. Retrieved from http://www.traumacenter.org/clients/Intertwining_Nature_of_Attachment_and_Trauma.pdf

Blaustein, M. E., & Kinniburgh, K. (2010). *Treating traumatic stress in children and adolescents: How to foster resilience through attachment, self-regulation, and competency*. New York, NY: Guilford Press.

Cook, A., Blaustein, M., Spinazzola, J., & van der Kolk, B. A. (Eds.). (2003). Complex trauma in children and adolescents. *National Child Traumatic Stress Network*. Retrieved from http://www.nctsnet.org

Duros, P., & Crowley, D. (2014). The body comes to therapy too. *Clinical Social Work Journal, 42*(3), 237–246. doi:10.1007/s10615-014-0486-1

Emerson, D., & Hopper, E. (2011). *Overcoming trauma through yoga: Reclaiming your body*. Berkeley, CA: North Atlantic Books.

Emerson, D., Sharma, R., Chaudry, S., & Turner, J. (2009). Yoga therapy in practice: Trauma-sensitive yoga: Principles, practice, and research. *International Journal of Yoga Therapy, 19*, 123–128. Retrieved from http://www.traumacenter.org/products/pdf_files/IJYT_article_2009.pdf

Gaskill, R. L., & Perry, B. D. (2012). Child sexual abuse, traumatic experiences, and their impact on the developing brain. In P. Goodyear-Brown (Ed.), *Handbook of child sexual abuse: Identification, assessment, and treatment* (pp. 30–47). Hoboken, NJ: Wiley.

Gil, E. (2016). *Posttraumatic play in children: What clinicians need to know*. New York, NY: Guilford Press.

Gomez, A. M. (2012). *EMDR therapy and adjunct approaches with children*. New York, NY: Springer Publishing Company.

Gomez, A. M., & Jernberg, E. (2013). Using EMDR therapy and theraplay. In A. M. Gomez (Ed.), *EMDR therapy and adjunct approaches with children*. New York, NY: Springer Publishing Company.

Goodyear-Brown, P. (2019). *Trauma and play therapy: Helping children heal*. New York, NY: Routledge.

Greenwald, R. (1999). *EMDR in child and adolescent psychotherapy*. Northvale, NJ: Jason Aronson.

Herman, J. L. (1992). Complex PTSD: A syndrome in survivors of prolonged and repeated trauma. *Journal of Traumatic Stress, 5*(3), 377–391. doi:10.1002/jts.24900050305

Kirkwood, G., Rampes, H., Tuffrey, V., Richardson, J., & Pilkington, K. (2005). Yoga for anxiety: A systematic review of the research evidence. *British Journal of Sports Medicine, 39*(12), 884–891. doi:10.1136/bjsm.2005.018069

Kleim, J. A., & Jones, T. A. (2008). Principles of experience-dependent neural plasticity: Implications for rehabilitation after brain damage. *Journal of Speech, Language, and Hearing Research, 51*, S225–S239. doi:10.1044/1092-4388(2008/018)

Korn, D. L., & Leeds, A. M. (2002). Preliminary evidence of efficacy of EMDR resource development and installation in the stabilization phase of treatment of complex posttraumatic stress disorder. *Journal of Clinical Psychology, 58*(12), 1465–1487. doi:10.1002/jclp.10099

McGuinness, V. (2001). *Integrating play therapy and EMDR with children*. Bloomington, IN: Author House.

Moroz, K. J. (2005). *The effects of psychological trauma on children and adolescents*. Vermont Agency of Human Services. Retrieved from https://kuswoyoaji.files.wordpress.com/2014/01/dmh-cafu_psychological_trauma_moroz.pdf

National Child Traumatic Stress Network. (2014). *Complex trauma*. Retrieved from http://www.nctsn.org/trauma-types/complex-trauma

Ogden, P., & Gomez, A. M. (2013). EMDR therapy and sensorimotor psychotherapy with children. In A. M. Gomez (Eds.), *EMDR therapy and adjunct approaches with children*. New York, NY: Springer Publishing Company.

Ogden, P., & Minton, K. (2000). Sensorimotor psychotherapy: One method for processing traumatic memory. *Traumatology, 6*(3), 149–173. doi:10.1177/153476560000600302

Ogden, P., Minton, K., & Pain, C. (2006). *Trauma and the body: A sensorimotor approach to psychotherapy*. New York, NY: W. W. Norton.

Perry, B. D. (2001). The neuroarcheology of childhood maltreatment: The neurodevelopmental costs of adverse childhood events. In K. Franey, R. Geffner, & R. Falconer (Eds.), *The cost of maltreatment: Who pays? We all do* (pp. 15–37). San Diego, CA: Family Violence and Sexual Assault Institute.

Perry, B. D. (2006). Applying principles of neurodevelopment to clinical work with maltreated and traumatized children. In N. B. Webb (Ed.), *Working with traumatized youth in child welfare* (pp. 27–52). New York, NY: Guilford Press.

Perry, B. D. (2008). Child maltreatment: The role of abuse and neglect in developmental psychopathology. In T. P. Beauchaine & S. P. Henshaw (Eds.), *Textbook of child and adolescent psychopathology* (pp. 93–128). New York, NY: Wiley.

Perry, B. D. (2009). Examining child maltreatment through a neurodevelopmental lens: Clinical application of the neurosequential model of therapeutics. *Journal of Loss and Trauma, 14*, 240–255. doi:10.1080/15325020903004350

Porges, S. W. (2004). Neuroception: A subconscious system for detecting threats and safety. *Zero to Three, 24*(5), 19–24.

Schaefer, C. E., & Drewes, A. A. (2013). *The therapeutic powers of play: 20 core agents of change* (2nd ed.). New York, NY: Wiley.

Shapiro, F. (1995). *Eye movement desensitization and reprocessing: Basic principles, protocols and procedures*. New York, NY: Guilford Press.

Shapiro, F. (2001). *Eye movement desensitization and reprocessing: Basic principles, protocols and procedures* (2nd ed.). New York, NY: Guilford Press.

Shapiro, F. (2018). *Eye movement desensitization and reprocessing: Basic principles, protocols and procedures* (3rd ed.). New York, NY: Guilford Press.
Siegel, D. J. (1999). *The developing mind: Toward a neurobiology of interpersonal experience.* New York, NY: Guilford Press.
Siegel, D. J. (2010). *The mindful therapist: A clinician's guide to mindsight and neural integration.* New York, NY: W. W. Norton.
Spinazolla, J., Rhodes, A. M., Emerson, D., Earle, E., & Monroe, K. (2011). Application of yoga in residential treatment of traumatized youth. *Journal of the American Psychiatric Nurses Association, 17*(6), 431–444. doi:10.1177/1078390311418359
Stolbach, B. C., Reese, M., Rompala, V., Dominguez, R. Z., Gazibara, T., & Finke, R. (2013). Complex trauma exposure and symptoms in urban traumatized children: A preliminary test of proposed criteria for developmental trauma disorder. *Journal of Traumatic Stress, 26,* 1–9. doi:10.1002/jts.21826
Telles, S., Singh, N., Joshi, M., & Balkrishna, A. (2010). Posttraumatic stress symptoms and heart rate variability in Bihar flood survivors following yoga: A randomized controlled study. *BCM Psychiatry, 10*(18), 1–10. doi:10.1186/1471-244X-10-18
van der Kolk, B. A. (2006). Clinical implications of neuroscience research in PTSD. *Annals of the New York Academy of Science, 107*(IV), 277–293.
van der Kolk, B. A. (2014). *The body keeps the score: Brain, mind, and body in the healing of trauma.* New York, NY: Viking.

RECOMMENDED FURTHER READING

Berger, D. L., Silver, E. J., & Stein, R. E. (2009). Effects of yoga on inner-city children's wellbeing: A pilot study. *Alternative Therapies in Health and Medicine, 15*(5), 36–42.
Drewes, A. A. (2005). Play in selected cultures: Diversity and universality. In E. Gil & A. A. Drewes (Eds.), *Cultural issues in play therapy* (pp. 26–71). New York, NY: Guilford Press.
Landreth, G. (2002). *Play therapy: The art of the relationship* (2nd ed.). New York, NY: Routledge.
Marteau, T. M., Hollands, G. J., & Fletcher, P. C. (2012). Changing human behavior to prevent disease: The importance of targeting automatic processes. *Science, 337*(6101), 1492–1495. doi:10.1126/science.1226918
Montessori, M. (1986). *Discovery of the child.* New York, NY: Ballantine Books.
Prevent Child Abuse. (n.d.). *Child abuse and neglect reporting guide.* Pawtucket, RI: Prevent Child Abuse.
Russ, S. W. (2004). *Play in child development and psychotherapy: Toward empirically supported practice.* Mahwah, NJ: Erlbaum.
Sara, S. J., & Bouret, S. (2012). Orienting and reorienting: The locus coeruleus mediates cognition through arousal. *Neuron, 76,* 130–141. doi:10.1016/j.neuron.2012.09.011
Schaefer, C. E. (1993). *The therapeutic powers of play.* Northvale, NJ: Aronson.
Siegel, D. J., & Payne Bryson, T. (2011). *The whole-brain child: 12 revolutionary strategies to nurture your child's developing mind.* New York, NY: Bantam Books.
van der Kolk, B. A. (2005). Developmental trauma disorder: Toward a rational diagnosis for children with complex trauma histories. *Psychiatric Annals, 35*(5), 401–408.
Yoga Journal. (2008). *Yoga in America.* Dublin, Ireland: Research and Markets.

12

The Pocket Smock as a Preparation Phase Resource

FAITH THOMPSON-LEE

INTRODUCTION

This chapter proposes the Pocket Smock as a Phase 2 intervention to facilitate the preparation process. The Pocket Smock is designed to be a visible and even tangible location to consolidate the child's acquired self-regulation resources. While it primarily serves to prepare the child for the trauma-resolution phases of the eye movement desensitization and reprocessing (EMDR) protocol, the Pocket Smock is suitable for use throughout the entire treatment process and beyond.

PHASE OF EMDR

Preparation (Phase 2)

MATERIALS

The following materials are introduced in this chapter: writing and coloring utensils; clothing items for smocks; preferred craft items; index cards; pocket smock template; office posters (see step-by-step instructions in this chapter); optional: electronic drafting applications, camera, and Velcro dots.

The materials required to create the Pocket Smock will vary according to the format and style preferred by the child; however, initially, the clinician and child are encouraged to draft the Pocket Smock with typical items found in the play therapy room, such as pencil and paper, dry erase board and dry erase markers, or chalk and chalkboard. Note that the tech-savvy child may be more engaged by drafting their Pocket Smock through a suitable app on personal electronic devices, but for safekeeping, the clinician is encouraged to retain a copy of the draft for subsequent sessions. This can easily be accomplished for any Pocket Smock draft by taking a picture of the child's work.

While it is suitable for the draft to suffice as the final product, creating a wearable Pocket Smock can lend similar benefits that the Safety Device (Greenwald, 1993) provides during trauma resolution, as it reinforces present safety and supplies tools to employ when the therapeutic work intensifies. Therefore, should the child decide to create a wearable smock, materials would include obtaining suitable garments, such as a T-shirt, dress, jersey, apron, or jumpsuit, and so forth. For the pockets, a *no-fuss* approach is encouraged; therefore, having felt fabric, fabric glue, stencils, and scissors on hand is recommended. Of course, sewing materials are welcomed, but this approach may not be time effective and can pose concerns for safety if the child does not already possess interest and experience with this creative method. Additionally, for wearable Pocket Smocks, the clinician may also want to have index cards available. These are placed inside of each pocket that is designated to store the child's self-regulation strategies recorded on them.

Lastly, the posters referred to in this chapter should be easily accessible or posted in the play therapy room for quick references, reminders, and reinforcers.

RATIONALE

Responsibility, Safety, and Control/Choice

The Pocket Smock enhances the EMDR protocol by facilitating the resolution of the three major topics integral to successful treatment, which are responsibility, safety, and control/choice (Shapiro, 2001). When children are able to integrate a balanced view of these concepts into the beliefs about themselves and in relation to others, therapeutic progress is more likely. These three issues usually emerge and resolve in this order, and incorporating the Pocket Smock supports this process. For example, as the child acquires self-regulation skills through use of the Pocket Smock, negative responsibility-themed beliefs of being damaged, stupid, and insignificant are confronted with indisputable evidence of their capacity for health, intelligence, and significance. This then leads to confidence in their judgment, ability to take care of themselves, and comfort with their emotions, all of which directly dispute lingering negative safety-themed beliefs as they approach mastery with their Pocket Smock tools. And finally, with mastery of self-regulation skills, negative control/choice-themed beliefs of being powerless, weak, and inadequate are undermined by acquired views of being powerful, adequate, and capable.

Lasting Protective Factors

Not only does the Pocket Smock enhance the EMDR protocol during treatment, it also continues to provide benefits after treatment termination. Effective termination plans include strategies for self-regulation and coping skills, which provide a solid foundation upon which a child can develop problem-solving skills, academic achievement, intellectual development, high self-esteem, and social skills (Collaborative for Academic, Social, and Emotional Learning, 2019; Youth. gov, n.d.). Each of these are individual protective factors for youth against adverse behaviors and external conditions (Youth.gov, n.d.). Referencing the Pocket Smock in the child's termination plan not only reminds them of their strategies but also serves as a symbol of success, healing, growth, and connection to positive adults, such as the child's clinician and caregivers who practiced and reinforced with the child the use of the Pocket Smock (see Modifications in this chapter). Through this single intervention, the clinician succinctly provides the child with protective factors in the three key areas identified for optimal youth development (Youth. gov, n.d.), which are (a) individual protective factors (i.e., the child's engagement with the Pocket Smock), (b) family protective factors (i.e., the caregivers' engagement with the child and Pocket Smock), and (c) community protective factors (i.e., the clinician's engagement with the child and Pocket Smock).

DESCRIPTION OF INTERVENTION

The purpose of the Pocket Smock is to organize, personalize, and provide a concise visual and even tangible reference for the child's resources that promote emotional regulation and stabilization. The intended result is for the child to feel equipped for trauma resolution. It is also a concise representation of the child's self-regulation skills consolidated into one place to be used throughout the duration of treatment and after termination to support relapse prevention.

Furthermore, the Pocket Smock is a framework that reinforces the idea of creating a new narrative regarding the trauma. The smock is intended to capture the preparedness of an artisan who is skilled and equipped (often with a smock) to take on the challenges of the journey ahead, in expectation and with confidence for a bright outcome. With the Pocket Smock, the artisan, or in this case the child, is prepared and equipped to reprocess mistakes, misfortune, and mistreatment into masterpieces.

STEP-BY-STEP INSTRUCTIONS

Before creating the Pocket Smock with the child, the clinician should have introduced "Our Thermostat System" (Figures 12.1A and 12.1B) to teach the child about their window of tolerance (Siegel, 1999). This allows the clinician to engage the child with a quick thermostat check that can be assessed with a wiggling thumbs-up to represent the too hot zone or hyperarousal, a still thumbs-up to represent the just right zone (window of tolerance), or a thumbs-down to represent the too cold zone or hypoarousal. It is important that the child is familiar with Our Thermostat System, as expanding the child's just right zone is the foundation of the preparation phase (Phase 2) and guides the use of the self-regulating resources of the Pocket Smock.

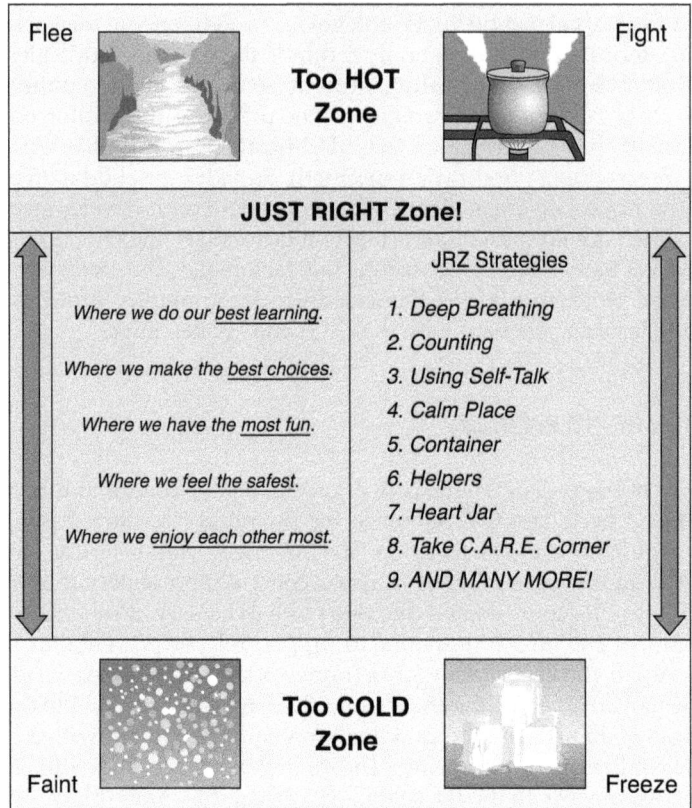

Figure 12.1A Our Thermostat System Poster with the Just Right Zone
Source: Adapted from the Modulation Model as cited in Ogden, P., & Gomez, A. (2013).
EMDR therapy and sensorimotor psychotherapy with children. In A. Gomez (Ed.),
EMDR therapy and adjunct approaches with children (p. 257). New York, NY:
Springer Publishing Company.

STEP ONE: EXPLAIN THE PURPOSE

The clinician first explains to the child the need to create a place to gather and store all of the self-regulating resources that the child has mastered. The child should understand that these need to be organized for quick access when it is time to *slay the dragon* (Greenwald, 2007) or trauma resolution. These are strengths that the child has gained and should be celebrated and emphasized with amazement! You might begin by saying, *"I was thinking about how smart you are and about all the just right zone strategies you have learned so far. You've learned so many! And I have an idea about how to organize them so that they're easy to remember when you need them."*

12. THE POCKET SMOCK AS A PREPARATION PHASE RESOURCE   329

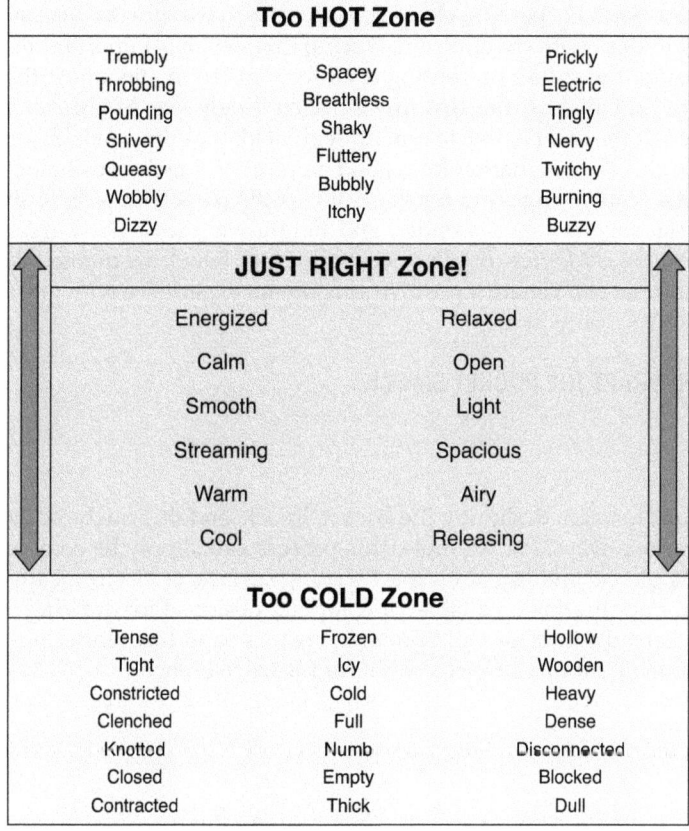

Figure 12.1B *Our Thermostat System Poster with Descriptors*
Source: Adapted from the Modulation Model as cited in Ogden, P., & Gomez, A. (2013). EMDR therapy and sensorimotor psychotherapy with children. In A. Gomez (Ed.), *EMDR therapy and adjunct approaches with children* (p. 257). New York, NY: Springer Publishing Company.

STEP TWO: PRESENT EXAMPLES

Next, the clinician displays what a smock is and what it is used for by showing various pictures of smocks and sharing office examples (see Modification Two in this chapter). It is essential that the clinician point out how the smock *protects* the wearer when their work gets messy and also *helps* to keep their most useful tools organized and close by for when the wearer needs them. For example, the clinician might say, "*Notice how the Pocket Smock protects the artist's clothes and how the most useful tools are in the pockets.*"

STEP THREE: BRAINSTORM IDEAS

At this point, the child may be excited to begin the next step, which is brainstorming ideas for their Pocket Smock, and likely may have already begun to share some of their ideas with the clinician. During this step, it is important that the clinician consider the child's presenting need for regulation and adjust the amount of structure provided during this process accordingly (see Modification One in this chapter). If the child is able to remain regulated, the clinician is encouraged to go with the child's imagination for a good amount of time because moments like these are likely to be engaging for the child, as the clinician reacts to their ideas with interest, surprise, awe, wonder, and lightheartedness. These moments are ripe for *Moments of Meeting* (Booth & Jernberg, 2010), which are moments when the clinician and the child share a positive attachment experience with one another.

STEP FOUR: DRAFT THE POCKET SMOCK

Designing

It is now time to begin designing the Pocket Smock, and this can be accomplished through various ways. For example, this process can simply be completed with any writing utensil and its counterpart writing surface, or electronically through an electronic application on a tablet or computer designed for drawing or sketching. Should an adventurous child prefer to create a sand tray rendering, it is vital that the clinician captures a picture of it for future reference.

Assigning

Also, during the drafting phase, the clinician should allow the child to assign functions to characteristics of the Pocket Smock, such as how each pocket will open and close (i.e., palm or finger scan, special word, double taps) and whether the material of the Pocket Smock has a significant empowering feature or purpose.

Structuring

This portion of the drafting process is perhaps the most crucial, as it enhances the usefulness of the Pocket Smock and the child's success with easily accessing the resources. Structuring should include labeling the pockets and categorizing the child's self-regulation strategies into each, as well as planning the strategic placement of the pockets. A few suggestions include (a) color coding the pockets according to the three information-processing channels (Gomez, 2013), which are the body, heart, and mind channels (see Figure 12.2), (b) placing pockets on the smock with body channel resources over or near areas of the body that experience negative sensations when the child is stressed, (c) separating calming strategies from stimulating strategies by color, location, or symbol on the smock,

Our Three Channels

Mind Channel	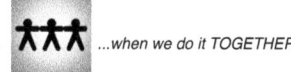	
	Thoughts in our minds.	
Heart Channel	😟 😐 😮 😊	
	Emotions in our hearts.	
Body Channel	🏃	*Our Thermostat System*
		Too Hot
		Just Right
	Sensations in our bodies.	Too Cold

We do it better... 👥 *...when we do it TOGETHER!*

Figure 12.2 Our Three Channels Poster

Source: Adapted from Gomez, A. M. (2013). *EMDR therapy and adjunct approaches with children: Complex trauma, attachment, and dissociation.* New York, NY: Springer Publishing Company

(d) identifying a pocket for "Go-To" strategies that signify the child's favorites, and (e) strategies that help to maintain dual awareness for children who are diagnosed or present with dissociative symptoms. (Note: If the child chooses not to create a wearable Pocket Smock, allow the child to fine-tune the draft with detailed personalization and then proceed to Step Six).

STEP FIVE: CREATE THE WEARABLE POCKET SMOCK

The child should now be ready and excited to proceed to the next step, which is to create the Pocket Smock. Prior to this point, the clinician takes steps to secure the materials needed to bring the child's draft to life by gathering or storing clothing items that typically would appeal to children, or actual aprons/smocks, such as clothes from thrift stores or T-shirts, aprons, or smocks purchased in bulk. The clinician could also prepare clothing garments that stay in the play therapy room that are reserved for Pocket Smock use and are adaptable to any child's pocket categorization. For instance, the clinician could place half of a pair of Velcro dots on a garment and the other half on index cards to suffice. The index cards could be designed with pockets on one side and have self-regulation strategies written on the opposite side.

STEP SIX: PRACTICE

Practice using the Pocket Smock completes the process. It is critical that the clinician expose the child to various scenarios for practice with returning to the just right zone, such as (a) hypothetical situations, based upon the child's previously identified triggers, (b) organic situations that the child may bring into and report during sessions, (c) reorienting after dysregulating moments in-session, for example with Calm Place and Safety Device (Shapiro, 2001), and (d) restoring dual awareness for children with dissociative symptoms, such as exposing them to the Constant Installation of Present Orientation and Safety protocol developed by Jim Knipe (2010) and revised for children by Eckers (2010) and Ana Gomez (2013).

MODIFICATIONS

MODIFICATION ONE: VOICE AND CHOICE

Clinicians must be mindful of and attuned to the child's needs, as too many opportunities for voice and choice can be triggering and dysregulating to some children. One modification to circumvent negative reactions to the amount of voice and choice that is inherent to creating a Pocket Smock is to provide a limited amount of choices. In Erik Erikson's Stages of Psychosocial Development (Feldman, 2014), the importance of supporting the child's *voice* and *choice* becomes apparent as development progresses through the following stages of development, which are autonomy versus shame (ages 1.5–3), initiative versus guilt (ages 3–5), industry versus inferiority (ages 5–12), and identity versus role confusion (ages 12–18) as shown in Figure 12.3. Through the optimal guidance of a caregiver with a secure attachment style, the positive outcome of each stage includes self-sufficiency, initiative, competence, and awareness of the uniqueness of self, respectively. Each of these involves the notion of nurturing the child's sense of voice or comfort with their opinion, and choice or confidence with pursuing their felt sense of direction.

Without the secure attachment with a co-regulating primary caregiver, negative developmental outcomes become more likely. These can include an apathetic, hypoarousal response or a pseudomature, hyperarousal response when the child's capacity for voice and choice is stretched beyond Vygotsky's zone of proximal development (Feldman, 2014; Jernberg & Booth, 1999; McLeod, 2018; Shabani, Khatib, & Ebadi, 2010; Siegel, 1999) (Figure 12.4).

In Theraplay®, the practice of *noticing* the child by the co-regulating clinician and expressing what is noticed to the child is nurturing, engaging, and communicates that the child is seen, heard, and felt (Booth & Jernberg, 2010). The child

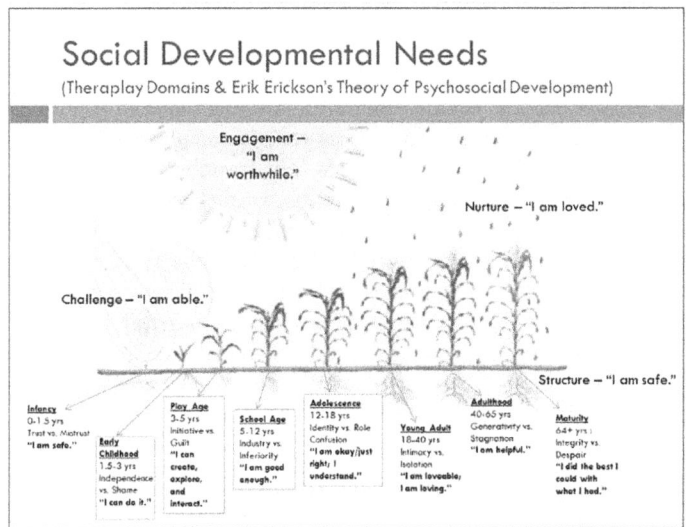

Figure 12.3 *Social and Developmental Needs Throughout Development*
Source: Adapted from Booth, P. J., & Jernberg, A. M. (2010). *Theraplay: Helping parents and children build better relationships through attachment-based play.* San Francisco, CA: Wiley; Feldman, R. (2014). *Development across the life span* (7th ed.). Upper Saddle River, NJ: Pearson; Shapiro, F. (2001). *Eye movement desensitization and reprocessing (EMDR): Basic principles, protocols, and procedures* (2nd ed.). New York, NY: Guilford Press

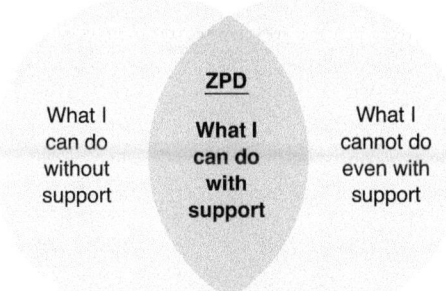

Figure 12.4 *Concept of Vygotsky's Zone of Proximal Development*
Source: Adapted from Shabani, K., Khatib, M., & Ebadi, S. (2010). Vygotsky's zone of proximal development: Instructional implications and teachers' professional development. *English Language Teaching, 3*(4).

will then begin to believe and feel valued and important to adults. Therefore, presenting the child with an abbreviated list of Pocket Smock themes and resources tailored to what the clinician has noticed about their interests can welcome the child to optimally participate. As a result, the child will likely begin to trust the support and rest within the guidance and nurturing of the clinician.

MODIFICATION TWO: PLAY THERAPY ROOM POCKET SMOCK

Another modification is for the *not yet motivated child* who may be uninterested in creating a Pocket Smock. Should the clinician still want to pursue the Pocket Smock framework as a succinct method of representing and storing the child's acquired self-regulation skills, providing a few standard Pocket Smocks in the Play Therapy room is another option to suffice until the child is motivated or expresses interest. For example, clinicians may want to create (or purchase) toy armor or a costume that a knight would use for battle. When providing office resources, the clinician should be mindful to provide gender-neutral and a variety of gender-specific options to avoid further resistance to the activity. The clinician may also choose to store the child's acquired self-regulatory resources on a blank template of a Pocket Smock until the child decides to move further with creating their personalized resource (Figure 12.5).

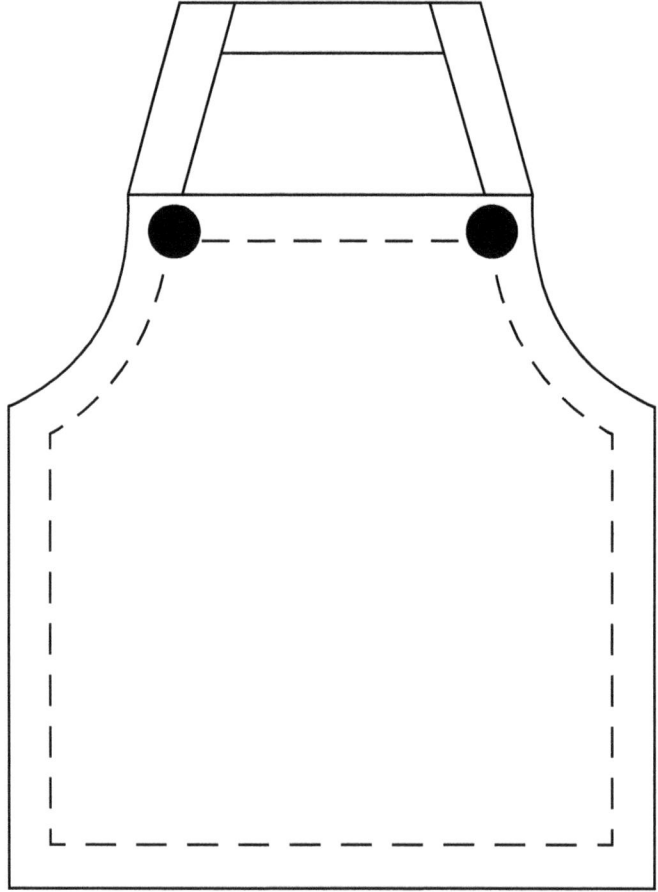

Figure 12.5 *Blank Pocket Smock Template*
Source: Copyright © 2019 Faith Thompson, MEd.

MODIFICATION THREE: CAREGIVER POCKET SMOCK

Generalization of the child's acquired self-regulation and stabilization skills from the play therapy room to other contexts and settings is an important goal of the therapeutic process and becomes vital during the trauma-resolution phases of the EMDR protocol. It is crucial then for the child's caregivers to be able to extend the role of co-regulating caregiver from the clinician and the play therapy room to themselves and the child's home environment. This involves attuning to the child's cognitive, emotional, and sensory needs in order to guide the child from a state of hyper-/hypoarousal to awareness, and then to self-regulation through modeling and coaching. Many parents, however, may need the co-regulating guidance of the clinician in order to achieve this. Clinicians, therefore, are urged to provide caregivers with an opportunity to create their own Pocket Smock during parent sessions with the clinician.

Powerful benefits of engaging in this activity with caregivers includes teaching self-awareness to caregivers, empowering caregivers to feel confident as models of healthy choices and communication, and creating the tone of teamwork for the family unit. As a result, the child is no longer viewed as the problem but rather seen, heard, understood, and considered worthy as the caregivers come alongside the child in the healing journey. The clinician, however, should take into consideration the child's presenting concerns and the family's dynamics to better inform the timing and implementation with the caregivers, sharing of the Pocket Smocks between the child and caregivers, and in-session modeling of how to use the resource at home. Competitiveness, criticism, and control over the child's Pocket Smock should be considered, as celebration, awe, wonder, and respect for the child's efforts and progress should be the focus for the caregiver.

CASE EXAMPLE

Hope* began receiving counseling services in kindergarten at the request of her parents. Transitioning into the classroom was challenging every morning and consisted of crying, clinging to her parents, and refusing to go any further than the entrance of her classroom once her parents left. When Hope did gather herself to join the class, she demonstrated antisocial behavior toward her peers and teachers. As a result of an early diagnosis of cancer and treatment regimens, Hope was not afforded much time for social interactions outside of her immediate family and support groups for cancer patients and later on fellow survivors in remission. Hope's traumatic memories were connected with her cancer treatment, as she remembered surgeries, medical diagnostic machines, being poked with needles to obtain blood samples, and being separated from her parents during some of these moments. She also remembered losing her hair and being stared at by other children. This greatly contributed to her dysregulation in social situations with peers. Hope excelled academically; therefore, treatment goals were primarily focused on social and emotional adjustments.

To ensure confidentiality, the identifying information has been modified and the Pocket Smock sample is a representation of the work completed with this client.

336 II. PLAY-BASED INTERVENTIONS FOR EMDR PHASES

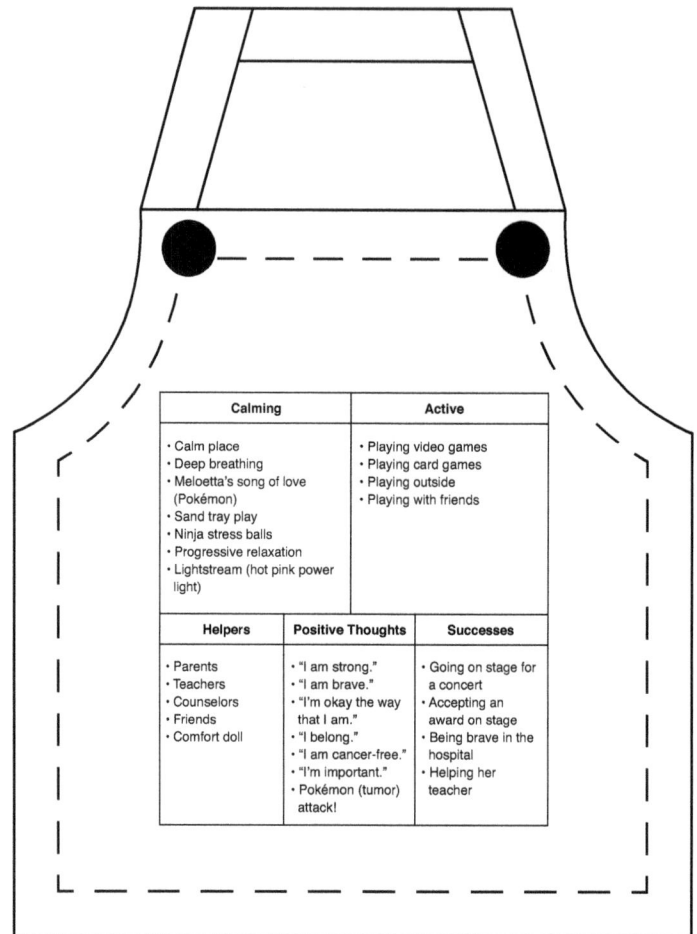

Figure 12.6 *Case Example: Hope's Pocket Smock*

Initially, Theraplay was solely used to address Hope's presenting concerns. Over time, her morning transitions to school improved, she began desiring social connections with her peers, and her ability to self-regulate improved. Hope also began spontaneously talking more about her experiences during her past cancer treatment and *fear* emerged as a primary theme. When her parents argued, this triggered memories of the tension in the home during her treatment, and she feared her parents would split up. Making mistakes triggered feelings of social inadequacies and fears of being different. Lastly, Hope feared that her cancer would come back, especially when she received news of the passing of a friend from her former cancer survivor group and when she had to return to the doctor's office for routine testing for those in remission.

The resources in Figure 12.6 show a draft of a Pocket Smock with Hope's self-regulation strategies. These were created and practiced to prepare her for reprocessing the traumatic experiences connected to her cancer treatment. Additionally, these strategies were integral to sessions dedicated to trauma resolution and consolidation of gains. At the end of treatment, Hope was able to use these strategies during moments of tension between her parents, and she was able to tolerate and learn from mistakes. Finally, Hope was able to implement plans that she created to deal with both the worrying thoughts about the cancer returning and the uneasiness she experienced during routine testing appointments.

REFERENCES

Booth, P. J., & Jernberg, A. M. (2010). *Theraplay: Helping parents and children build better relationships through attachment-based play*. San Francisco, CA: Wiley.

Collaborative for Academic, Social, and Emotional Learning. (2019). *What is SEL: Competencies*. Retrieved from https://casel.org/core-competencies/

Eckers, D. (2010). The method of constant installation of present orientation and safety (CIPOS) for children. In M. Luber (Ed.), *Eye movement desensitization and reprocessing (EMDR) scripted protocols: Special populations* (pp. 51–58). New York, NY: Springer Publishing Company.

Feldman, R. (2014). *Development across the life span* (7th ed.). Upper Saddle River, NJ: Pearson.

Gomez, A. M. (2013). *EMDR therapy and adjunct approaches with children: Complex trauma, attachment, and dissociation*. New York, NY: Springer Publishing Company.

Greenwald, R. (1993). *Using EMDR with children*. Pacific Grove, CA: EMDR Institute.

Greenwald, R. (2007). *EMDR: Within a phase model of trauma-informed treatment*. Binghamton, NY: The Haworth Press.

Jernberg, A. M., & Booth, P. J. (1999). *Theraplay: Helping parents and children build better relationships through attachment-based play* (2nd ed.). San Francisco, CA: Jossey-Bass.

Knipe, J. (2010). The method of constant installation of present orientation and safety (CIPOS). In M. Luber (Ed.), *Eye movement desensitization and reprocessing (EMDR) scripted protocols: Special populations* (pp. 235–241). New York, NY: Springer Publishing Company.

McLeod, S. A. (2018, August 5). *Lev Vygotsky*. Retrieved from https://www.simplypsychology.org/vygotsky.html

Shabani, K., Khatib, M., & Ebadi, S. (2010). Vygotsky's zone of proximal development: Instructional implications and teachers' professional development. *English Language Teaching*, 3(4). Retrieved from https://files.eric.ed.gov/fulltext/EJ1081990.pdf

Shapiro, F. (2001). *Eye movement desensitization and reprocessing (EMDR): Basic principles, protocols, and procedures* (2nd ed.). New York, NY: Guilford Press.

Siegel, D. J. (1999). *The developing mind: How relationships and the brain interact and shape who we are*. New York, NY: Guilford Press.

Youth.Gov. (n.d.). *Mental health: Risk and protective factors*. Retrieved from https://youth.gov/youth-topics/youth-mental-health/risk-and-protective-factors-youth

13

The "Lemon Squeezies" Metaphor for EMDR Processing With Children

KRISTEN HURVITZ

INTRODUCTION

This intervention was designed to support and assist children and adolescents in developing negative cognition (NC) and positive cognition (PC) in the assessment, desensitization, and installation phases using a creative intervention of "making lemonade" and turning "sour" thoughts into "sweet" thoughts. This intervention integrates eye movement desensitization and reprocessing (EMDR) and play in the processing of traumatic material.

PHASES OF EMDR

Assessment (Phase 3), desensitization (Phase 4), and installation (Phase 5)

MATERIALS

- Paper (yellow or pink) cut out as lemon slices
- Visual aids for SUDS (Subjective Units of Disturbance Scale) and VOC (Validity of Cognition) Scale. Templates for creating these are offered at the end of this chapter.
- Pitcher
- Wooden spoons
- Yellow and white felt balls or pom-poms
- Stress balls that are yellow (The therapist may substitute Play-Doh or other tactile media that are lemon-like and other expressive art materials for the creation of lemonade, if needed.)

RATIONALE

Creativity and modifications to the standard EMDR protocol have been used to great success by the leading child and adolescent therapists in the field. The combination of play and metaphors with EMDR can meet the developmental needs of children and adolescents with trauma histories. Integrating play and EMDR can support children and adolescents in the creation of new neural networks and connections, which can improve therapeutic outcomes and processing of traumatic memories (Gomez, 2013). Play is critical in the formation and growth of healthy brain organization as well as the creation of neural connections that support continued brain development (Brown, 2009).

A metaphor can help children and adolescents process traumatic memories, creating distance and reducing the flow of emotions. Additionally, metaphors may be helpful as children and adolescents struggle to identify and verbalize their feelings. For example, developmentally a young child would realistically be unable to verbalize "I am unlovable." However, the young child could verbalize "No one can love this puppy because this puppy is bad" through play.

Lastly, metaphors can also motivate children and adolescents to reprocess traumatic memories (Wesselmann, Schweitzer, & Armstrong, 2014). A metaphor is a right brain process that generates new meaning and understanding in an imaginative and creative way with children and adolescents (Mills & Crowley, 2014). As play is primarily a right brain process, children and adolescents can explore sensations and emotions stored in implicit memory. The "Lemon Squeezies" intervention is a modification of the standard EMDR protocol that combines play and the use of metaphors, which supports children and adolescents in processing traumatic memories and creating new neural pathways.

DESCRIPTION OF INTERVENTION

Lemon Squeezies is a modification of the standard EMDR protocol in the assessment, desensitization, and installation phases when working with children and adolescents. The standard protocol will be followed for history and treatment planning, preparation, body scan, closure, and reevaluation. The therapist may use sandtray, play therapy, expressive arts, or other techniques in order for the child or adolescent to create and explore the worst part of the memory from the identified target. The therapist will describe the metaphor of making lemonade in a playful way by using a pitcher, wooden spoons, and yellow felt balls and pretend to add sweetener with white felt balls in order to explore the idea of how a child or adolescent can change their "sour" NCs to "sweet" PCs. The use of lemon stress balls or other mediums for bilateral stimulation (BLS) to target the worst part of the memory creates a tactile experience of squeezing juice from the lemon in the metaphor of making lemonade.

STEP-BY-STEP INSTRUCTIONS

Step 1: The therapist will describe to the child or adolescent the process of creating lemonade: collecting lemons, pitcher, spoons, juicer, and sweetener and using lemons, which are sour, to make sweet lemonade! The therapist can demonstrate playfully with the child or adolescent the process of making lemonade using an actual pitcher, spoons, yellow felt balls to represent the lemons, and white pompoms to represent the sugar, in order to change NCs or "sour" thoughts into PCs or "sweet" thoughts. See Figure 13.1, which features a nonclient volunteer demonstrating the intervention.

Assessment Phase:

Step 2: Once the child or adolescent is able to express the worst part of the image from the target, the therapist will introduce the yellow and pink lemon slices, which have PCs and NCs prewritten.

Special Considerations: When writing both NCs and PCs, the developmental age of the child must be considered. For children under the age of 5, simplifying the PC and NC can be helpful. The therapist may also leave one yellow and one pink slice blank in the event the child or adolescent identifies a cognition that is not listed.

Step 3: The therapist begins by explaining that when an individual experiences trauma, the body and mind create an adaptive response to protect, which may be unconsciously triggered by sight, smell, touch, or other events. Often when thinking of the trauma, the child or adolescent may have "sweet" or "sour" thoughts about themselves. Using the metaphor of making lemonade, the therapist will describe the process. A person chooses a lemon, cuts it in half, and then begins to squeeze the lemon for the juice; then they add the sweetener in order

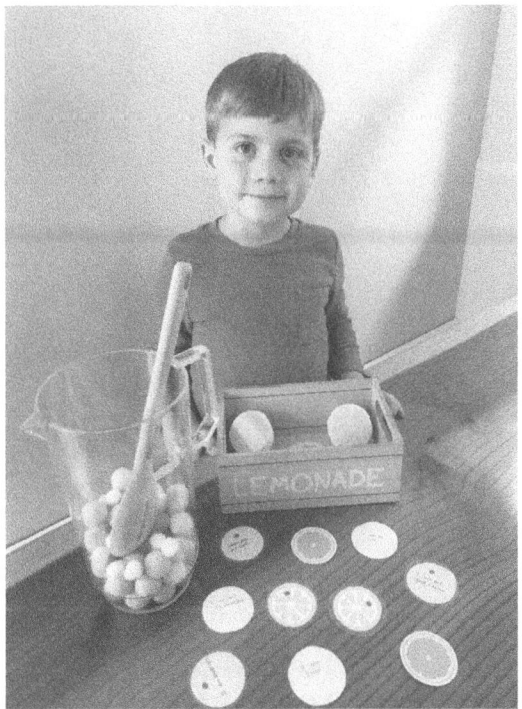

Figure 13.1 *Lemon Squeezies Setup With Supplies Used for Intervention*

to make lemonade. The child or adolescent will be working to change the "sour" lemon thoughts into "sweet" lemonade thoughts.

Step 4: The therapist will show the child or adolescent the pile of "sour" lemon thoughts (NCs) and ask for the child or adolescent to pick a "sour" thought related to the target and held negative beliefs about the self. If the child or adolescent is unable to pick an NC from the "sour" pile, the therapist can introduce the blank slice and invite the child or adolescent to create a "sour" thought that feels most appropriate.

Step 5: The therapist will then ask the child or adolescent where they identify the "sour" thought in their body.

Step 6: Once a child or adolescent is able to identify the worst part of the memory, the "sour" NC thought, and the location in the body, the therapist will introduce the "sweet" or PC pile of lemon slices.

Step 7: The therapist again will invite the child or adolescent to choose a "sweet" thought that they would prefer to believe about themselves now. Again, if the child or adolescent is unable to identify a "sweet" PC, the therapist can invite the child or adolescent to identify their own on the blank slice. See Figure 13.2.

Step 8: Once the "sour" NC and "sweet" PC have been identified, the therapist will then introduce the VOC form to the child or adolescent to pick a spoon: The smallest spoon (1) represents feeling completely false and the largest spoon (7) represents feeling completely true.

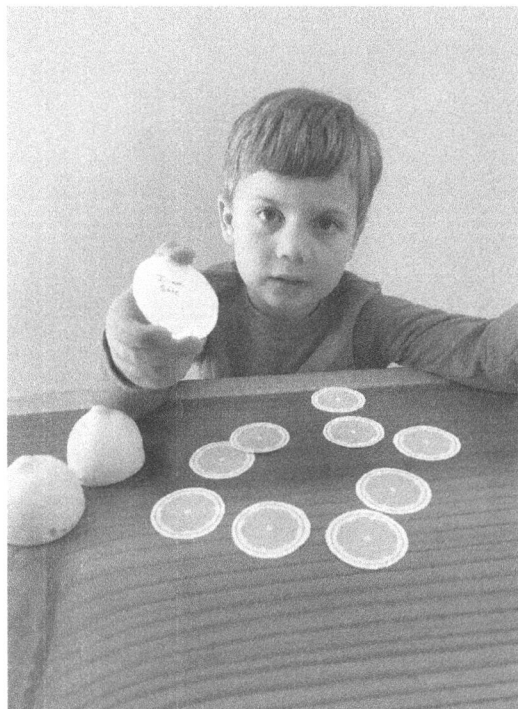

Figure 13.2 *"Sweet" Positive Cognitions, With Paper Lemon Slices Used to Identify Positive Cognitions*

Step 9: Then using the SUDS form, the child or adolescent will choose a lemon slice (0–10) in the pitcher, where 0 is no disturbance and 10 is the most disturbing. The therapist will then ask the child or adolescent what emotions do they feel when they bring up the worst part of the memory and "sour" NC thoughts. The therapist can use feelings flashcards, charts, or other tools in assisting children or adolescents in identifying emotions.

Step 10: Last, the child or adolescent will explore and identify where they feel those "sour" or negative thoughts in their body. If the child or adolescent is struggling to name or locate those sensations in the body, the therapist could introduce a body scan, movements such as yoga, or mindfulness.

Desensitization and Reprocessing Phases:

Step 11: The therapist will ask the child or adolescent to create or, if able, verbalize together (a) the worst part of the memory, (b) where the child or adolescent feels the sensations in their body, and (c) the "sour" or NC thought.

Step 12: The therapist will give the child or adolescent lemon squeezies (one for each hand) for BLS. The therapist could also use Play-Doh, stress balls, or other BLS tools. See Figure 13.3.

Step 13: The therapist will direct the child or adolescent in BLS, remaining attuned for any affect or change. It is important to remember when processing traumatic memories that the child or adolescent is grounded in the present while exploring the past. The therapist may introduce mindfulness techniques, yoga, or sensory interventions to the child or adolescent.

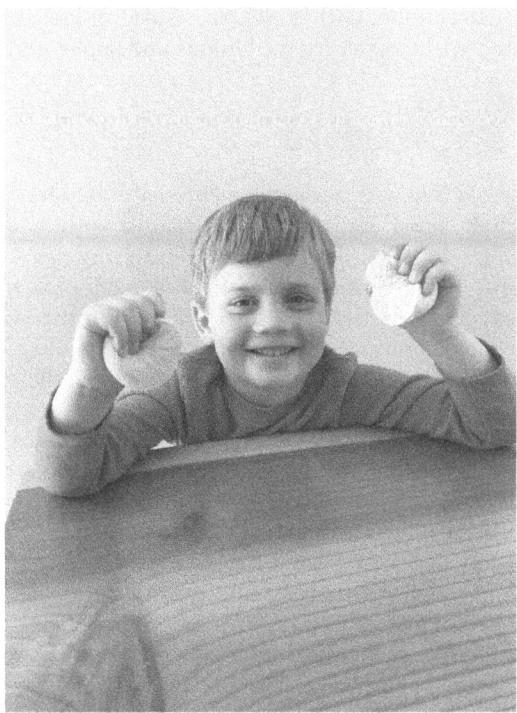

Figure 13.3 *Lemon Stress Balls Squeezed Alternatively for Bilateral Stimulation*

Installation Phase:

Step 14: Once the target memory has been processed, where the SUDS is 0 and VOC is 7, the therapist can reintroduce the "sweet" thought PC for installation. The standard EMDR protocol is then followed for body scan, closure, and reevaluation.

MODIFICATIONS

Modifications to the EMDR standard protocol should only be made to accommodate the developmental needs of each age group (Tinker & Wilson, 1999). For example, in younger children under the age of 8, PCs and NCs can be difficult to identify, and the use of games or metaphors can be helpful in naming and simplifying NC and PC. Additionally, the therapist can help the child or adolescent form both an NC and PC with the assistance of the prewritten lemon slices in the Lemon Squeezies intervention.

CONSIDERATIONS

If the child or adolescent does not like lemonade, the therapist may substitute another metaphor using their best clinical judgment. For example, they may substitute another sour and sweet food recipe, such as a berry pie. Additionally, the therapist may use other materials as needed to represent the "ingredients" in the Lemon Squeezies intervention: with Play-Doh instead of lemon stress balls, with crumpled yellow and white paper for the lemons and sugar, and the like.

CASE EXAMPLE

Michael* is a 7-year-old boy with a diagnosed anxiety disorder. His adoptive parents' concerns include sleep disturbances, difficulty with transitions and new events, somatic complaints, excessive worries, and struggles with separation—particularly from his adoptive mother. Michael was adopted from Russia at 18 months. Prior to adoption, he lived in three different orphanages. His prenatal history is unknown: His adoptive parents report that he was found beside a dumpster at 1-day-old. The adoptive parents report that Michael required surgery at 9 months to correct the shape of his skull. Michael was brought to play therapy because he was (a) having difficulty separating from his adoptive mother to attend school, (b) leaving his room multiple times at night, and (c) complaining of stomach aches. Michael has missed over 20 days of school, and his adoptive parents are concerned that he is falling behind and will need to repeat first grade.

Over the first few sessions, I built rapport with Michael through somatic interventions such as yoga, drumming, and creating obstacle courses. Michael struggled while separating from his adoptive mother at the beginning of the sessions, refusing to let her leave the room. Playful and somatic interventions helped

---

* In order to protect client confidentiality, the information in this case example has been modified.

Figure 13.4 *Lemon Paper Slice Template, Used to Create Lemon Slices Used for Negative and Positive Cognitions*

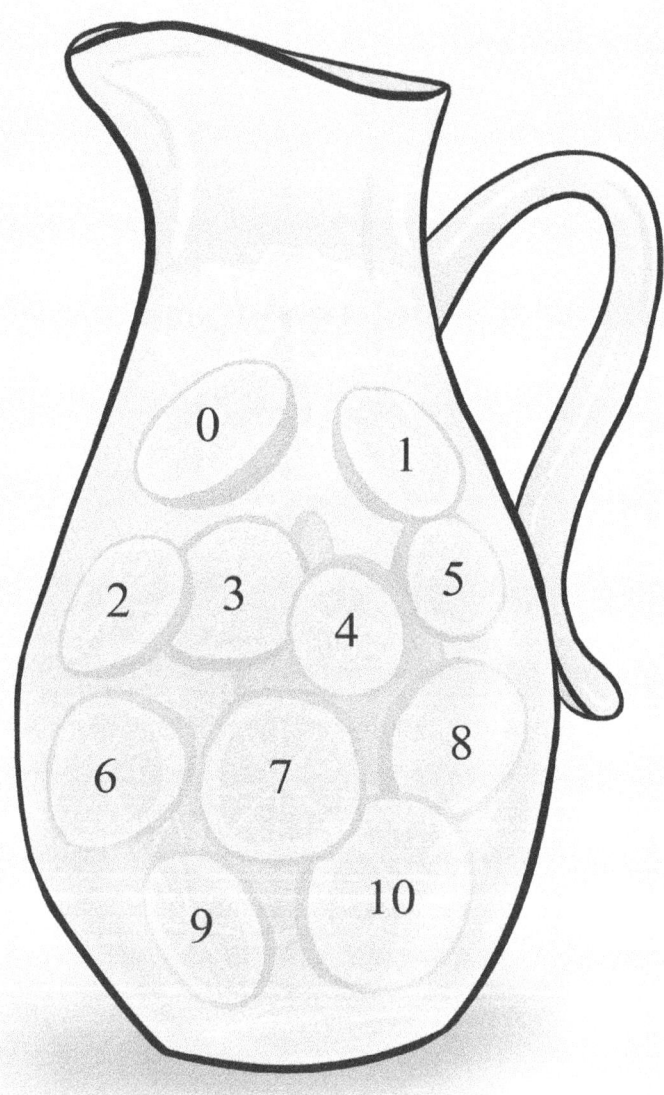

Figure 13.5 *Subjective Unit of Disturbance Scale (SUDS) Form, Used for Measuring Disturbance*

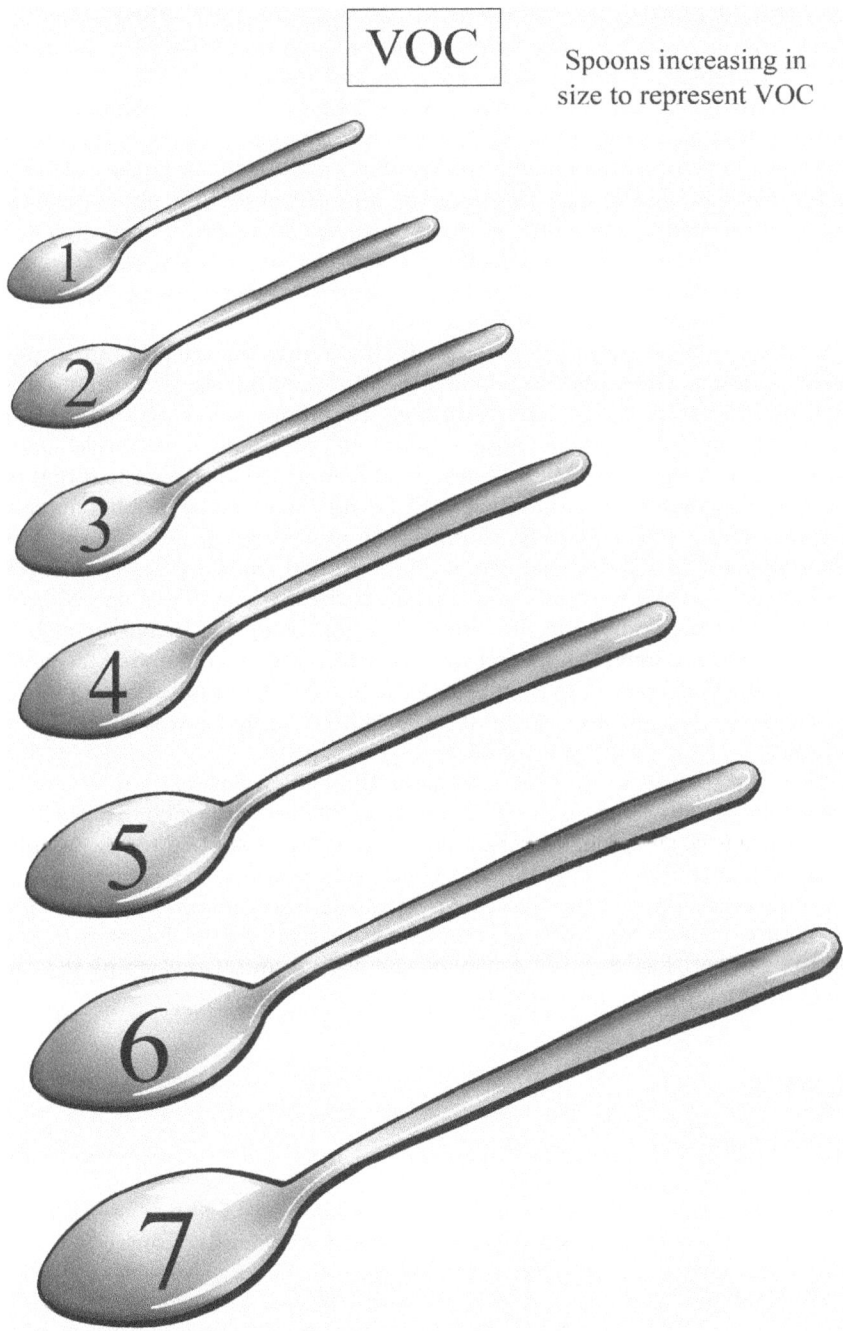

Figure 13.6 *Validity of Cognition (VOC) Scale*

calm and regulate Michael, and eventually, he was comfortable letting his mother exit the session. I was then able to introduce the standard EMDR protocol beginning in the preparation phase using safe place and containment.

First, Michael created a sand tray of the worst part of his memory, which was himself alone in the tray with *"no one else who cares about me."* The Lemon Squeezies intervention was next introduced in the assessment phase of EMDR. The playful metaphor of making lemonade introduced the concept of NCs and PCs. We discussed the metaphor of making lemonade, where lemons are cut in half to squeeze the sour juice into the pitcher, and sugar is added to sweeten the lemonade for drinking. We further explored the metaphor of "sour" and "sweet" thoughts by pretending to make lemonade.

Michael enjoyed putting the yellow felt balls into the pitcher and using a wooden spoon to "mix" the lemonade. I then brought out the prewritten paper lemon slices with NC "sour" and PC "sweet" cognitions (see template for lemon slices in Figure 13.4). Michael chose a "sour" NC of *"I don't deserve love"* and a "sweet" PC of *"I am loved."* Michael described feeling sad and identified that the feeling was located in his stomach. The SUDS for the worst part of his memory was an 8, and the VOC was a 3 (see Figures 13.5 and 13.6 for SUDS scale and VOC scale templates). In the desensitization phase of the Lemon Squeezies intervention, Michael was able to recall the worst part of the memory, the "sour" NC, and the location in his body from the "sour" thought. Using the lemon stress balls for BLS, Michael completed several rounds before the session ended, at which point his SUDS decreased to 3 and his VOC to a 5. Due to the session ending, a container exercise, as used in the standard EMDR protocol, was utilized with Michael.

Over the span of several sessions using the Lemon Squeezies intervention, Michael was able to decrease the SUDS of the worst part of the memory to a 0 and his VOC to a 6. The Lemon Squeezies intervention was then used for the installation phase to install the "sweet" PC. Standard protocol was then used for the body scan and closure. After using the Lemon Squeezies intervention, Michael's adoptive parents reported that Michael was able to separate from his adoptive mother with less distress, had decreased somatic complaints, and was sleeping through the night with minimal interruption.

REFERENCES

Brown, S. L. (2009). *Play: How it shapes the brain, opens the imagination, and invigorates the soul.* New York, NY: Penguin.

Gomez, A. M. (2012). *EMDR therapy and adjunct approaches with children: Complex trauma, attachment, and dissociation.* New York, NY: Springer Publishing Company.

Mills, J. C., & Crowley, R. J. (2014). *Therapeutic metaphors for children and the child within.* New York, NY: Routledge.

Tinker, R. H., & Wilson, S. A. (1999). *Through the eyes of a child: EMDR with children.* London, UK: W. W. Norton.

Wesselmann, D., Schweitzer, C., & Armstrong, S. (2014). *Integrative team treatment for attachment trauma in children: Family therapy and EMDR.* New York, NY: W. W. Norton.

14

EMDR-Infused Theraplay®

FAITH THOMPSON-LEE

INTRODUCTION

This chapter demonstrates how the gains acquired through Theraplay® can be leveraged for healing by infusing eye movement desensitization and reprocessing (EMDR) into Theraplay treatment. Infusion in the preparation phase will be the primary focus; however, considerations for infusing EMDR and Theraplay are offered for application within the assessment, desensitization, installation, and body scan phases of the EMDR protocol.

PHASES OF EMDR

Preparation (Phase 2), assessment (Phase 3), desensitization (Phase 4), installation (Phase 5), and body scan (Phase 6)

MATERIALS

The following materials are introduced in this chapter:

- Theraplay materials
- Child-friendly bilateral stimulation (BLS) tools
- Office posters

The materials found within a standard play-therapy room, including sand and water trays, as well as typical arts and crafts materials, can likely be incorporated into treatment with EMDR and Theraplay; however, the clinician must structure the room to ensure that these materials are inaccessible for the child and out of sight, yet still easily accessible for treatment activities. Successful Theraplay treatment does not require much space; however, ideally there should be enough room for essential items, such as large floor pillows (or a beanbag chair) and small throw pillows (Booth & Jernberg, 2010). Next, the clinician should be sure to have key items that are commonly used within each Theraplay dimension. These include but are not limited to (a) cotton-balls, bubbles, and toilet tissue for activities designed to reinforce structure, (b) lotion, powder, face paint, snacks, and soft blankets for activities targeting nurture, (c) foil, stickers, and marshmallows for activities geared for engagement, and (d) balloons, feathers, and newspaper for activities planned for challenge. The clinician should note that not every Theraplay activity will require materials and that most Theraplay materials are useful for multiple activities across each domain.

Another tool that is great to have on hand are finger puppets for BLS, which can be used for EMDR resourcing and reprocessing. They add a sense of fun to EMDR-infused Theraplay, which can set a child at ease for therapeutic work. Finger puppets are inexpensive to make or purchase and lend themselves to easy adaptation for use with tappers and wands when providing BLS with children.

Lastly, the posters referred to in this chapter should be easily accessible or posted in the play-therapy room as quick references, reminders, and reinforcers.

RATIONALE

Fundamental Therapeutic Differences and Professional Training

The goal of Theraplay is to create positive and restorative experiences for the child through healthy, co-regulating adult relationships to repair early unmet attachment needs. Theraplay differs from child-centered and traditional forms of play therapy in that Theraplay is clinician-directed and not child-directed. Theraplay clinicians model the behaviors of caregivers with secure attachment styles attuned to the child's mental, emotional, and physical needs. They also adhere to the therapeutic format of Theraplay sessions. Therefore, it is recommended that EMDR be infused into Theraplay, as EMDR is adaptable to various therapeutic approaches. Attempting to infuse Theraplay into EMDR would compromise the integrity of Theraplay's therapeutic approach. Clinicians seeking to maximize the benefits of Theraplay should receive professional training from The Theraplay Institute (2018).

A Common Foundation

Theraplay and EMDR form a strong therapeutic alliance because they are both rooted in attachment theory. The pioneers of human attachment theory, John Bowlby in 1951, and later Mary Ainsworth in 1978, believed that children depend upon the emotional bonds with primary caregivers for their survival. These bonds are a *home base* from where they begin to develop a view of themselves and others, and ultimately how they approach the world. A child needs a strong emotional bond with at least one primary caregiver with a secure attachment style for optimal development (Feldman, 2014). Theraplay is modeled after primary caregivers with secure attachment styles, who are in tune with the needs of their children and provide them with a healthy and balanced home base characterized by the dimensions of structure, nurture, engagement, and challenge (Booth & Jernberg, 2010). The human body is naturally inclined to heal from physical and emotional wounds (Shapiro, 2001), and for some children, Theraplay is all that is needed to support the child's natural emotional healing process from early attachment trauma. This is because the multisensory positive experience of Theraplay leverages the strengths of the child's right brain. As a result, it promotes the regulation of the child's limbic system and provides the material the child needs to integrate into their own neural networks for adaptive information processing (Trevarten, 1990, as cited in Gomez, 2013; Shapiro, 2001). Coupled with other protective factors (i.e., talking with friends, receiving compassion and guidance from primary caregivers at school, and making healthy life choices with regard to sleeping, eating, and exercising), memory networks that contain traumatic experiences have an increased likelihood of being completely worked through to resolution (Greenwald, 2007).

A Natural Progression of Therapeutic Intervention

Still, some children will need more support, like the intensive therapeutic intervention that EMDR provides. As with Theraplay, EMDR also relies upon a multisensory experience and when infused or provided through a tiered approach for therapeutic intervention, the two provide an ideal combination of interventions that further supports the body's inherent healing process from early emotional wounds. Based upon the response-to-intervention tiered approach for providing academic intervention in schools (Hatch, 2014), Figure 14.1 suggests a tiered conceptualization of therapeutic interventions that support the body's natural

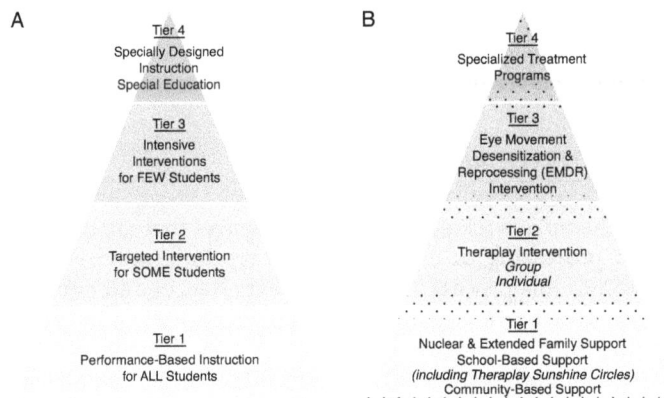

Figure 14.1 *Tiered Conceptualization of Therapeutic Interventions, Inspired by the Response to Intervention Model*

Source: Left image from Hatch, T. (2014). *The use of data in school counseling: Hatching results for students, programs, and the profession.* Thousand Oaks, CA: Corwin.

healing process. It is important to note that upward movement through the tiers signifies the need for additional support and not the irrelevance of the therapeutic interventions prior.

A Seamless Phase 2 Fit

Greenwald (2007) provides a simple way of conceptualizing Phase 2, which is the preparation phase. He separates the phase into two major components by categorizing the phase's stabilization measures as fence around preparation and the phase's self-management measures as personal training preparation. Approaching the preparation phase with Theraplay seamlessly supports both of these components. The first line of security and safety for children is through their caregivers. A caregiver with a secure attachment style is likely in tune with their child's needs and is able to provide the necessary emotional, mental, and physical stabilization that the child craves. Caregivers who are not adept with stabilization in this manner, perhaps because of their own attachment traumas or because their child may be presenting with concerns that are outside of their present co-regulating abilities, will benefit from the caregiver training that is embedded within Theraplay. There are also times when pressing external matters can compete with the caregivers' capacity for attunement, and support and intervention from the Theraplay clinician can provide an additional level of fence around preparation.

With adequate external preparation, triggers that impact both the caregiver and the child are greatly reduced, which gives the child a safe space to begin the self-management aspect of the preparation phase. This primarily involves increasing the child's capacity for emotional regulation, providing the child with the foundation to develop strengths in the form of social skills, decision-making skills, self-reflection, self-esteem, and self-efficacy. Theraplay's four dimensions of treatment, which are structure, nurture, engagement, and challenge, provide the child with an ideal climate to develop in these areas and afford the child with an optimal preparation experience.

DESCRIPTION OF INTERVENTION

Treatment with Theraplay yields reparative experiences that can be used for adaptive information processing during the trauma-resolution phases of treatment. Infusing EMDR into this process allows these experiences and subsequent positive feeling states to be harnessed as resources through EMDR-specific strategies. Additionally, this infusion provides the child with the benefit of being familiar with EMDR terms and procedures before desensitization and reprocessing begin. For example, clinicians can seamlessly infuse Subjective Units of Distress Scale (SUDS) ratings, Validity of Cognition (VOC) Scale ratings, and BLS (Shapiro, 2001) into any Theraplay session. The following steps demonstrate how these strategies can be used for resource gathering and installation, and the Considerations section later in this chapter explains how to infuse EMDR into Theraplay for target gathering or assessment (Phase 3) and reprocessing (Phases 4–6).

STEP-BY-STEP INSTRUCTIONS

STEP ONE: CROSS-REFERENCING CLIENT HISTORY SOURCES FROM BOTH THERAPEUTIC APPROACHES

Theraplay treatment planning is informed by the information gathered from the Marschak interaction method (MIM) assessment. This assessment is a structured observation technique designed to assess the quality and nature of the relationship between the child and each primary caregiver (Booth & Jernberg, 2010). Feedback from the MIM should be cross-referenced with the child's EMDR case formulation information gathered during Phase 1 (client history and treatment planning). Cross-referencing allows the clinician to be strategic about choosing Theraplay activities most likely to create opportunities for moments that are exceptions (Jong & Berg, 2013) to the child's negative experiences and maladaptive cognitions for adaptive information processing. Exceptions are the primary ingredients for successfully infusing EMDR resource gathering and installation into Theraplay.

STEP TWO: NOTICING AND COMPLIMENTING

Early on, it is recommended that sessions remain pure Theraplay sessions, as Theraplay alone provides an optimal preparation opportunity for EMDR treatment. Theraplay requires the clinician to notice the child and express to the child what is noticed. In a standard Theraplay session, the practice of *noticing* is significant during the check-up activity, but noticing by an attuned clinician occurs throughout the session. The expressions of noticing communicate to the child that they are seen, heard, and felt (Booth & Jernberg, 2010) and lend to the beginning of the child believing and feeling valued and important. Noticing is a vital reparative ingredient as "the most profound trauma comes when a neglectful environment gives nothing for the child to work with and when the material for constructing an image of oneself is oneself alone" (Sleed & Fonagy, 2010, as cited in Gomez, 2013, p. 15). To introduce the child to EMDR terms as well as to prepare them for desensitization and reprocessing, the clinician should begin to notice and compliment the child's accomplishments, skills, and strengths. For instance, a common way to begin an active Theraplay activity is with a *special word* to signal "Go!" (Booth & Jernberg, 2010). To engage or reinforce structure with the child, the clinician would propose a special word, or a short list of special word options, from a category of one of the child's interests or preferences. Once decided, the child cannot begin the activity until the clinician or caregiver says that special word. Should the special word be *purple*, the child's favorite color, the clinician would say a few other incorrect colors to maintain optimal engagement and structure. When the child successfully ignores the incorrect colors and responds only to the color that is correct, the clinician should notice this and compliment the child by saying things like, (a) "You have such good ears," (b) "Wow! You are so good at ignoring distractions," or (c) "I should've known I couldn't trick you. You are becoming an expert at following directions!" Noticing identifies exceptions to the child's negative experiences and maladaptive cognitions, while complimenting these exceptions helps to magnify the moment.

STEP THREE: WONDER

Noticing can be linked with expressions of wonder about the child's experience. Expressions of wonder guide and invite the child to notice their own internal states and provide an opportunity to teach and reinforce the principles of Our Thermostat System (Figures 14.2A and 14.2B), which is based upon Siegel's window of tolerance (1999).

For example, should face painting (Booth & Jernberg, 2010), which is primarily a nurturing activity, be planned for the child, as the clinician is painting the

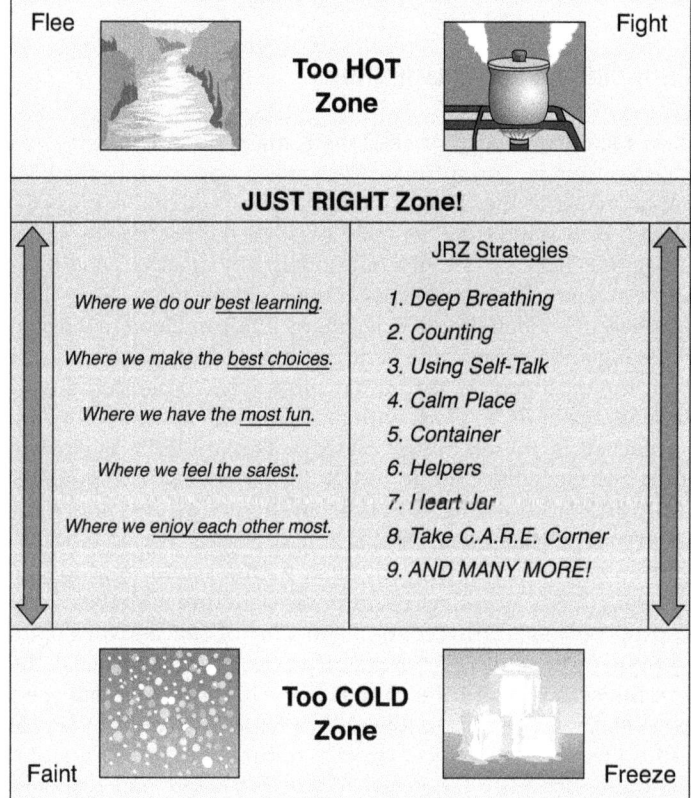

Figure 14.2A *Our Thermostat System Poster with the Just Right Zone*
Source: Adapted from the Modulation Model as cited in Ogden, P., & Gomez, A. (2013). EMDR therapy and sensorimotor psychotherapy with children. In A. Gomez (Ed.), *EMDR therapy and adjunct approaches with children* (p.257) New York, NY: Springer Publishing Company.

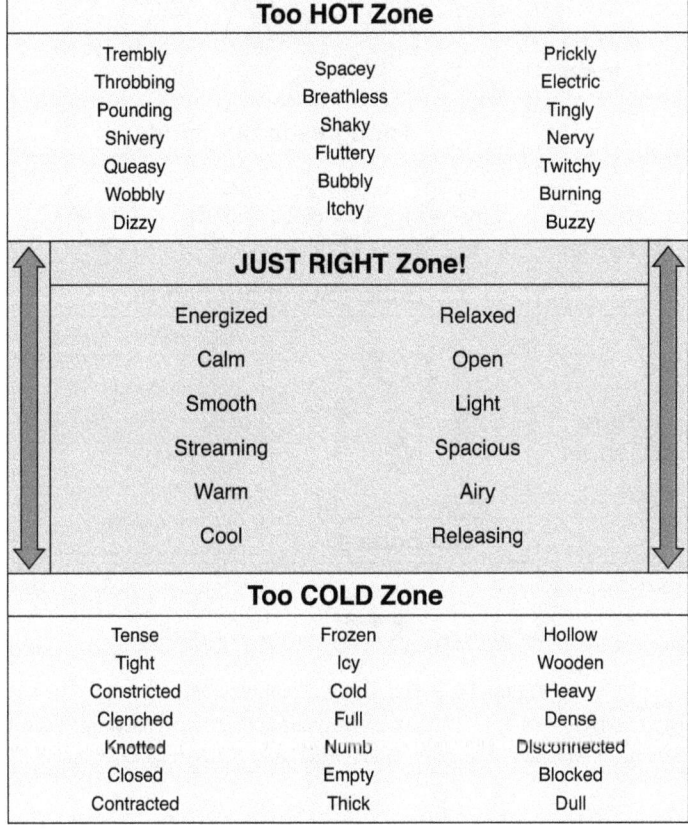

Figure 14.2B *Our Thermostat System Poster with Descriptors*
Source: Adapted from the Modulation Model as cited in Ogden, P., & Gomez, A. (2013). EMDR therapy and sensorimotor psychotherapy with children. In A. Gomez (Ed.), *EMDR therapy and adjunct approaches with children* (p. 257). New York, NY: Springer Publishing Company.

clinician should notice and describe the child's wonderful cheeks, lovely eyebrows, and beautiful freckles, and so forth. However, as the activity nears the end, for instance, when the child is admiring their painted face in the mirror and before cleanup from that activity, the clinician could say, *"You seemed to really enjoy getting your face painted. Your body channel appeared to feel safe and relaxed. I wonder, is that what your body channel was speaking to you?"* Allow the child to agree or disagree and to provide their own description of that experience on their body channel. If the experience was positive and enjoyable, the clinician should attune to that and connect that experience to the just right zone or the window of tolerance. The clinician could then go on to say, *"I wonder what your heart and mind channels were speaking?"* A child already adept with the language of Our Three Channels (Figure 14.3) will be able to ascribe an emotion and cognition (an "I am"

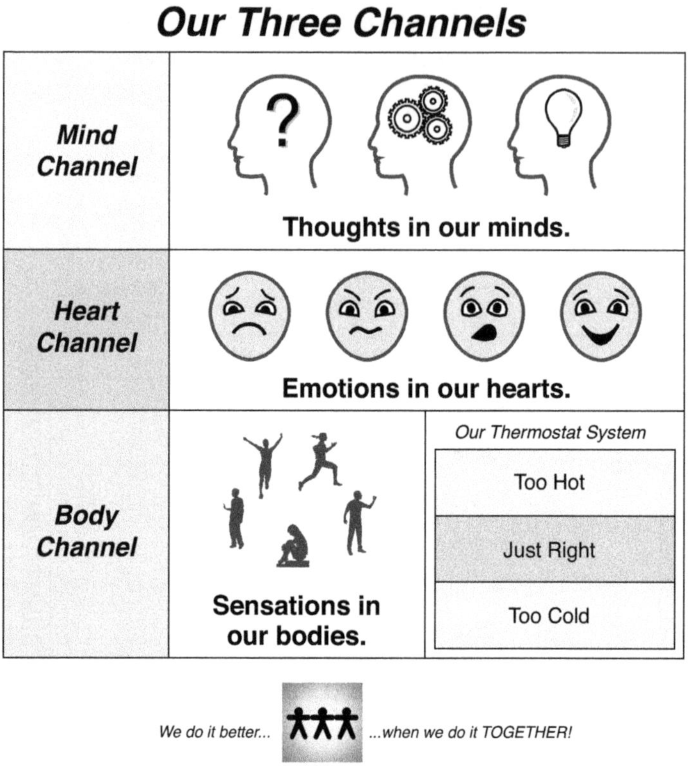

Our Three Channels

Mind Channel		Thoughts in our minds.
Heart Channel		Emotions in our hearts.
Body Channel	Sensations in our bodies.	Our Thermostat System — Too Hot / Just Right / Too Cold

We do it better... ♦♦♦ ...when we do it TOGETHER!

Figure 14.3 Our Three Channels Poster
Material adapted from Gomez, A. M. (2013). *EMDR therapy and adjunct approaches with children: Complex trauma, attachment, and dissociation.* New York, NY: Springer Publishing Company

statement). Those who are not will require additional guidance and support in the form of a menu of options that explain what each channel might have been speaking to the child (Gomez, 2013; Greenwald, 2007).

STEP FOUR: ADD BLS

To install this positive experience as a resource to aid adaptive information processing, the clinician should explain that *"it's important to notice moments like these to help us remember them forever and ever."* BLS can be introduced as a way to help the child's whole brain experience and notice the moment with both hemispheres. Referring to a developmentally appropriate office poster depicting the functions of both sides of the brain could provide a visual connection for the child, in addition to examples of relatable and enjoyable activities where *"experiencing them is better to do with two sides."* For example, watching a movie with both eyes open, using the controls to a video game with two hands instead of one, or having two working earbuds for listening to music on their smartphone. The clinician should tell the child that both sides of the brain are turned on by following a hand signal from side to side, listening to alternate sounds from ear to ear, tapping on both sides of the body, or alternating gentle squeezes between hands, knees, or toes. While eye movements are preferred, the clinician should use their clinical judgment and introduce BLS through a mode most likely to connect with the child's comfort level. After explaining BLS, the clinician should say,

> *"We will try a few ways, but first I'm going to tap your knees. While we're sitting knee to knee, I want you to think about how enjoyable the face painting was for you. Remember how calm your body channel was, how happy you felt on your heart channel, and how you thought in your mind channel, 'I am safe and relaxed.' I'm going to continue to softly tap your knees one at a time, and all you have to do is remember and focus on all of that goodness."*

The clinician should proceed to apply short and slow sets of BLS taps of about four complete passes to enhance the resource and to prevent the child from accessing disturbing material (Gomez, 2013).

STEP FIVE: ASSESSING FOR VOC

Once BLS has been provided, the clinician can assess for the VOC. You could say, *"I wonder how true 'I am safe and relaxed' feels to you?"* While demonstrating by adjusting your hands horizontally from wide to narrow, say, *"Can you show me how true that sounds with your hands stretched very wide for ver-r-r-y true, or with your hands stretched sort of wide for sort of true, or with your hands close together for not so true?"* (It is important to assess the child's VOC with horizontal hand movements to differentiate its meaning and association from the vertical hand movements used during the case formulation [Greenwald, 2007] to depict large and small amounts of distress.) Once the child reports the VOC with their hands, the clinician could link this to a poster of The Thought Scale (Gomez, 2013) for an actual VOC rating number and then provide one more set of short and slow BLS to complete the resource installation. If the child's VOC report remains less than a 6 or 7 (Shapiro, 2001) after two sets of BLS, the clinician should stop the resource installation activity, make a note of this for target planning, and wrap up the activity with a connecting compliment, by saying, *"You're really good at paying attention to yourself. Let's see what's next* (turning the attention to the clinician's stash or bag of Theraplay materials organized for the remainder of that session)."

NOTES

Once the child and the clinician become well versed with the terminology of this resource-installation process, it can occur briefly during the respective goal-related activities of The Session Proper (see Exhibit 14.1 for Theraplay session sequence). An alternative place for this resource installation to occur is just before the child is situated for the session's standard nurturing activities, which are the feeding and song activities of The Session Proper, just before the closing. As the clinician or the caregiver is holding the child, or the child is situated in a comfy chair, or wrapped in a soft blanket, the clinician can outwardly wonder about the child's favorite activity, proposing one or two and describing the child's channel responses as reasons for their suspicions. Once the child expresses their favorite, the clinician can employ this resource-installation process.

Exhibit 14.1 *Typical Sequence of a Theraplay Session**

<u>The Opening</u>
Greeting
Entrance
Checkup

<u>The Session Proper**</u>
*(3 to 4 Goal-Related Domain Activities)****
Structuring activities
Nurturing activities
Engaging activities
Challenging activities

Feeding Song
<u>The Closing</u>
Gathering and Parting
Transition to the "outside world" and return to caregivers

* Typically lasts 40–50 minutes.
** Caregiver typically enters where planned. (Note: When there is a history of trauma, the caregiver may be included from the beginning.)
*** Subject to change to meet the child's presenting needs.

Source: Adapted from Booth, P. J., & Jernberg, A. M. (2010). *Theraplay: Helping parents and children build better relationships through attachment-based play.* San Francisco, CA: Wiley.

MODIFICATION: PREDICTABILITY

Predictability is a vital component of Theraplay. It provides structure for the child, reinforces a felt sense of safety and trust within the clinician's care, and provides the child with an opportunity to self-regulate in preparation for the conclusion of an activity that they may not want to end. For example, when a tossing activity is concluding, the clinician should say, *"Let's take 10 more tosses,"* with subsequent warnings that the activity is coming to an end at *"five more"* and then *"two more,"* and so forth, as opposed to *"alright, time's up"* without warning. When moving to the next activity, the clinician should explain what the activity is and could say, *"Let's have a shoe and sock race to gather our things today,"* as opposed to abruptly beginning a competitive race with the child. Likewise, touches should be thoughtful, predictable, and announced. It reinforces and models respect for the child's personal space and avoids activating possible memory networks that contain traumas connected to touch. For instance, the clinician can say things like, (a) *"I'm going to help you take your shoes and socks off as we get comfy and settled in,"* (b) *"I'm going to softly touch your cheeks with this cotton ball,"* or (c) *"I'm going gently tap your knees to help us remember this moment forever and ever."*

For a child initially uncomfortable with the clinician applying the BLS for resource installation, the butterfly hug created by Lucina Artigas (Artigas & Jarero, 2014) is an effective alternative. Mirroring the clinician, the child can be guided to self-administer BLS with their hands crossed over their chest while alternating taps near their shoulders, or alternatively taping either sides of their knees or alternating squeezes between their thumbs that are hiding in their gently clenched fists. Furthermore, the butterfly hug is great for every child and caregiver to know for enhancing self-soothing or use as self-regulation resources for the child outside of the therapeutic setting.

CONSIDERATIONS

CONSIDERATION ONE: STORYTELLING (PHASES 3–6)

Storytelling can be a nurturing experience and a brief story of triumph to install a positive feeling state achieved during the session. It can easily be incorporated into a Theraplay session. Either before both the feeding and the song, or just before the song, the clinician tells a story about the child's positive experience. Using Joan Lovett's (1999) storytelling template for EMDR processing with children, this story should have a beginning, middle, and end. Using the face painting example, the beginning could provide a description of the child and their excitement for the activity. The middle could describe how the paint brush felt ticklish to the child at first, but then it became very calming and the child felt relaxed, happy, and believed that they were safe. Lastly, the end of the story would connect this positive feeling state resource to a lasting skill or strength that the child is developing in line with their treatment goals, such as becoming an expert at paying attention to themselves.

Reprocessing through the security and nurture of storytelling is very powerful, and a clinician could also restructure a Theraplay session to allow enough time for in-depth trauma resolution work using this approach. To accomplish this, the clinician selects one or two of the child's favorite activities to begin The Session Proper, preferably those that provided a positive feeling state and that have previously been installed as a resource. The first activity is conducted without the caregiver's presence, and the second takes place once the caregiver has entered the session, followed by the reprocessing storytelling activity. The story is created by the clinician and the caregiver during parent feedback sessions. The entire story surrounding the traumatic event is told by either the clinician or the caregiver with the opposite adult providing the BLS. For moments in the story that describe traumatic or bothering content, the standard 24 complete passes of BLS that are as fast and intense as the child can tolerate are provided, or until the child affirmatively motions that the bothering feeling is not there anymore. For portions of the story containing resources, strengths, and installations, short and slow sets of BLS with about four passes are provided, or until the child verbally or nonverbally expresses that they feel calm and safe (Gomez, 2013; Lovett, 1999). A Theraplay activity that the child has enjoyed with the clinician and the caregiver for containment ends The Session Proper. The Theraplay session would then conclude according to standard Theraplay procedures. Depending upon the capacity of the child and the nature of the trauma or its complexity, the story can be told over the course of a few sessions with strategic planning to end on a positive note in the story for containment.

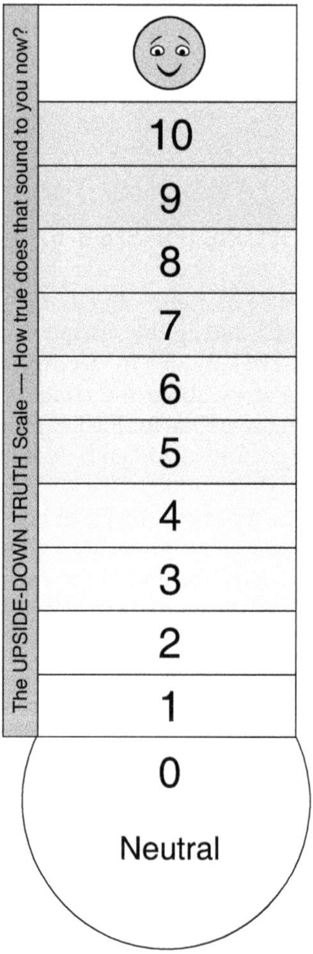

Figure 14.4 *The Upside-Down Scale for the Feeling-State Addiction Protocol*
Source: Miller, R. (2012). Treatment of behavioral addictions utilizing the feeling-state addiction protocol: A multiple baseline study. *Journal of EMDR Practice and Research*, 6(4), 159–169. doi:10.1891/1933-3196.6.4.159

CONSIDERATION TWO: THE UPSIDE-DOWN SCALE (PHASES 3-6)

The Upside-Down Scale (Figure 14.4) is a tool utilized to measure the strength of an addictive feeling state, which according to Robert Miller (2012) is a fixation of feelings (sensations, emotions, and cognitions) and unhealthy behavior. It is a child-friendly name for the Positive Feeling Scale (PFS) that assesses the strength of the feeling state in the Miller's Feeling-State Addiction Protocol (FSAP). This protocol is intended to remove the desire to make unhealthy choices for self-regulation. Though outlined to treat clients with addictions, this scale and the protocol can also be useful in identifying the desire behind a child's nonsubstance-related compulsive, reactive, or high-risk maladaptive choices.

Upon the family's arrival to therapy, the clinician may find a planned Theraplay session to be in competition with the need to address concerns provided by the caregiver about *an event* involving the child's poor choices. Use of the Upside-Down Scale allows the issue to be seamlessly addressed within a Theraplay session in a way that respects the caregiver's concerns, attunes to the child's needs, and enriches the therapeutic process. Attuning is part of the standard check-up Theraplay activity and lends well to providing the space needed for a brief check-in when the Upside-Down Scale is needed.

CASE EXAMPLE

Once the parent left the room, the clinician said,

"*You know, I think the choices that people make are always meant to help them in some way. Like, it makes them happy, or gives them relief, or makes them feel better about themselves. When you put your head down during math and stopped working, I wonder, did it make you feel safe or relieved to get away from math for a bit?*"

In this actual example, the child* affirmed. The clinician went on to say, "*I wonder what thoughts might be connected with that feeling?*" In this situation, the child identified "*I am popular*" and "*I am powerful/ruling*" as being associated with the desire and choice to shut down in class. The clinician went on to assess the strength of this feeling state using the Upside-Down Scale. Once the child provided the rating, the clinician asked the child to focus on the behavior and its associated positive feelings while a standard set of BLS was provided. When the feeling state addiction protocol (FSAP) is used with adults, the clinician reassesses the PFS (Upside-Down Scale) rating after every set of BLS to measure for a decreasing or weakening association between the feelings and the behavior of the targeted feeling state. However, with children (especially for those who present with defiant behavioral patterns), it is recommended that the clinician reassess once or maybe twice later in the session, for example, just before the feeding and song activities of The Session Proper when the clinician might review the child's favorite moments from the session. Another suggestion would be to reassess the Upside-Down Scale rating the following session, once again during the check-up. Alternatively, a session dedicated solely to more work with the protocol could be planned. Before moving on with

---

In order to protect client confidentiality, the information in this case example has been modified.

the remainder of the Theraplay session, the clinician offered a containing statement after BLS has been applied, such as, *"Okay, let's set this aside for later."*

With the child presented in this case example, before the following session, the teacher reported that he had returned to class the following school day referring to himself in the past as the *Old Ryan* and as the *New Ryan* in the present. She also reported that she observed an increased effort on his part to self-regulate and self-advocate when challenged by his class work. Additional EMDR sessions involved work with the rest of the FSAP protocol that included targeting events where he felt *stupid* and *weak*, which corresponded to underlying negative cognitions of *"I am a failure"* and *"I'm not good enough,"* respectively. These events included being picked on, almost drowning, and grief surrounding events from a previous school year when his teacher abruptly resigned. Lastly, the negative beliefs about himself that developed as a result of making maladaptive choices in the past to survive were targeted, such as *"I'm bad"* and *"I'm unlovable."* When the reprocessing work with the FSAP was completed with this child, the positive cognitions included, (a) *"I'm cool when I accept challenges and try my best to reach my goals,"* (b) *"I now have choices,"* (c) *"I can tackle big problems by breaking them down into small problems," "I can take care of myself," "I can ask for help when I need to,"* and *"I am deserving."* By the end of treatment, Ryan's grades had improved, and he was expressing remorse, in addition to taking an active leading role in making amends and finding solutions whenever needed. The most profound evidence of improvement was noticed when his mother said, *"I don't know what you did to my son, but he skipped to the bus this morning. He likes going to school now."* The combination of EMDR and Theraplay shifted the trajectory of the school experience for both Ryan and his family.

CONSIDERATION THREE: THE REAL DEAL REEL

As the child accumulates positive resources gained from Theraplay sessions, the clinician will be presented with the need to create a place to store them all. The Real Deal Reel is a place to store positive images that represent these true ("Real Deal") moments about the child and the adults who care for them. Stored in one place, the child can revisit all of the accomplishments, skills, and strengths they learned, and the mere fun they had as well. This metaphor is connected to the EMDR analogy of watching a videotape or movie of the traumatic event from a safe place, with the ability and choice to stop it at will (Shapiro, 2001). When presented as such, the Real Deal Reel represents another choice that the child has with regard to what they choose to believe about themselves and how they view themselves in relation to others, ultimately with the goal of integrating both narratives in a healthy way. The Real Deal Reel is best suited for sessions not dedicated to Theraplay or when a planned Theraplay session cannot be completed because of unforeseen circumstances. For instance, the clinician could have a session dedicated solely to consolidating resources or if the time allotted for the planned Theraplay session is limited to due to the family's late arrival, an image or two could be created for the Real Deal Reel instead. The child's Real Deal Reel images can be stored in a PowerPoint or a folder with images of the child's artwork for future therapeutic use.

REFERENCES

Artigas, L., & Jarero, I. (2014). The butterfly hug method for bilateral stimulation. *EMDR Research Foundation*. Retrieved from https://emdrresearchfoundation.org/toolkit/butterfly-hug.pdf

Booth, P. J., & Jernberg, A. M. (2010). *Theraplay: Helping parents and children build better relationships through attachment-based play*. San Francisco, CA: Wiley.

Feldman, R. (2014). *Development across the life span* (7th ed.). Upper Saddle River, NJ: Pearson.

Gomez, A. M. (2013). *EMDR therapy and adjunct approaches with children: Complex trauma, attachment, and dissociation*. New York, NY: Springer Publishing Company.

Greenwald, R. (2007). *EMDR: Within a phase model of trauma-informed treatment*. Binghamton, NY: The Haworth Press.

Hatch, T. (2014). *The use of data in school counseling: Hatching results for students, programs, and the profession*. Thousand Oaks, CA: Corwin.

Jong, P. D., & Berg, I. K. (2013). *Interviewing for solutions* (4th ed.). Belmont, CA: Brooks/Cole, Cengage Learning.

Lovett, J. (1999). *Small wonders: Healing childhood trauma with EMDR*. New York, NY: The Free Press.

Miller, R. (2012). Treatment of behavioral addictions utilizing the feeling-state addiction protocol: A multiple baseline study. *Journal of EMDR Practice and Research*, 6(4), 159–169. doi:10.1891/1933-3196.6.4.159

O'Shea, K., & Paulsen, S. (2009). *When there are no words: EMDR for early trauma and neglect held in implicit memory*. Retrieved from https://emdr-belgium.be/wp-content/uploads/2017/12/When-There-Are-No-Words.-EMDR-for-Early-Trauma-and-Neglect-Held-in-Implicit-Memory.-Katie-OShea-M.S.-2009.pdf

Shapiro, F. (2001). *Eye movement desensitization and reprocessing (EMDR): Basic principles, protocols, and procedures* (2nd ed.). New York, NY: Guilford Press.

Siegel, D. J. (1999). *The developing mind: How relationships and the brain interact and shape who we are*. New York, NY: Guilford Press.

The Theraplay Institute. (2018). *Professional training*. Retrieved from https://www.theraplay.org/training

15

Resource Wand for Bilateral Stimulation in EMDR Therapy

ANNIE MONACO

INTRODUCTION

Resource Wand is an intervention that is designed to give added support to a child during the reprocessing of a memory that has the potential for overwhelming or flooding. It is used to manage levels of arousal and affect in Phase 4 of EMDR: Desensitization. A resource wand is a play-based item such as a magic wand or stick that has a picture (real or drawn) of a support person, animal, or object on it. During eye movements, the child follows the wand with the picture while processing the target.

PHASES OF EMDR

Assessment (Phase 3) and desensitization (Phase 4)

MATERIALS

- Picture of the support person (caregiver or other person), animal, superhero, or symbol; this can be a printed photo, actual photo, or a drawing of the person or the symbol
- Wand, stick
- Tape

RATIONALE

EMDR therapy accesses cognitive beliefs, emotional states, and somatic experiences. Children with limited internal resources struggle to tolerate Phase 4 without significant preparation of external and internal resources. In the preparation phase, children are often provided with many tools such as a safe place, container, and other resource-development interventions (Shapiro, 2001; Tinker & Wilson, 1999). Yet, some children still struggle with emotional regulation and the ability to tolerate negative thoughts and emotions that emerge not only during the desensitization phase but throughout the entire eight phases of EMDR. This population is what Ana Gomez (2013) refers to as Type 2 and Type 3 individuals, which include children who have complex trauma characterized by chronic and repeated exposure to multiple and prolonged traumatic events. The events can consist of but are not limited to foster care, adoptions, late-age adoptions, severe neglect, abuse, and inconsistent caregivers. These are children who are the products of parents with insecure attachment and severe traumatic histories themselves. Due to the disrupted attachment, they are difficult to engage in therapy and struggle to tolerate any emotions or discussion of the traumatic events. With their pervasive dysregulation, they have limited ability to stay within the window of tolerance and often require the therapist to work very hard to keep them grounded, present, and engaged in the EMDR therapy (Gomez, 2013). Phobia of the memory and the trauma work is common with these children; they often utilize all of their defensive behaviors to create obstacles to participate in desensitization of their memory. They may refuse to participate or utilize repetitive avoidance behaviors such as aggression or dissociation, so as not to experience the horrific memory and emotional pain. This intervention helps to manage the child's arousal during processing by promoting increased safety in the playroom and encouraging connection to the child's caregiver or perceived supports, which can include an animal or own inner strength symbolized by a superhero.

DESCRIPTION OF INTERVENTION

During history taking and the preparation phase, the therapist and child should identify the supports that exist in the child's life. This intervention then uses these identified supports during desensitization. It requires a picture or drawing of the caregiver, animal, superhero, or superhero's powers, which is then placed on an item that is used for eye movements like a magic wand or rain stick. This intervention provides children with the opportunity to be following the wand during bilateral stimulation (BLS) while gazing at a picture that feels supportive to them.

STEP-BY-STEP INSTRUCTIONS

Step 1: In Phase 1, history taking and treatment planning, identify supports and resources in the child's life, including extended family, other caregivers, teachers, or animals. Another idea is to identify any superheroes or superpowers that resonate with the child and are positive or supportive in nature. Paying attention to what the child plays with in the playroom may offer possible options as well. It is important that these supports or resources are consistent, predictable, and safe.

Step 2: In Phase 2, the preparation phase, discuss with the child who they want supporting them through the processing of the traumatic memory. If needed,

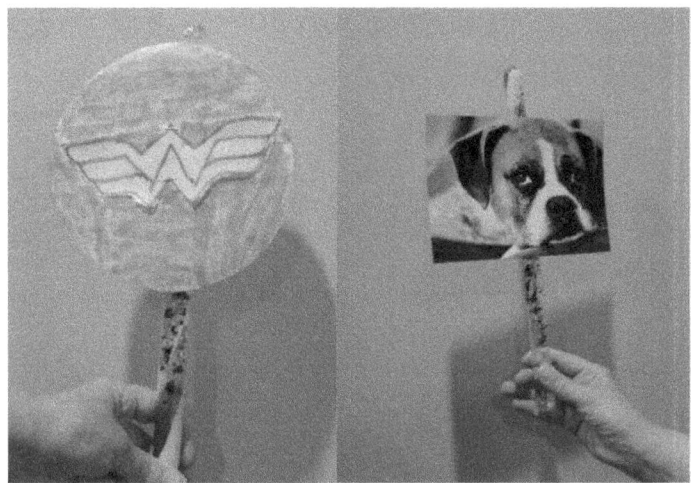

Figure 15.1 *Samples of Superhero and Pet Resource Wands for Bilateral Stimulation*

offer suggestions that were obtained from history taking. Then you can collect or create a picture of the supporter. If possible, you may obtain a picture from the caregiver or use a digital photo. Otherwise, or if it may have an added therapeutic benefit, the child can draw the supporter during session.

Step 3: Tape the picture to the wand/stick to be used for eye movements. Sometimes having several pictures allows for choice and can be used at different times during processing. You may also choose to have multiple wands to ease the use of multiple pictures. See Figure 15.1 for some examples.

Step 4: In Phase 4, the desensitization phase, utilize the wand during BLS. If more than one supporter/picture is being used, have the child choose which one to start with.

MODIFICATIONS

Cognitive interweaves with complex trauma cases are essential to help make the adaptive neuro-network connection "by using the cognitive interweave the clinician attempts to change the client's perspective somatic reactions, and personal references...to the adaptive perspective" (Shapiro, 2001, p. 252).

If the child is still struggling during the processing of the memory, you can say:

"*What would* (in picture) ___ *say to you?*"

"*Do they think you are a good girl or good boy?*"

"*Does* _____ (in picture) *want you to be happy? Or get stronger? Or be able to handle this?*"

"*Do they believe you can handle this memory?*"

"*Can you see them here with you and can they put an arm around you or hug you?*"

"Can you see your dog licking your face, wagging its tail… and if it could speak what would the dog say to you?"

"Have the superhero protect you or give you superpowers to make you stronger and handle this memory. Can you imagine it? Feel it? What does the superhero want you to know about doing this memory?"

Knipe (2018) stresses the importance of the Constant Installation of Present Orientation and Safety (CIPOS) with his dissociative adult clients. The resource wand can be used as a prompt during reprocessing to reorient children to the present moment between sets of reprocessing with BLS by using questions that engage the child's awareness of the resource such as the ones mentioned earlier.

CONSIDERATIONS

When choosing a person, consider how much of a support or hindrance they are to the child. It is important to make sure the individual is mostly consistent, predictable, and able to provide internal support for the child. It's important to have a person that the child feels truly supports them and that the child is able to visualize or internally feel this support. If it is a conflictual relationship, the therapist should explore other options. It is risky to choose a caregiver as the child may hear their negative statements while processing the memory. If the child does not have a supportive homelife, consider identifying an extended family member, even if the child does not see them often. Consider using a teacher, teacher's aide, school counselor, caseworker, in-home or after school worker, or neighbor.

A supportive person who is deceased is an option, depending on the child and how much they have coped with the loss of that person. This choice tends to be riskier, especially if the supportive person died tragically, if the death was not handled well, or when the child did not get a chance to say goodbye. However, if the child is able to talk about it, this option can yield great results.

If choosing an animal, make sure the child feels connected to them and has not been harmed by the animal. It should be an animal that is primarily connected to them and not another family member instead. Using an animal that is kind and gentle is key! Identifying and using a superhero is typically the best and safest option. Another option is identifying the superpower that gives them strength to handle the memory. In this case, the superhero's badges or weapons can be the identified image that makes the child feel strength through the processing.

CASE EXAMPLE

Keith* was a foster child placed in his final adoptive home after two foster homes and removal from his teenage birth parents. Keith and his adoptive mom did filial therapy with a play therapist in the local area. Once the attachment was more secure, the therapist asked if I could help make the transition to EMDR

---

*In order to protect client confidentiality, the information in this case example has been modified.

therapy, as Keith was avoidant about his past neglect and witnessing the physical abuse of another child in one of the foster homes. Keith had many problematic behaviors at home, at school, and in the playroom. If an intolerable emotion came up, he would go to great lengths to avoid the feeling in his body and often would become dissociative and disruptive. If past traumas surfaced during play therapy in the sand, he often flung rubber bands at me, threw toys, or broke items in the playroom. I struggled to assist him to tolerate difficult emotions and body sensations, and he challenged me to find new and creative ways to help him cope. I hung in there with him, and he eventually made improvements in tolerating emotions. I was still concerned about him as we were nearing the possibility of utilizing EMDR for reprocessing. I entertained the idea that he could come to my home office with my therapy dog to offer additional regulation. The fear was that he would harm the dog and it would be a failed experience. My dog, Sadie, was immediately drawn to him and sat on his lap (all 60 lb [27.22 kg]) to decrease his anxiety and hyperactivity. Keith was so kind and caring to Sadie that his mom was taken aback, as it was a rare occasion to see him gentle and loving. Two months later, his mother got him a dog! He soon was attached to his dog, and it was then that Resource Wand was developed. I asked his mother for a picture of the dog as well as a picture of him and her at a park (also his favorite place). We taped the picture of his dog onto a magic wand and then used a rain stick for the picture of him and his mom. He got to choose which picture to start with and he chose his dog. When it became so difficult and he wanted a change, he would ask for the picture of his mom. With Sadie by his side and a picture of his dog and mom used for BLS, Keith was able to tolerate the processing of many memories.

Cognitive interweaves were common in our work together as this was an opportunity to help Keith make the adaptive connection. Since he had a significant history of neglect, it was common that Keith would sink into a more depressive state, dissociate, and become hypo-aroused when reprocessing of memories. For cognitive interweaves I would say to him: *"What would your dog (or mom) say to you about this bad thing that happened? What is Sadie by your side trying to tell you right now? What would they want you to know right now as you struggle to go through this memory? Do they think you can get through the memory?"*

Keith liked the changing of pictures, and over time we accumulated several funny dog pictures, different fun times with his mom, and various badges of superheroes. To help with regulation, we often did two or three sets of eye movements and then would stop and do different activities to manage the emotional regulation: *"Tell me about this picture. What is your dog doing? What are you and your mom doing?"* He would often playfully yell out his answers, and we were able to stay in the window of tolerance. We also smelled scents, did yoga, or played with Sadie to aid with regulation. Many different preparation interventions were used to help soothe and increase safety. His regulation improved over time, but it took significant and ongoing effort to keep the dissociation to a minimum. Resource Wand was one of the most effective strategies I used with him in order to help Keith process with EMDR.

Resource Wand is an intervention that is playful to make and use during the reprocessing of a memory. It offers any child an opportunity to feel safe during the desensitization phase.

REFERENCES

Gomez, A. (2013). *EMDR therapy and adjunct approaches with children.* New York, NY: Springer Publishing Company.

Knipe, J. (2018). *EMDR toolbox: Theory and treatment of complex PTSD and dissociation* (2nd ed.). New York, NY: Springer Publishing Company.

Shapiro, F. (2001). *Eye movement desensitization and reprocessing: Basic principles, protocols, and procedures.* New York, NY: Guilford Press.

Tinker, R. H., & Wilson, S. A. (1999). *Through the eyes of a child: EMDR with children.* New York, NY: W. W. Norton.

16

Using the Superhero Shuffle for Bilateral Stimulation in EMDR With Children

TYNE POTGIETER

INTRODUCTION

The Superhero Shuffle is a playful intervention that is designed to work best with high-energy children and children who have low tolerance for exposure to trauma or engaging in the bilateral eye movements of eye movement desensitization and reprocessing (EMDR) therapy. Superhero figurines are utilized to assist with bilateral eye movements for desensitization and installation as well as to serve as inspiration for resource development in the preparation phase and cognitive restructuring in the installation phase. The effectiveness of this intervention relies on the therapist's ability to maintain a playful, fast-paced approach to meet the child's energy levels for maintaining concentration and participation.

PHASES OF EMDR

Preparation (Phase 2), desensitization (Phase 4), and installation (Phase 5)

MATERIALS

Superhero figurines (minimum of two recommended)

RATIONALE

This play-based intervention was designed specifically for the child who is unable to sit still and concentrate for long periods of time. Symptoms of trauma may include hyperarousal, sensory-seeking behaviors, inattention, and low tolerance for exposure to anything related to processing the trauma (Solomon & Siegel, 2003). Because of this, a typical approach to EMDR may result in setting the child up for failure, as the expectation to sit still and participate for an extended period of time is unreasonable. This intervention is most effective when conducted in a fast-paced, playful approach. Instead of expecting the child to achieve a calm and controlled state, this approach allows the therapist to meet the child where they are at in terms of energy levels. Doing this encourages participation, removes real or imagined barriers or unobtainable expectations that the child may feel, promotes and strengthens the therapeutic alliance, and encourages the child to process in a way that they find safe and achievable. This modification helps children to have a more positive experience with EMDR and bilateral eye movements, therefore being more willing to continue with the protocol, even when challenged with having to revisit the negative feelings and experience of the trauma.

Superheroes are used as motivational props in this intervention. Most children seem to be in a despondent frame of mind as a result of the experienced trauma and therefore find resource development very challenging. Resourcing requires more of an optimistic view that sometimes may feel unobtainable for the child. By removing the personalization and exploring resource development and cognitive restructuring for traumas using a "what would the superhero do" approach, children seem more likely to participate and identify coping skills, support systems, and thoughts or behaviors for the superheroes. This would then later be applied to their own personal growth and therapy process. This can assist the child in overcoming the negative self-view that they may have developed and instead instill a sense of hope that change could take place.

Another significant element of this intervention is the level of control that the therapist provides the child. By allowing the child to make choices and participate in reciprocal play throughout the EMDR treatment, the child may be more willing to engage. This feeling of control is of utmost importance for a young child, as the experience of trauma may have rendered them feeling powerless to their environment and others, and may be an underlying theme for possible triggers. Providing the child with this feeling of power and control may assist them in feeling safe and secure and therefore more willing to persist through the "tough stuff" in order to continue with the EMDR treatment.

DESCRIPTION OF INTERVENTION

This intervention incorporates the use of superhero figurines for Phase 2, resourcing; Phase 4, desensitization; and Phase 5, installation, of the EMDR protocol. Rather than using one's fingers to assist the child in engaging in bilateral eye movements for processing, the therapist uses a superhero figurine that the child is asked to follow back and forth with their eyes (Figure 16.1). Using the figurines encourages participation, assists in building tolerance for exposure to the thoughts and feelings of the trauma, and provides the child with a role-model character upon which to develop resourcing and cognitive restructuring. When challenged to identify a positive cognition during target setup, which may occur when working with young children, it is helpful to prompt the child to identify a superhero quality that they would like to have.

16. USING THE SUPERHERO SHUFFLE FOR BILATERAL STIMULATION   373

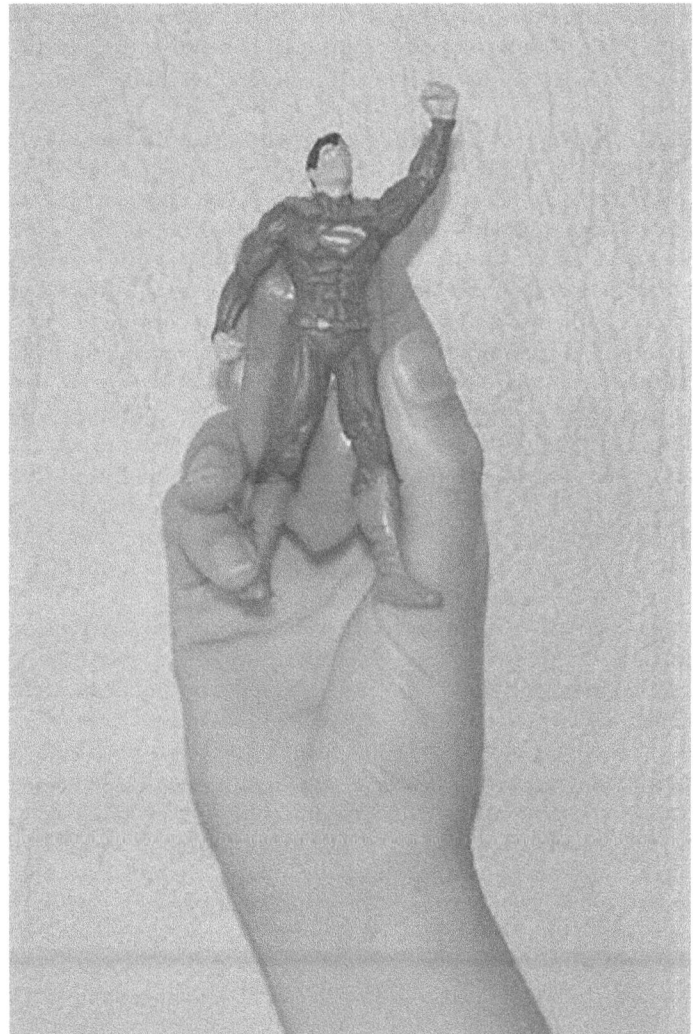

Figure 16.1 *Superhero Shuffle for BLS*
BLS, bilateral stimulation.

STEP-BY-STEP INSTRUCTIONS

Step 1: After completing Phase 1, client history and treatment planning, the therapist would then move to Phase 2, preparation. This phase includes establishing a strong therapeutic alliance and exploring therapy objectives and desired outcomes, and also explains the use of EMDR as a treatment modality and initiates resource development and strengthening of relaxation techniques (Greenwald, 2012). The therapist may introduce the use of the figurines during preparation to test the child's eye movement capabilities and assist in resource development. The therapist may choose to introduce the character as an additional assistant to the therapeutic process and can initiate resource development using the superhero figurine to explore different qualities and skills. See the sections "Modifications," "Considerations," and "Case Example" for more on resource development.

Step 2: Once the therapist and child have identified sufficient information for target setup by moving through client history (Phase 1), preparation (Phase 2), and assessment (Phase 3), then desensitization (Phase 4) can take place (Shapiro, 2018). During this phase, the therapist will set up for eye movements by using the chosen superhero as an object for the child to follow for bilateral eye movements. It is important that the therapist monitor the child's responses during this phase, as a child may indicate the need for a break by behaviors including becoming disengaged or defiant. It is recommended that the therapist have adequate knowledge of the child's ability to tolerate "tough stuff" and be prepared to implement play breaks for managing dysregulation and then redirect the child back to eye movements when ready. Should the child seem to become distracted altogether from the original target processing, the therapist may find it helpful to implement a quick break and then verbalize the target setup to begin eye movements again. Asking a young child to place a hand on the location of the feeling during processing may also assist in keeping the target feelings and thoughts as the focus for processing.

Step 3: Phase 5 will focus on cognitive restructuring and will require the therapist to return to the original positive cognition and ensure that the Validity of Cognition (VOC) feels true when concentrating on the traumatic incident. It is recommended that the therapist utilize visual scales to assist a younger child in grasping the abstract scaling concept. Once the positive cognition has been selected, the therapist will initiate short sets of eye movements using the superhero figurine again to install the cognition. The therapist may also choose to use installation to encourage reciprocal play, whereby the child can mimic the therapist's hand movements using the superhero figurine. This will allow the therapist to model tracking and positive cognitions. The therapist may find that verbalizing positive cognitions allows a young child to identify positive cognitions that resonate with them. The therapist will then continue with Phase 6, body scan, and Phase 7, closure, in order to complete the EMDR process (Shapiro, 2018). It is important that the therapist ensure sufficient time is allocated to these phases so that the child is able to achieve a level of closure and leave the session in a calm, controlled, and safe manner. It is suggested that a certain amount of free playtime be allowed once EMDR has been completed for that session. It allows the child time to continue processing the trauma through play and ground before leaving the office.

MODIFICATIONS

It is recommended that breaks are provided between desensitization sets in order to increase tolerance and maintain the playful, fast-paced approach that is suggested. The quantity and duration of breaks will need to be modified according to the child. These breaks need not be long or complex, but can instead be a quick diversion from the process. This can include things such as shaking wiggles out of one's body, doing jumping jacks, scribbling on paper as fast as one can, and so on. The therapist may choose to use the superheroes to initiate the breaks by having superhero races (from one side of the room to the other) and then quickly returning to eye movements.

The child may not hold any regard for superhero figurines, at which point the therapist will be required to present additional objects to the child as options to use in the EMDR process. It is suggested that the therapist identify characters that the child naturally gravitates toward and that have positive qualities or attributes that can be used to assist the child in resource development and cognitive restructuring. It is most effective when the figurines utilized have personality traits, but should this not be possible, it is recommended that the therapist aid the child in personifying the chosen object. For example, the child may choose to use the figurine of a dog and the therapist could explore traits such as loyalty, respect, listening skills, and nurturance.

CONSIDERATIONS

1. First and foremost, after any mention of "tough stuff" related to trauma or the child's negative thoughts, feelings, or behaviors, it is recommended that the therapist initiates play with the child by providing a menu of options in which to engage. This is important as it will assist in increasing the child's tolerance for trauma exposure, ensures that the child continues to regard therapy and EMDR as a positive experience, and allows the child to continue processing after EMDR through the means of play. It also allows the therapist to navigate the child between play and trauma processing, therefore maintaining a fast-paced, high-energy approach that will aid in keeping the child engaged. Using play at the end of each session also provides the child with a level of incentive to revisit the "tough stuff" and to return and continue in the therapy process, knowing that there is the opportunity to engage in fun afterward.
2. The therapist should have a strong therapeutic relationship and knowledge of the child's verbal and behavioral responses in order to monitor tolerance for strong emotions that may cause the child to become disengaged. By monitoring the child's reactions, the therapist is able to switch to another activity prior to exceeding the child's tolerance, therefore ensuring that it does not become unbearable and result in later resistance to EMDR.
3. When choosing superhero figurines, the therapist may find it best to have a number of different figurines available and allow the child to choose two of their favorite characters. This is important for a number of reasons: It allows the child a level of choice and control, the buy-in from the child will be improved as choosing the figurines creates a level of responsibility for participation and, finally, the character qualities are used during Phase 5, installation, and it is useful if the characters are ones that the child has some knowledge of and that they resonate with them. It is recommended that the therapist carefully select the figurines that are presented to the child, as there are some characters that embody a "bad" persona. A child who has experienced trauma may have adopted this negative self-view as a result of thoughts, feelings, and behaviors experienced

or expressed. The therapist should attempt to avoid presenting characters as options for this intervention that may perpetuate this negative self-view.
4. The therapist may choose to prompt the child to select a figurine while the therapist verbalizes the target setup. The therapist may find it helpful that the child remains busy during target setup by engaging them in figurine selection and again briefly before starting eye movements. This may result in the child being more willing to engage and less threatened by the information that had just been presented.
5. The therapist should present a minimum of two superhero figurines as options and allow the child to choose which they would like to use for eye movements. The therapist may want to suggest that the child may choose a figurine to hold during eye-movement sets for a number of reasons. First, holding a figurine may provide the child with some level of nurturance and means to release energy by fiddling with the object. Second, it allows the child to "take turns" by moving the figurine in an identical manner so that the therapist may engage in eye movements. This reciprocal play strengthens the therapeutic alliance, allows for the therapist to model eye-movement tracking to the child, and provides the child with a feeling of power and control.
6. When setting up the target for processing, the more information the therapist is able to gather without utilizing direct questions, the better. The therapist may find that younger children are more responsive to reflective statements than direct questioning (Landreth, 2012). This is true especially if this is a child who has adopted a self-view of being "bad," as they are most likely accustomed to lots of direct questioning regarding behaviors and may tend to become subdued, disengaged, and unresponsive as a result.
7. When asking a young child for a VOC and Subjective Units of Distress Scale (SUDS) rating, it is suggested that the therapist demonstrate these using two different visual scales that show varying quantities associated to the numbers. Anything that shows a range of size or quantities is useful to lessen the abstract nature of a rating scale for a young child.

CASE EXAMPLE

The following is a case example transcript of a session with a 7-year-old child to illustrate the use of the Superhero Shuffle intervention. Identifying information has been changed with respect to client confidentiality. During intake and treatment planning, Phase 1 of EMDR treatment was completed utilizing a comprehensive biopsychosocial assessment, trauma assessment, medical history questionnaire, adverse behaviors and/or symptoms checklists, and the creation of a safety plan, and desired treatment outcomes were explored. The first 4 months of therapy were spent engaging in nondirective play therapy in order to establish and strengthen the therapeutic alliance and become familiar with the client's themes and views of self and others.

> Therapist: *So, I remember that you told me about Superman being really brave during that one rescue. He must have been scared when that happened.*

Client: *He was! But he's big and strong and brave.*

Therapist: *Brave, hmm. That sounds like when you told me about helping your friend take the spider off her desk at school. That was brave of you.*

Client: *Kind of, I guess. Spiders don't scare me.*

Therapist: *They do scare some people. It sounds to me like you were brave! I wonder how that makes you feel when you think about being brave.*

Client: *I feel proud. Proud of me.*

Therapist: *You were brave and felt proud. I wonder if we can stand just like Superman* (gestures to figurine) *in a brave and proud way. Does standing with your body that way show that you felt brave and proud?*

Client: *Yes.*

Therapist: *Great! Let's bring Superman in and think about feeling brave and proud. Maybe we can stay standing like that. I'm going to have Superman fly back and forth like we practiced okay? Head still, eyes watching him and thinking of those feelings in our Superman stand, ready?* (Resource development and installation)

Eye movements using superhero figurine: Short set. Repeated.
Allowed break for child to engage in play.

Therapist: *So, when you arrived here today, your mum told me that something happened at school the other day. Maybe something that didn't feel too great?*

Client: *I got into trouble at school for being bad.* (Negative cognition)

Therapist: *It seems like something may have upset you.* (Reflective listening)

Client: *Yes, the teacher said I did the wrong page in my book and everyone at my table laughed at me. I had to start all over again and so I pushed the table over because I didn't want to do even more work.* (Image/picture)

Therapist: *I'm wondering how that made you feel?*

Client: *Stupid. And angry.* (Emotion/feeling)

Therapist: *And it doesn't make our bodies feel good when we experience those sorts of feelings. I wonder where in your body you felt that.*

Client: *My belly and my hands because I made them into fists.* (Body sensation/location)

Therapist: *You mentioned that you felt like you were bad at school because of what happened. I wonder what you would like to think about yourself instead.*

Client: *I'm smart and brave.* (Positive cognition)

Therapist: *And when you think of being laughed at and say I'm smart and brave, how much do you believe that? Believe it lots or a little?* (VOC checked using a visual scale)

Client: *A little bit.* (Child pointed to number 2 on visual scale)

Therapist: *And when you think about it now, is there a lot of bad feeling or no bad feelings at all?* (SUDS; use visual scale)

Client: *Lots.* (Child pointed to number 8 on visual scale)

Therapist: *Okay, so what do you think about bringing in Superman to help us fly through that situation. What do you think? Can you fly him in here?*

Client: *Okay.* (Child flew Superman figurine to therapist)

Therapist: *Alright, Superman. I wonder if you can help us out. We're going to think about that situation that we just spoke about, feeling bad, feeling angry and stupid in our hands and belly and we're going to watch you fly back and forth. Ready?*

Eye movements using superhero figurine were done while monitoring the child's response and repeated so long as the child was able to remain engaged. We followed the EMDR protocol by checking for SUDS for no change on channel, no change and no distress or no change and SUDS of 0, while allowing for breaks for the child to engage in play.

Therapist: *So how does "I'm smart and brave" sound? Is that still the best thing to say or do you want to say something else instead?* (Installation)

Client: *Brave, smart, and strong.*

Therapist: *So, when you think of being laughed at, all those feelings, and say "brave, smart, and strong" out loud, does it feel lots or a little bit true?*
(Using VOC visual scale)

We continued with eye movements in short sets to no change, and VOC of 7, body scan, and closure as needed. The Superhero Shuffle was helpful in keeping this child engaged enough to benefit from the EMDR protocol.

REFERENCES

Greenwald, R. (2012). *EMDR within a phase model of trauma-informed treatment.* Hoboken, NJ: Taylor and Francis.

Landreth, G. L. (2012). *Play therapy: The art of the relationship.* New York, NY: Routledge.

Shapiro, F. (2018). *Eye movement desensitization and reprocessing (EMDR) therapy: Basic principles, protocols, and procedures* (3rd ed.). New York, NY: Guilford Press.

Solomon, M. F., & Siegel, D. J. (2003). *Healing trauma: Attachment, mind, body, and brain.* New York, NY: W. W. Norton.

17

"Splatting" Out the Trauma With Movement in EMDR Processing

ALICE STRICKLIN

INTRODUCTION

This play-based intervention addresses the challenge of providing EMDR to early elementary school–aged boys. Their energy level, restlessness, and need to engage physically can at times get in the way of reprocessing a traumatic memory. "Splatting" Out the Trauma has built in resourcing, social engagement, and organic trauma response completion that can help facilitate the desensitization and installation phases of EMDR.

PHASES OF EMDR

Assessment (Phase 3), desensitization (Phase 4), and installation (Phase 5)

MATERIALS

- Paper
- Markers
- Splat ball (Splat balls are squeezable, sticky, rubbery textured balls filled with filtered water. You can purchase them in various forms including eggs, emojis, animal characters, or regular balls. When thrown against the wall or floor, it will splat out and then pull back together into a ball.)
- Tape
- Optional materials: paint, crayons, colored pencils

RATIONALE

Children with higher energy levels often need interventions that are shorter in time and are more hands-on to engage them physically. Additionally, children with a history of trauma tend to demonstrate higher levels of hyperactivity, fidgeting, and inattentiveness, which may appear as high energy. Peter Levine (2007) explains that chronic hyperarousal in children looks very much like symptoms of attention deficit disorder with hyperactivity (ADHD), and often teachers will describe this hyperarousal in the classroom as fidgeting, restless legs, compulsive talking, constantly getting out of their seat, looking around the room at others, or looking for a fight. Generally, boys have more externalized symptoms when it comes to trauma, which looks like acting out, being more aggressive, or doing dangerous activities, while girls tend to have internalized trauma symptoms where their anger is turned inward, which looks like anxiety, aches and pains, depressed affect, and negative self-talk (Levine, 2007; van der Kolk, 2014). Boys who specifically come to treatment for trauma can be difficult to engage long enough to do much in the way of interventions. Eliana Gil (2006) describes two behavior responses as the basic instinctual drives that children use to help regulate emotional injuries. She describes these two responses as the drive to have mastery over painful or confusing experiences and the drive to avoid or suppress what is painful (Gil, 2016). Splatting Out the Trauma allows the child to have mastery over the painful by making it easier for them to engage in the intervention as it is done physically. This intervention also challenges the instinctual drive of avoidance by creating a safe and fun way to engage in trauma content that was too scary to address before.

Unprocessed trauma memories are stored in fragments (van der Kolk, 1994; van der Kolk & Fisler, 1995). This is supported by the behavior, affect, sensation, knowledge (BASK) model of dissociation, which states that traumatic events cause varying levels of dissociation varying from localized to generalized (Braun, 1988). We see this dissociation in children when the therapist begins to activate a target memory and the child becomes fidgety, gets up and moves away from eye movements, shows signs of aggressive agitation, or begins staring into space with a "faraway" look in their eyes. Shapiro (2001) hypothesizes that bringing into focus the disturbing imagery, sensations, cognition, and emotion begins the integration process of this fragmentation. This intervention addresses the fragmentation that happens with trauma and the way it gets stored in the maladaptive networks in this fragmented state. The intervention also takes into consideration the need for short interrupted exposure experiences, while also allowing the system to experience positive adaptive present-day counter-conditioning in the therapeutic setting.

Shapiro (2001) discusses the need to get creative when using dual attention stimuli (DAS), also called bilateral stimulation (BLS), with children and cites Wilson, Tinker, Hofmann, Becke, and Marshall (2000) as evidence for this creativity. She goes on to describe other pioneering clinicians who adapted Phase 3 to include drawing the picture of the worst part of the incident then adding the Butterfly Hug as the BLS in Phases 4 to 6 (Artigas, Jarero, Maurer, López Cano, & Alcalá, 2000; Boel, 1999; Jarero, Artigas, Mauer, López Cano, & Alcalá, 1999; Wilson, et al., 2000). The work of these pioneers who creatively adapted DAS with children informed the development of this intervention.

The splat ball technique originated with an idea to engage children physically through running while activating a traumatic memory. Running allows the BLS to occur in a natural way, while inviting the child to look at the picture on the wall incorporates dual attention. The use of both running in place and maintaining external focus away from the therapist allows the child to feel a sense of control and reduces the possible overstimulation from engaging in eye contact with the therapist. The physical engagement as well as the dual focus of this intervention appears to work well with boys and girls who display higher levels of energy. The splat ball portion of this technique is modified from the splat balls play therapy technique also referred to as "egg splat balls" commonly used in Level 3 of release play therapy (Shaefer, 2011).

DESCRIPTION OF INTERVENTION

Splatting Out the Trauma is introduced during Phase 3, assessment. The child is asked to draw a picture of the worst part of the identified memory to be processed. The picture is then lightly taped on the therapist wall. The child is invited to look at the picture and run in place. After running in place, the therapist cues to the client to stop and throw the splat ball. The client throws the splat ball at the picture, trying to make it stick and pull the picture off the wall. Once the picture is pulled off the wall, the therapist has the client redraw the image that represents the worst part of the trauma now. Once the trauma memory has been desensitized and the memory reprocessed, indicated by changes in the child's drawing and reduced Subjective Units of Disturbance Scale (SUDS) rating, the therapist will then move on to Phase 5, installation. The therapist invites the child to state their positive cognition (PC) out loud while running in place. Phase 5 is completed when the child indicates a Validity of Cognition (VOC) of 7.

STEP-BY-STEP INSTRUCTIONS

Step 1: This step begins in Phase 3, assessment, with inviting the child to draw the image that represents the worst part. The language that can be used with small children may be, *"When you imagine this bad memory now, I wonder if you could draw me a picture of what you see now when you imagine it?"* or *"When you remember that time we talked about that was so scary, could you draw me a picture of the part of that day that was the worst part?"* Having a variety of materials such as markers, crayons, colored pencils, and paints to use is best, but whatever the therapist has available will suffice.

Step 2: The therapist invites the client to help tape the picture up on the wall. For best results, tape the picture so it will be able to come off easily.

Step 3: The therapist will have the child stand about 20 steps away from the wall. Adjust depending on the client, making sure they are far enough to throw the ball and close enough to hit the target. Then demonstrate to the child what they will be doing. *"I'm going to stand this far away from the picture. I'm looking at the picture and remembering how bad that day felt. I'm running in place as I look at that picture and remember. When I hear the word 'splat,' I stop and throw the splat ball at the picture and try to get it to come off the wall."* After demonstrating, hand the child the splat ball and have them do a test run of running in place and throwing the splat ball at the picture when the therapist says *"splat."*

Step 4: Invite the client to look at the picture and try to remember the worst part of the memory. The therapist should try to use the client's words. If they describe it as a *"thing,"* say *"That thing that happened."* If the client describes it saying *"the bad day,"* the therapist should use those words.

Step 5: Ask the child if they have a bad thought that comes up when they remember the worst part. The therapist should use the negative cognition (NC) that the client identified in Phase 2, preparation, if the client has a hard time identifying one in Phase 3. A therapist can say, *"Before, when we talked about that day, you said it felt like 'I'm bad,' do you still have that thought now as you remember it?"* The therapist should go with whatever the client gives.

Step 6: Ask for the PC, *"What is the good thought you wish you had?"* Then continue with the traditional steps of assessing the VOC, the emotion, SUDS rating, and finally body sensations using all the tools you introduced to the client in Phase 2.

Step 7: Ask the client to *"Look at the picture, remember the worst part about that day, the thought "I'm bad"* (or whatever their NC is) *and run in place."*

Step 8: After the client has run in place for about 15 to 20 seconds, the therapist will say *"splat."* The therapist should wait for the client to throw the ball and offer encouragement with whatever the result of the throw. Some examples the therapist could offer are *"Wow, look how strong you are, you are splatting out that picture"* or *"That's it! You are good at splatting out that bad memory."*

Step 9: If the client has not done so, invite them to go pick up the splat ball and invite them to stand back where they were. Ask them to look at the picture again and run in place. Again, after about 15 to 20 seconds, say *"splat."*

Step 10: After they retrieve the splat ball, invite them to stand back where they had been running in place. Ask them to look at the picture and say, *"Now when you look at that picture, and remember that day, what do you remember now?"* The therapist is assessing for change. If the client reports change to the memory, continue doing the sequence. If the client does not report change, you may add some additional resourcing, such as cognitive interweaves in the next few sets. Some examples may include *"You are doing a great job, just looking at the picture and remembering"* and *"It's all over with now. We are just looking back on something that already happened."* After 15 to 20 seconds, the therapist will say *"splat."* Assess for change by asking the client, *"When you look at the picture and think of that day now, what do you notice?"*

The therapist may even offer some resource affirmations between sets. These should be empowering and offer a counter both physically and emotionally to their experience (e.g., feeling weak to feeling strong, feeling powerless to feeling powerful, feeling helpless to feeling in control). The therapist may even have the client say out loud an affirmation that connects with the memory. This is a way to build in resourcing interweaves that can help them connect with adaptive networks. Some examples may be, *"You can't hurt me anymore,"* *"I am not scared of you anymore,"* *"I am a good boy/girl,"* and *"My _____ loves me."*

Step 11: When the client is able to pull the picture down with the splat ball, invite the client to now remember the memory and draw what feels like the worst part of it now. The therapist is assessing again for change in the memory and also giving the child's system time to shift into a slower paced activity. This can help with short attention spans by offering a different way to process.

Step 12: When it is evident to the therapist that the image is changing, the therapist should reassess the SUDS rating. If the SUDS is above 1, repeat steps 7 to 10 until the client splats the picture off of the wall again.

Step 13: When the client indicates a SUDS of 1 or 0, then invite the client to hang the most recent picture on the wall. The therapist then asks the client to remember the memory and see if the good thought *"I am good"* (or the PC the client indicated in Phase 3) feels true. If the client indicates that the PC feels true, invite them to run in place repeating the PC out loud. Ask them to again throw the ball when the therapist says splat. Have them run in place for 10 seconds. The therapist should assess the VOC in between throws until the client indicates the VOC is 7.

MODIFICATIONS

There may need to be some modification if the picture does not change. Sometimes when the clinician has the child draw how they see the memory now, the child either responds with *"It looks the same"* or draws something very similar to their first drawing. This is an indicator that the reprocessing is blocked in a fragmented channel (Braun, 1998; van der Kolk, 1994; van der Kolk & Fisler, 1995). The therapist may assess if the client is using running in place as a distraction to get out of the disturbing exposure experience. This is easy for children to do because their systems naturally want to move away from the pain and disturbance (Gil, 2006). If this is the case, you may first ask the client what bothers them still about the memory. Then ask them to focus really hard on that part that really bothers them, ask them if they feel something in their body as they focus hard on the disturbance. If they do, hand them a piece of paper with a body outline drawn on it. Ask them to choose a color that seems to go with that place they feel in their body and color in where they feel it on their body on the piece of paper. Then have them tape that up on the wall. Then ask them to think of that bad part of the memory, then point to where they feel it in their body. While looking at the picture, focus this time on the body part while they run in place. The clinician could also have the client put their hand on the body part that hurts or feels bad when they remember the memory, then the clinician could tap on the client's shoulders or feet bilaterally while they look at the picture. When the therapist stops tapping, say *"splat"* and the client can then throw the splat ball at the picture. This adaptation can be used both when the picture doesn't seem to be changing and when it seems that the running in place is more of a distraction for the client than helpful.

While originally created to work with high-energy boys, this intervention has been used with girls as well. Girls with higher levels of energy and who seem to be more competitive by nature seem to respond well to this intervention. Some modifications may need to be made in the distance to the wall for some girls. It is recommended to do a few practice throws before beginning the bilateral running in place, to measure the distance that will be most effective.

CONSIDERATIONS

There are some considerations and possible adjustments that may need to be made with this intervention depending on the client's needs and abilities. One consideration is what to do if the client has a physical disability that does not allow them to run in place. If this is the case, the therapist may encourage the client to clap on their legs bilaterally while looking at the picture, and then when the therapist says *"splat,"* they then pick up the splat ball from their lap and throw. The client may need to be closer to the wall and picture for this adaptation.

Another consideration that often happens with children who have experienced trauma is a negative self-talk cycle. For these children, if the picture is not falling off after 1 or 2 times, this may cause a response of anger, sadness, or disengagement. Usually this comes from a negative internal self-talk of *"I'm not doing this right"* or *"There is something wrong with me."* It's important to remember that this is common, and may actually be what they experienced at the time of the trauma. The first response from the clinician should be offering a different response. This includes the therapist considering what the client needed but didn't get. For example, if the child was being criticized at the time of the incident, you may say something like, *"Did you know that I have done this activity with a lot of kids and it usually takes a lot of throws before it comes down?"* Offering them an interweave of normalizing their experience and offering that they are like other children can be a subtle way to also let their brain make the same associations with the trauma memory. Another possible interweave is to validate what the child is feeling in the moment. Again, offering an experience they may not have gotten at the time of the trauma and offering it now in the moment of activation helps allowing the system to move toward healing. This may look like offering an interweave similar to, *"It looks like you are upset that the picture hasn't torn down yet. Your arms are crossed and you have a mad look on your face. Can you tell me what you are feeling right now?"*

If the client indicates they are feeling mad, the therapist may assess further with, *"I'm wondering if you are feeling mad at yourself or mad at the picture?"* This begins the validation process while also assessing where the child is stuck in reprocessing (e.g., locus of control being stuck internally *"I should have done different"* or externally *"They did something wrong and let me down"*). It is from here that the clinician can then offer the client a different experience and invite integration. The important thing for the clinician to remember is whatever the child's experience in the office with the intervention, it is a manifestation of a fragmented part of the memory.

CASE EXAMPLES

CASE EXAMPLE 1

Joe* is an 8-year-old child who had a history of physical abuse by a stepparent. His parents divorced when he was 4 years old, and both parents remarried within the next year. Joe is the second oldest in a sibling group of four. He experienced physical abuse by a stepparent from the ages of 5 through 7, when reports were

---

*In order to protect client confidentiality, the information in this case example has been modified.

made and legal action was taken to forbid contact between Joe and that stepparent. His presenting problems included rage outbursts at home and school and a recent development of major fear of storms. During the history-taking phase, Joe and the therapist identified a few memories of physical abuse by his stepparent that continued to bother him as well as a bad thunderstorm he had experienced. Joe had a slight reduction of symptoms in Phase 2 of EMDR, as he began to learn emotional intelligence to express his internal experience to the caretaker adults in his life. He also learned how to do body scans regularly by practicing progressive muscle relaxation at home and in the classroom.

The first target that the therapist and Joe agreed to work on was the first time the stepparent was physically abusive by punching him in the mouth when Joe had told the stepparent no. The incident had been done in the presence of the biological parent with no intervention from them.

> Therapist: *"Joe, let's remember the time that _____ punched you in the mouth. And when you remember it right now, I wonder if you could draw me a picture of what is the worst part about it that seems to come up in your mind."*
>
> Joe: *"What should I draw?"*
>
> Therapist: *"Whatever seems to be in your mind right now when you think about that day."*

Joe bent over his paper and began drawing a picture using the colors red, black, and blue. He drew a picture of a large stick figure with an angry face in red and a smaller stick figure with an angry face in red. He drew a green couch with black marks on the ground around the couch. Then he drew another stick figure with an angry face in the far corner of the picture and drew this figure with the black marker. He looked up at me and nodded his head indicating he was done. The therapist invited Joe to help her tape the picture to the far wall of the therapy room where there were no other items to block the way. The therapist checked the tape to make sure it was lightly taped on. Then the therapist had Joe back up about 10 steps from the wall.

> Therapist: *"Now let's do a little test throw so you can get used to what we are going to do."* The therapist showed Joe the splat ball and explained that it's sticky on the outside and squishy on the inside. The therapist let Joe feel the ball while she still held on to it. The therapist then explained, *"When you throw the splat ball against the wall, it splats out in what looks like a blob, then peels itself off the wall and falls to the floor."* The therapist demonstrated by throwing the ball against the wall (not the picture) to show Joe what happened when it hit the wall. The therapist asked Joe if he'd like to give it a try.
>
> Therapist (after Joe nodded and threw the splat ball hard against the wall): *"Wow, you are pretty good at throwing! Would it be okay if we try it from a few steps farther back?"* Joe nodded and took three steps back and practiced throwing again. The therapist then asked for the splat ball back and explained what will happen next.
>
> Therapist: *"Joe, we are going to do a little game that can help your brain work through this bad memory so it doesn't bother you as much anymore. I'm going*

to explain the game and show you how it works first, and then I'll let you have a try at it." The therapist saw that Joe was watching her and seemed attentive, so she continued, "See that picture on the wall of the memory we decided to help your brain work through?" Joe nods.

Therapist: *"So how it works is I'm going to have you look at that picture, and remember how bad it felt when you were there. And when you start feeling some of that bad you let me know and I'm going to ask you some questions. After you answer the questions, I'm going to say, 'okay let's run in place' and then when I say 'splat,' you get to throw that ball as hard as you can at the picture and try to pull it off the wall with the splat ball. Now don't worry, it usually takes a lot of throwing the ball before it comes off the wall. After you throw it one time, I'll get the splat ball, then I'll have you think of the bad day again, look at the picture, run in place then when I say 'splat' throw the ball again. We will do that a few times until I say 'stop.' Any questions?"*

Therapist: *"I'm thinking of that day and how bad it felt."* The therapist pauses and gives the examples while running in place: *"I remember the mean faces, I feel my tummy hurting right now, and my hands want to make a fist, I feel scared and mad."* Then the therapist said "splat" and stopped running and aimed and threw the ball at the picture.

Joe (laughing out loud and running to get the splat ball): *"That was cool. I'm ready to try."*

Therapist: *"Remember that day that you were punched. Is there a bad thought that comes up for you about that day?"*

Joe: *"I'm in trouble."*

Therapist: *"Is there a good thought you want to have about that day?"*

Joe: *"I am a good boy."*

Therapist: *"Do those words 'I'm a good boy' seem true right now when you think of that memory?"*

Joe shook his head no.

Therapist: *"Look at the picture and remember that day and see if you have a feeling about it right now."*

Joe paused and then stated, *"Mad. "*

Therapist: *"How bad does this memory feel right now as you look at the picture?"* (The therapist offered Joe the 0 to 10 SUDS rating that was introduced in Phase 2, and he pointed to 8.)

Therapist: *"As you look at that picture, does your body feel tight or uncomfortable anywhere right now?"*

Joe pointed to his stomach.

Therapist: *"Okay, Joe. Look at that picture and focus on all the things that feel bad right now and run in place."* Joe started running in place with a determined look on his face. He alternated between looking at the floor and his feet and the picture.

17. "SPLATTING" OUT THE TRAUMA WITH MOVEMENT

> Therapist (after about 10–15 seconds): *"Okay, splat."*
>
> Joe stopped and looked hard at the picture and threw the splat ball as hard as he could. He caught the top left corner of the picture. The splat ball stuck, then rolled off the wall.
>
> Therapist: *"That was a great throw. Let's keep working on splatting out that memory."* The therapist retrieved the splat ball, then handed it to Joe. The therapist then invited Joe to look at the picture and remember the day again and start running in place. Joe ran in place at a faster pace this time and looked at the picture with a mean, determined look on his face. The therapist observed in silence.
>
> Therapist (after about 10–15 seconds): *"Splat."*

Joe stopped and threw the splat ball at the picture again this time, catching the middle of the picture. He smiled and watched the ball roll off the picture after sticking for a few seconds.

> Therapist: *"Okay, remember that day again and whatever you remember then run in place again."*

Joe looked at the picture, then started running in place. The therapist observed that Joe did not have the glaring mad look on his face any longer but more of a determined look. The therapist also observed that Joe's running in place did not seem as fast or as hard of a run.

> Therapist (offered as Joe ran): *"You're doing a great job Joe, remembering that this happened a long time ago."* (15–20 seconds of letting Joe run). *"Splat."* Joe stopped and threw the splat ball at the picture and caught the bottom corner. The picture ripped slightly from the tape. Joe got a huge smile on his face.
>
> Therapist: *"That's a great job, Joe. You are in charge of this memory now and are slowly tearing it away. Keep focusing on it and it will keep tearing away."*

Joe's shoulders relaxed a little as the therapist gave the splat ball back to him.

> Therapist: *"Would you like to do it again?"*

Joe nodded.

> Therapist: *"Okay, look at the picture and remember whatever still feels bad about it then start running in place."*

Joe looked at the picture and started running in place. The therapist observed him running faster and harder again only without the angry look on his face.

> Therapist (after 20 seconds): *"Splat."*

Joe stopped and, panting, he squinted his eyes at the picture, reared his arm back, and threw the splat ball as hard as he could. The splat ball caught the bottom half of the page and ripped it off the wall. Joe started jumping around celebrating. The therapist joined him in celebrating and jumping around the room.

> Therapist: *"That was so good! How do you feel?"*
>
> Joe: *"Happy!"*
>
> Therapist: *"Are you ready to draw another picture of that day now?"*
>
> Joe nodded.
>
> Therapist: *"Okay, as you remember that day again, draw what you remember now."*

Joe started drawing a picture of his house in blue and orange and a yellow sun shining in the sky above the house. He drew a picture of a large stick figure in black, and four smaller stick figures on the grass around the house. The stick figures had either smiles or straight lines for their mouth in the picture. All the figures were drawn in black.

The therapist asked Joe if this picture was something else that happened that day. Joe shook his head and said, no; it was his parent and siblings playing kickball in the front yard last week.

The therapist asked Joe if there was anything else about the memory that bothered him. Joe shook his head and smiled saying *"I splatted it out."* The therapist showed Joe the SUDS and asked Joe to identify how bad the memory felt to him when he thought about it. Joe pointed to the 1 and the 0. The therapist asked Joe if, when he thought of that memory, did the words *"I'm a good boy"* feel true. Joe nodded and pointed to the new drawing. He told the therapist that the parent had told him on this particular day that he was a good boy while they were playing outside. The therapist asked Joe if he wanted to hang the new picture up and do some more running in place. Joe looked confused and said *"I don't want to splat it out."* The therapist agreed with Joe and asked if he'd like to do something different with it. Joe agreed and the therapist and Joe hung up the picture.

> Therapist: *"Okay, Joe. As you look at the new picture, how about you saying the words 'I'm a good boy' out loud this time while you run in place."*

The therapist let Joe know we would not use the splat ball this time, but just run in place saying those great words. He stood up and looked at the new picture with a smile on his face. The therapist had him think of the first memory and then run in place saying *"I'm a good boy"* while looking at the new picture. The therapist had Joe stop after 10 seconds

> Therapist: *"How true do those words 'I'm a good boy' feel right now when you remember that day."* (The therapist showed Joe the VOC scale previously introduced in Phase 2.)
>
> Joe quietly pointed to 7 on the scale.

Therapist: *"So now when you remember the old memory again and say those words 'I'm a good boy' out loud, see if there is anything that feels uncomfortable in your body."*

Joe paused and seemed to be thinking, then looked at therapist and smiled and said *"No, I feel great."*

He then ran over to the new picture and took it off the wall and asked if he could take it to his parent waiting in the waiting room.

CASE EXAMPLE 2

In another case example, a young boy who had had an allergic reaction and been rushed to the hospital processed that memory. He described and drew the worst moment when he had to have IV therapy and the nurse missed the vein causing

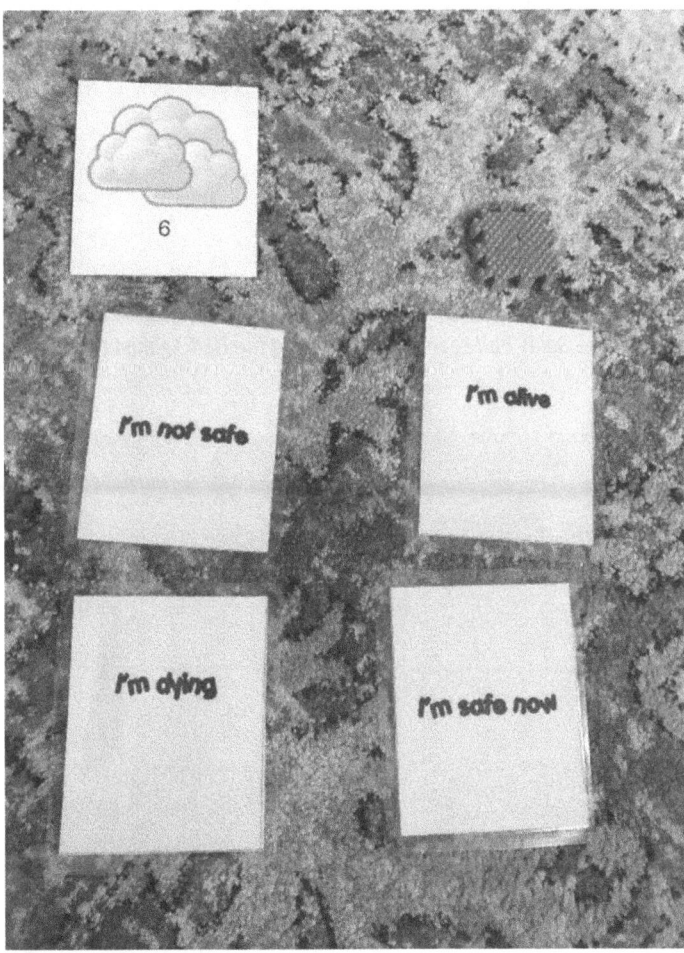

Figure 17.1 *Assessing the Target With the Negative and Positive Cognitions*

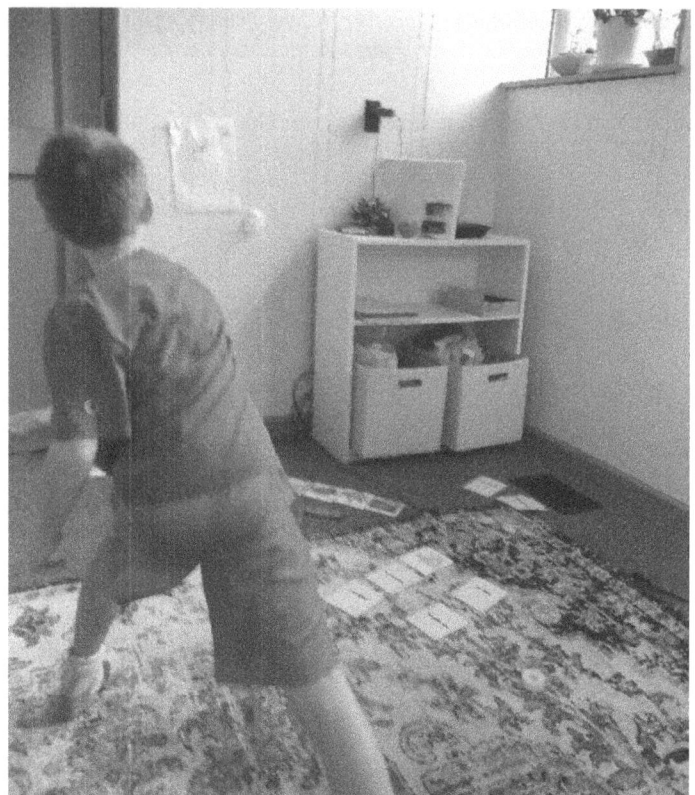

Figure 17.2 *The Splat Ball Technique: Throwing the Ball Against the Bad Image*

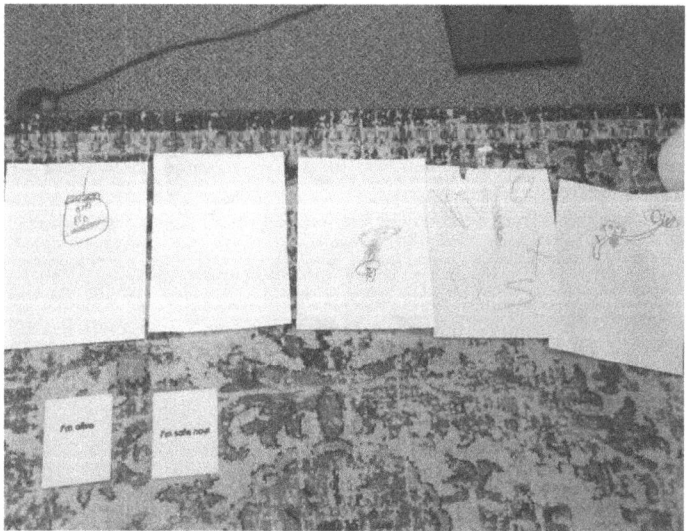

Figure 17.3 *Images (From Right to Left) From the Spat Ball Processing Session*

blood to spurt onto the sheets. He identified the NC of *"I'm dying"* and *"I'm not safe"* and the PC he wished for as *"I'm alive and I'm safe now"* with a VOC 4 and SUDS 6 (Figure 17.1).

He began by throwing the splat balls against the first picture of himself getting a shot (Figure 17.2), and BLS from running in place was encouraged.

In between sets, he drew the additional images that emerged (Figure 17.3), including throwing up and feeling like he couldn't breathe. In the fourth picture, a related memory emerged of another allergic reaction where he needed an injection and finally a picture of the EpiPen where, between splats, he came up with the adaptive idea that *"It hurt but it saved my life."*

Using this splat ball process activates the child's full body and provides for the need of expressive options to make EMDR processing more interactive and accessible for younger children.

REFERENCES

Artigas, L. A., Jarero, I., Maurer, M., López Cano, T., & Alcalá, N. (2000, September). *EMDR and traumatic stress after natural disasters: Integrative treatment protocol and the butterfly hug.* Poster presented at the EMDRIA Conference, Toronto, ON, Canada.

Boel, J. (1999). The butterfly hug. *EMDRIA Newsletter, 4*(4), 11–13.

Braun, B. G. (1988). The BASK model of dissociation. *Dissociation, 1,* 4–23.

Gil, E. (2006). *Helping abused and traumatized children.* New York, NY and London, UK: Guilford Press.

Jarero, I., Artigas, L., Mauer, M., López Cano, T., & Alcalá, N. (1999, November). *Children's post-traumatic stress after natural disasters: Integrative treatment protocols.* Poster presented at the annual meeting of the International Society for Traumatic Stress Studies, Miami, FL.

Levine, P. A. (2007). *Trauma through a child's eyes: Awakening the ordinary miracle of healing.* Berkeley, CA: North Atlantic Books.

Shaefer, C. E. (2011). *Foundations of play therapy* (2nd ed.). Hoboken, NJ: Wiley.

Shapiro, F. (2001). *Eye movement desensitization and reprocessing: Basic principles, protocols, and procedures.* New York, NY: Guilford Press.

van der Kolk, B. A. (1994). The body keeps the score: Memory and the evolving psychobiology of posttraumatic stress. *Harvard Review of Psychiatry, 1,* 253–265. doi:10.3109/10673229409017088

van der Kolk, B. A. (2014). *The body keeps the score.* New York, NY: Penguin Group.

van der Kolk, B. A., & Fisler, R. (1995). Dissociation and the fragmentary nature of traumatic memories: Overview and exploratory study. *Journal of Traumatic Stress, 8,* 505–525. doi:10.1002/jts.2490080402

Wilson, S., Tinker, R., Hofmann, A., Becke, L., & Marshall, S. (2000, November). *A field study of EMDR with Kosovar-Albanian refugee children using a group treatment protocol.* Paper presented at the annual meeting of the International Society for the Study of Traumatic Stress, San Antonio, TX.

18

Using the Color Hands Approach to Bilateral Stimulation

TYNE POTGIETER

INTRODUCTION

This intervention was designed to work best with children who may be sensory seeking, seem hesitant or cautious when discussing the trauma, have low tolerance for exposure to the trauma, or find bilateral eye movements challenging. It requires that children engage in bilateral stimulation and eye movements by physically tapping different color hand images for desensitization and installation. The effectiveness of this intervention relies on the level of control and independence that the child has, the bilateral stimulation and sensory experience that they gain from the tapping motions, and the increased feeling of safety for children who tend to be more guarded when exploring their trauma experience.

PHASES OF EMDR

Desensitization (Phase 4) and installation (Phase 5)

MATERIALS

- Colored paper
- Sticky tape
- Blank wall space
- Scissors
- Additional decorations to add to hand images

RATIONALE

Color Hands is a creative, play-based intervention for Phase 4, desensitization, and Phase 5, installation, of the eye movement desensitization and reprocessing (EMDR) protocol (Shapiro, 2018). It was designed specifically for children who constantly seek sensory input and find it difficult to engage in conversation or therapeutic interventions regarding trauma because of the shame the child has associated with the incident. Because of this, any attempt to address the trauma in a direct manner may result in the child becoming dissociative or dysregulated, which may present as behavioral outbursts or efforts to receive tactile stimulation (Solomon & Siegel, 2003). When using this intervention, the child may be more willing to engage and verbalize their thoughts and feelings related to the trauma due to the feeling of safety and the nonconfrontational environment this intervention creates. The child may also experience an increased level of independence and control, and therefore be more open to doing the trauma work while also attaining the sensory input desired during bilateral stimulation.

This modification to the desensitization and installation phases of the EMDR protocol allows the child to engage in a way that feels less threatening than having to face a therapist and do the work in a more direct manner. The real or imagined feelings of threat and judgment are reduced, and participation is more likely. The child may also be more willing to engage for longer periods because of the physical movement required, ensuring that kinesthetic and tactile needs are met. Finally, this intervention allows children to participate in the setup, which provides a sense of control, increases willingness to participate, and allows conversations regarding the EMDR process to take place so the child is more informed and at ease. Another significant element of this intervention is the level of control that the therapist provides the child. By allowing the child to make choices throughout the set up and execution of this EMDR intervention, the child is provided a sense of control and safety. This may encourage resistant children to participate and will provide them with a sense of independence and authority, which will in turn have positive impacts on participation and result in a strengthened therapeutic relationship.

DESCRIPTION OF INTERVENTION

This playful intervention uses colorful hand cutouts that are used to complete bilateral eye movements and hand-tapping motions for Phase 4, desensitization, and Phase 5, installation. Different colored papers are helpful in terms of explaining the process of alternating "high-fives" for the BLS.

STEP-BY-STEP INSTRUCTIONS

Step 1: The therapist may choose to involve the child in the creation of the intervention materials. This may include choosing different colored papers, tracing hands, decorating them, and sticking them up at eye level on a blank wall. It is

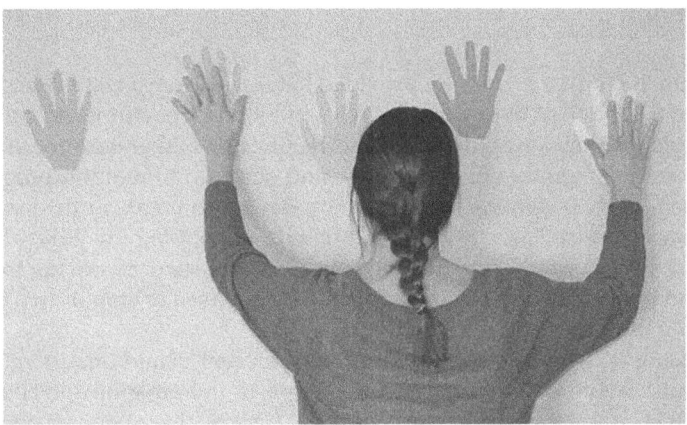

Figure 18.1 *High-Fives With the Color Hands for Bilateral Stimulation Demonstrated*

recommended to encourage choice and creativity during this time, as the more the child feels attached to and proud of the created product, the more likely the buy-in to be involved during the later desensitization phase.

Step 2: The therapist sets up for eye movements by prompting the child to tap or "high-five" the different color hands one at a time. The child will be prompted to tap their left hand on one color hand cutout followed by their right hand on a different color cutout (Figure 18.1). They will repeat this alternating pattern until told to stop by the therapist, who will be counting sets all the while. The child may also be asked to keep their head still and follow each tap with their eyes. It is important that the therapist monitor the child's responses during this phase, as they may indicate the need for a break behaviorally, such as becoming disengaged or defiant.

Step 3: This intervention can be used again during Phase 5, installation, to focus on cognitive restructuring and will require the therapist to return to the original positive cognition (PC) and ensure that the Validity of Cognition (VOC) feels true when concentrating on the traumatic incident. The therapist will then instruct the child to resume the alternative tapping motions for short sets to install their cognition. The therapist may also choose to use installation to model PCs and for resource development by taking turns to demonstrate the tapping and allowing reciprocal play to take place (see Consideration #4). The therapist will then continue with body scan and closure in order to complete the EMDR process (Greenwald, 2012). It is important that the therapist ensure that sufficient time is allocated to these phases so that the child is able to achieve a level of closure and leave the session in a calm, controlled, and safe manner. It is suggested that free playtime be allowed once EMDR processing has been completed for that session. Play may be promised as an incentive for the child to work through the EMDR protocol. Moreover, it allows the child time to ground and express additional thoughts or feelings that may arise from the EMDR process.

MODIFICATIONS

It is recommended that breaks are provided between desensitization sets in order to increase tolerance of exposure. Breaks can be an opportunity to utilize play for soothing and managing dysregulated feelings. It is therefore recommended that the therapist monitor client response and check in to monitor progress and remind them of their options to use a safety device, to break, or to stop entirely. Using a safety device (Greenwald, 2012) or safe place (Shapiro, 2018) allows the client the opportunity to access feelings of safety and security during the EMDR process and provide them with the opportunity to pause or stop if they feel overwhelmed by the experience.

The therapist may also choose to utilize different visual images rather than hand cutouts. This is only limited by the therapist's imagination and could range from pictures that the client has drawn, book/movie characters, or patterns. By making this fun, playful, and client-centered, the child is more likely to connect with the therapist, feel ownership over the process, and engage in the EMDR protocol.

Should the child be extremely sensory seeking, the therapist may choose to utilize a consistent shape but different materials for the visuals in order to increase the tactile experience. For example, cutouts could be blanket material, cotton rounds, paper, tissue, sandpaper, string, plastic, metal, and so forth. This again is limited by the therapist's imagination and any sensory aversion the client may have.

Rather than providing visual scales for rating Subjective Units of Distress Scale (SUDS) and VOC, the therapist may choose to use the displayed hand cutouts for the client to use. This would then provide the child with a level of control while demonstrating the responses. For example, the therapist could prompt the child to demonstrate the response by choosing hand colors that are near or far apart. The tapping could then be done as a representation of that. For example, the therapist instructs the child, *"So if we start with one hand on green, how big is that feeling when you think about the incident now? Does it go from the green hand to the red one? Or all the way to the blue one? Let's use those colors to do our tapping."*

CONSIDERATIONS

1. It is recommended that the therapist monitor the child's reaction in order to initiate play should they need a break from processing. This is important as it assists in increasing the child's tolerance for trauma exposure, ensures that they continue to regard therapy and EMDR as a positive experience, and allows the child to continue processing through play. Using play at the end of each session also provides the child with a level of incentive for EMDR, knowing that there is the opportunity to have fun afterward.
2. With regard to the created visuals used during this intervention, it is recommended to steer clear of any image that may evoke a strong emotional reaction that could create a "stuck point" for the child. For example, a picture of an animal may be too closely linked to the recent traumatic loss of a pet and therefore

interrupt the trauma processing. It is important that the therapist take into account the entire trauma history of the client prior to providing a menu of options for the visuals that may be created.
3. During Phase 3, assessment, the therapist may also choose to involve the child in an activity when reviewing this information, such as sticking the hand cutouts to the wall. This will ensure that the child does not start to feel overwhelmed or threatened when hearing the target information verbalized by the therapist, especially if the child seems resistant to trauma processing to begin with.
4. The therapist may allow for reciprocal play to occur during the EMDR process to model the bilateral hand tapping and eye movements. It may be helpful for the therapist to initially demonstrate the motions and then instruct the child that it is their turn. Should the child need a break, the therapist can use this to switch roles and model the movements again while the child provides instructions. This reciprocal play strengthens the therapeutic alliance and provides the child with a feeling of power and control.
5. When setting up the target for processing, the more information the therapist is able to gather without utilizing direct questions, the better. The therapist may find that younger children are more responsive to reflective statements than direct questioning (Landreth, 2012). This is especially true if the child has associated a level of shame with the trauma. Using reflective listening, tentative statements, and monitoring play themes may feel less threatening for the client and may reduce the resistance that direct questioning evokes (Landreth, 2012).

CASE EXAMPLE

The following is a case example transcript of a session with a 10-year-old client to illustrate the use of the Color Hand intervention. Identifying information has been changed with respect to client confidentiality. During client intake and treatment planning, Phase 1 of EMDR treatment was completed utilizing a comprehensive biopsychosocial assessment, trauma assessment, medical history questionnaire, adverse behaviors and/or symptoms checklists, and the creation of a safety plan. Desired treatment outcomes were explored. The first 2 months of therapy were spent engaging in nondirective play therapy in order to complete Phases 1 and 2 of the EMDR process. Techniques such as nondirective play therapy and reflective listening (Landreth, 2012) were used to explore the client's emotions experienced and overall themes for PC and negative cognition (NC). Having knowledge of the client's automatic cognitions regarding their belief of self and others will allow the therapist and client to identify cognitions that resonate for later in the EMDR process.

> Therapist: *So, the last few sessions, we've spent some time making lots of different colored hand cutouts. I think you're cutting out the last one now. Do you think we're ready to stick them up on the wall today? Maybe we can practice those high-fives that I was telling you about. I know it may seem a little bit funny, but when we think about things that have happened, and high-five with our hands*

in a special way, it can help our brain and body figure out how to feel better. Would you like to give it a try today? (referencing the preparation phase that took place regarding EMDR process).

Client: *Okay.*

Therapist: *Okay, well let's stick them up on the wall. You may choose which order the colors go in. And let's spread them out so that your hands can reach the ones on each end.*

The therapist will indicate height as it is best to have them at eye level to promote eye movements as tapping takes place. The therapist may choose to review information for target setup, while client sticks hand cutouts to wall. This information may have been gathered from previous sessions utilizing nondirective play therapy techniques.

Therapist: *So, I remember we briefly spoke about that one time something happened at school with your friend. I know it can be difficult, but today we're just going to think about that for a little bit and try our tapping. Remember, you can always say stop when you need a break. And, you don't even need to look at me. You'll just be looking at the wonderful hands you've made.*

Client: *Okay.*

Therapist: *So, thinking about that time at school. And that you felt sad. And in your head, you heard your voice say, "I am bad." And all you wanted was to feel safe.* (Emotion, NC, and PC parts of the target were acquired through nondirective play therapy techniques in previous sessions.)
When you think about it now and say, "I am safe," does it feel true? Can you show me with your hands, how true does it feel? From the green hand all the way until which color hand? (VOC scaling)

Client: *Until the red hand.*

Therapist: *And when you think of the sad feeling, how big is that feeling right now? From the green hand until which color hand?*

Client: *The blue hand.*

Therapist: *So, still a really big feeling then. And where do you feel that in your body? Some people feel it in their head, shoulders, legs, hands. Where is it for you?* (body sensation/location).

Client: *My head and my belly.*

Therapist: *Okay, so now we're going to do our hand tapping. Which colors would you like to tap?*

Client: *Pink and blue.*

Therapist: *Okay! Maybe we can take turns. I'll show you with my hands first. I'm going to tap the pink with my left hand and the blue with my right hand and I'll keep doing that until you tell me to stop. Ready, go.*

Therapist tapped in alternating motion to model bilateral movements.

> Client: *Stop!*
>
> Therapist: *That was great. Well done. Okay, let's switch. So, I want you to think of that time at school feeling sad and "I am bad," feeling it in your head and belly. Ready to tap?*

Bilateral tapping sets. Monitor client response. Repeat if the client is able to continue to engage. Follow the EMDR protocol by checking for SUDS for no change on channel, no change and no distress, or no change and SUDS of 0. Allow for breaks for client to engage in play.

> Therapist: *So how does I am safe sound? Is that still the best thing to say or do you want to say something else instead?* (installation)
>
> Client: *I am safe is the right thing.*
>
> Therapist: *So, when you think of that time at school, and say "I am safe," can you show me now how true that feels? From the green hand until which one?* (VOC)
> *Let's think about that time at school, say "I am safe" out loud and try some of our tapping. Maybe from the green hand until the pink one this time?*

BLS is continued with short sets to no change and VOC of 7. It is continued with body scan and closure as needed. In conclusion, the Color Hands method of movement-oriented BLS has proven helpful in adapting the EMDR protocol for children.

REFERENCES

Greenwald, R. (2012). *EMDR within a phase model of trauma-informed treatment*. Hoboken, NJ: Taylor and Francis.

Landreth, G. L. (2012). *Play therapy: The art of the relationship*. New York, NY: Routledge.

Shapiro, F. (2018). *Eye movement desensitization and reprocessing (EMDR) therapy: Basic principles, protocols, and procedures* (3rd ed.). New York, NY: Guilford Press.

Solomon, M. F., & Siegel, D. J. (2003). *Healing trauma: Attachment, mind, body, and brain*. New York, NY: W. W. Norton.

19

Play Therapy Targets for EMDR Processing: How to Get a "Bulls-Eye"

VICTORIA MCGUINNESS

INTRODUCTION

The playroom provides a range of materials that can aid in eye movement desensitization and reprocessing (EMDR). Blending both cognitive and experiential therapies for children helps to reduce anxiety in children. Introducing a child to EMDR in a room full of toys, art, sand, and other creative avenues for EMDR processing is challenging and requires skill and an age-appropriate explanation. This chapter illustrates ways to both introduce and engage a child in EMDR even for a limited amount of time such as 5 to 10 minutes during play therapy. The interweaving of EMDR and play is also illustrated in a case study. Within the eight phases of EMDR processing, the five stages of experiential play therapy are woven together, led by the child and supported by the therapist.

PHASES OF EMDR

All phases, with an emphasis on preparation (Phase 2), assessment (Phase 3), and desensitization (Phase 4)

MATERIALS

- Chalk board
- White board
- A target with metallic darts

- A thera-tapper (a device therapists use for bilateral stimulation, comprised of two wires with small handles at each end that vibrate alternately, generally held in the client's hands; with children, this is often referred to as "the buzzy thing")
- A fully equipped playroom will also aid in this intervention

RATIONALE

Experiential play therapy is based on Dr. Byron Norton's model (Norton & Norton, 1997) and has served thousands of children in the past 30 years. Grounded in a developmental perspective, there are five stages of experiential play that allow children to redo or complete portions of their development that may have gone wrong or are incomplete. The first two stages are the exploratory stage and testing for protection, or the establishment of trust (Norton & Norton, 1997). A fully equipped playroom is important in this approach. The room should contain miniature objects and people of different ethnicities, medieval characters, monsters, swords, castles, a doll house, baby dolls, a sand tray, and art supplies (including clay, Model Magic, paint), puppets, musical instruments, a kitchen, and toy food (Landreth, 2012). Because there are so many choices in a playroom, it is revealing to the therapist how the child interacts with the playroom during the exploratory stage, and this can help the therapist identify memory targets. Also, installing a safe place with positive beliefs coincides with the establishment of trust.

The third stage of experiential play therapy is the working stage that reflects the expression of the child's needs (Norton & Norton, 1997). Here, the therapist is a witness to the child's journey and works with negative cognitions (NCs), honoring the child's feelings, and reframing their role in the experience. The working stages of play can present a treasure trove of targets for EMDR processing. It is also a good time to use a safe place, especially after a challenging session, to ground them and anchor in the trust of the process.

As the child moves into the fourth stage of experiential play, therapeutic growth, many developmental struggles would have already been smoothed out (Norton & Norton, 1997). This presents an opportune time to install the positive growth experience and positive cognitions (PCs) about self. As the therapist and child move through the empowerment stage, we come to the fifth stage of play therapy, or termination/friends saying goodbye (Norton & Norton, 1997). The therapist and child process separating. Some children feel sad, and some feel glad. It may be a bit of a celebration or graduation of the child's work. The parents are encouraged to find another outlet for the child such as art, sports, or spending that hour together every week.

Depending on the needs of the child, the introduction to EMDR and preparation for it varies in both the timing and method. Sometimes, children literally burst into their play and it would be counterproductive to introduce a cognitive, therapist-led process. Discernment of a child's readiness for the combination of the two methods is something to assess starting with the first session with the child. In other words, most children are ready to process through play but not always with EMDR.

There are eight basic phases in using EMDR in therapy (Shapiro, 2018). Letting go of the adult protocol is necessary for working with children, but there is still a structure for this process (Tinker & Wilson, 1999). One of the major goals of experiential play therapy is to discover the true motivation for a child's behavior and process any maladaptive motive to an adaptive and positive one. EMDR processing takes the play process to another level as it seems to anchor the experiential changes in a more balanced brain. The creative experience of guiding a child to find a safe and/or powerful place inside their own minds is an important part of preparing the child for EMDR.

STEP-BY-STEP INSTRUCTIONS: EXPLAINING EMDR

Step 1: Providing the child with a visual and verbal explanation of EMDR and bilateral stimulation (BLS) helps them to want to engage in the process. The explanation varies with the age and developmental stage of the child. One possibility is drawing the brain on a white board. I divide a circle into two halves and label one Right Side and one Left Side. I draw big red blobs on the Right Side to represent fears, dreams, traumas, self-perception and explain that it is where emotional events are stored and stuck. For the Left Side, I use a different color marker to draw squares to explain how this side is about science, logic, problem-solving, and the part that helps to calm down the upset Right Side of your brain. Drawing arrows from the Right Side to the Left Side, we discuss the possibility of having these two sides of the brain *meet* and exchange information. I might ask an older child what they think might happen or what they would like to see happen to help ascertain the child's understanding of the process and willingness to try it.

Step 2: The therapist gives a short verbal summary to the child that provides protection and validation for the child's experience and their willingness to move forward.

> Therapist: *The left side of your brain knows that you have lived through it all already, it knows that monsters are not real and that you did nothing wrong! And the buzzy thing helps you to claim that good feeling in your body when both sides of your brain can talk to each other and find a solution. Does this make sense to you?*

It generally may not make sense yet, but these steps tickle a child's curiosity and readiness to heal in a deeper way. It is helpful for the therapist to remember that finding targets with younger children can be subtle, and the child may or may not be consciously aware that the therapeutic focus is a target at all.

STEP-BY-STEP INSTRUCTIONS: IN THE ASSESSMENT PHASE

Therapists will be sleuthing for EMDR targets during these sessions, preparing the child to identify NCs and PCs.

Step 1: The child's NCs and PCs can be discovered during exploratory play in both literal and symbolic manners. This may be done through use of colors, good guys/bad guys, identifying with a broken toy, scary feelings versus safe feelings, liking oneself or not, feeling included, liked by peers and teachers, and so forth.

Step 2: For younger children, use hands spread apart as measurements for a belief in a positive feeling the child has for themselves (PCs) and the child's Subjective Units of Distress Scale (SUDS). This step involves the child indicating with any amount of space between their hands the intensity of either PCs or SUDS. For older children or kids with a love of numbers, the therapist can use the adult protocol for measuring PCs and SUDS.

Step 3: This step tests the options for BLS. The child is introduced to theratappers for processing; with children I call this *the buzzy thing*. The first introduction indicates how the physical vibration feels to the child. Some start to relax immediately when they feel the vibration and others find the stimulation uncomfortable or ticklish. If the child is not comfortable with it, we try another way of using the EMDR processing such as hand taps, a puppet (of the child's choice) on each hand, or a sound in each ear.

Step 4: Construct a safe and powerful place. In order to measure the child's response to the stimulation while they hold the tappers, we start with the child focusing on their safe or powerful place. Most children need some direction to include all the sensory data they can come up with such as images, sounds, tastes, odors, and companions. The construction of this place in the child's psyche provides an opportunity for body scans and identifying the transforming feelings in the child's body.

Step 5: Install a safe place. The therapist then reads back the description of the child's creation and asks them to see themselves there. The therapist walks the child through their senses and keeps an eye on the physical response of the child. Most children start to smile and relax. If something unwelcome or uninvited shows up unexpectedly, remind the child that they are "safe in the playroom" and ground them in their body. I generally suggest they have special rocks or other items to ground them.

Playing, creating art, or finding treasure in the sand after installing a safe place might enhance and anchor these feelings of safety, control, and security. It creates a whole-body expression that reinforces the safety that grounds the processing. This step can lead to new feelings and more adaptive perceptions that result in integrating the opposing feelings.

CONSIDERATIONS

The creation of a safe or powerful place might reveal targets to the therapist. If home is the safe place, it is a good indication that this child has a solid foundation in life. Good body sensations and positive cognitions can be nurtured through almost any safe place. Yet choosing home is the most helpful because it is based in the reality of their lives. Children sometimes choose the playroom as their safe place or a completely constructed fantasy of their own. Paying attention to who is not in a child's safe place, who is, how protected this place needs to be, and who can get in and out without the child's permission are all components of this internal place that illustrates a child's fears and defenses against those fears. When there is no safe place, the therapist should discard EMDR processing until deeper trust is established.

CASE EXAMPLE

During the initial session, George's* mother disclosed that during the past 3 years, George had been forced to go out of town to his father's home each summer and every other weekend. George's father had a teenage son from a previous marriage who lived with him and was George's sexual abuser. George tried to disclose this abuse to his mother, but she struggled to believe it despite George crying, screaming, and hiding in his closet begging not to go with his father. The last time George's father dropped him off at his mother's home, he told George he would never see him again. This flat-out rejection by his father after being sexually abused by his half-sibling escalated George's acting-out behaviors. At the time of intake, his mother described it as simultaneous relief and hurt. He was angry with her for not protecting him, but happy to never have to see his biological father again.

George came to therapy when he was 6-1/2 years old. He did most of his play and EMDR work standing at the sand table and creating moving sand trays, providing specific targets for EMDR processing. George was receptive to the white board explanation of the bilateral nature of our brains, and I followed the steps as outlined earlier. Because of his need for the sensory experience during processing, we agreed to keep the tappers in his pockets or socks for BLS.

George agreed to construct a safe and powerful place. His cooperation showed a clear desire to heal and his willingness to trust. As George discovered a safe place of his own using a place he constructed in his mind, I collected the sensory data. George quickly constructed a distant planet surrounded by a huge plastic bubble. He could see out, but no one would see in. First, George stored up pizza, tacos, and candy. I narrated back to him and encouraged him to smell and taste the candy and food and engage all of his senses. Then, I told him that no one could get into his bubble unless they know the password. Did he want any company? He invited his best friend Ace and their combined electronics, games, and imaginary iPhones. George was in control of who called or who could "get through the plastic." The absence of adults in George's safe place pointed to a lack of trust in adults and his needing freedom from their inconsistent behaviors.

To install the safe place, I repeated the data he provided while installing the feeling of safety and control over his personal space with the tapper. Because his favorite color was green, he agreed to fill his plastic bubble with a soothing green color he chose. Filling a child's body with a sparkle-version of their chosen color, starting in the sky and moving through their body from the top of their heads and out their toes, is a way of installing positive feelings and cognitions in a child. George was visibly relaxed after installing his safe place, and he headed to the sand table with tappers in each pocket. Sometimes, he was silent and sometimes he narrated his story referring to his self-object in the third person.

---

*In order to protect client confidentiality, the information in this case example has been modified.

STEPS IN THE REPROCESSING AND INSTALLATION PHASES

Step 1: Support the child's experiential play related to the target. By referring to his self-object, a male child figure about 1.5 inches tall, in the third person, George was able to distance himself from the immediate confusion and pain he was experiencing in his life and in his body. His play focused around the "boy" being in a "blue sleeping bag" in a dark room. He created this "picture" in the sand, thus providing a pivotal out-picturing of the place of abuse as a possible target. Knowingly or not, George has revealed the first significant sensory target: the blue sleeping bag.

In the sand tray, a toy police officer was stuck in the corner upside down (perhaps a symbol indicating the upside-down values of the authority figures in his life). George's fear was represented by a two-headed dinosaur whose big body would land heavily next to the sleeping bag. George starting growling as he became the monster as well as the boy in the sand. He stomped the two-headed dinosaur over to the bump in the sand that hid the child and stepped on the bump like the child was nothing but part of the "dirt."

> Therapist: *That boy needs to hide from the monster; he doesn't want to be found.*

At his point, George covered the boy's head in sand. I asked where the boy was now in the story and George said he was at his grandparents and that he hated the blue sleeping bag. This dissociative experience followed by his ability to land himself at his grandparents, a safe place for him, let me know we had reached a tipping point and that now, this session, George kept himself safe. I asked him to show me a measure with his hands as to how bad he felt about having to sleep in the blue sleeping bag. Arms opened to about shoulder-width, which might be construed to measure SUDS at about 6/7 or approximately midway through this phase.

Clearly, George was in the working stages of play therapy and EMDR simultaneously. His need for control became evident by starting out with such small objects, distancing by referring to himself in the third person, processing and validating his feelings that felt claustrophobic with emotions we worked on self-regulation.

Step 2: Boundary setting. A request for limit-setting reinforces practice with boundaries, respect for authority, and emotional regulation. George did his best. When sand spilled out over the side of the table…

> Therapist: *This kid is so sad; he is really scared and confused. But it's still your job to keep the sand in the sand table. Sometimes there is just too much to keep in. Sometimes there is just too much sand (or feelings) to keep in a box.*

Step 3: Body scanning. The feedback to George validates that he has too many emotions, feelings too big to contain in his little body. While George continues his moving sand tray, the tapper is doing its job stimulating bilateral brain functions. At the end of this session, we did a super-quick body scan by asking George what colors were in his body now.

Child: *Mostly green, some brown, a little blackish in the back.* George was "done" for the day, having exhausted himself in this session.

Around his tenth session, the sand began to be filled with skeletons, gravestones, gargoyles, and skulls and bones with a skeleton claw reaching out. Metaphorically, bones and graveyard images could be references to a frightening past and/or a part of this child that is passing away. Interpretation of play is variable, archetypal, or subjective. The bones also may indicate that these experiences have become an integral part of the structure of his being.

Processing and reprocessing with both methods continued in further sessions.

Step 4: The therapist acts as the witness.

Child: *He is asleep; he doesn't know…someone is in the room.*

Therapist: *He is a sound sleeper! How does he know someone is there with him?*

Child: *He is frozen; he can't move.*

Therapist: *Can he move his eyes?*

Child: *I don't know. Only one eye can open, see?*

George brushed a tiny bit of sand off his toy self-object's face, revealing who is in the sleeping bag, coming awake, perhaps coming to terms with what happened. George moved the two-headed dinosaur very close to the child and said, "He stinks! He's hungry; he wants to eat the kid and kill him." Again, George revealed his target: the two-headed dinosaur. The stepbrother abused George while he was in the blue sleeping bag, but during the day, they played video games together and sometimes seemed to enjoy each other's company.

Therapist: *That's just how it went for that boy; he was half-frozen, and no one could see him or hear him or anything at all. He must be terrified and lonely…. He is very brave and he is safe now. He could not tell how he felt about the ones that were sometimes fun and nice and other times terrifying and hurtful; it was just too confusing.*

George let that sink in.

Step 5: The therapist provided closure and containment of fears between sessions.

Therapist: *We have 10 minutes left for today. Let's put this boy in a safe place.*

As a part of reprocessing his fears, George had piled the sand on top of the child figure. He now took the two-headed dinosaur to "jail" and locked the creature in jail thus containing his fears. George was experiencing a more pronounced feeling of control and mastery over his own body, his fear, and his feelings of powerlessness by taking action like locking the two-headed dinosaur in jail. He has the power to contain the fears and he has done so to the extent of his developmental ability. The main target is still the blue sleeping bag; the boy is buried under a pile of sand (feelings) keeping him down but invisible.

Therapist: *Where is the boy now at the end of the story for today?*

Child: *Can I take these out now?* (dangling the handles of the tapper to the floor)

Therapist: *Yes, of course, you played really hard today. Let's go back to your own safe place.*

George cooperated, and that session ended.

Step 6: Processing continues in further sessions.

Around session 16, George had reprocessed his feelings of powerlessness, anger, hurt, and confusion. I noted that he discarded his father symbol and distanced from him during the entire process. Focusing on the targets provided by the child, the blue sleeping bag, his feelings/colors, and the two-headed dinosaur were his chosen, yet unconscious targets. If I had insisted on inserting the father, the entire process might be disrupted. George can deal with his father when he is ready, when he is older.

More often during the working/growth stages of play therapy, George chose to process through art, which allowed him to express and distance from his feelings simultaneously. He was drawing rockets that blew up, exploding. Then, he did something new. He grabbed a green baby bottle and started drinking from it with his eyes closed. I stayed quiet, as silence is often the path to targets and verbalizations!

Child: *We played the rocket game; his rocket exploded in my face.*

That moment was the disclosure of the abuse. He tore up the rocket drawing and threw it in the trash. George's awareness of these significant targets had increased, although I never consciously identified them for him.

Step 7: The therapist asked questions to help the child with changing NCs during the working/growth stage of play.

Therapist: *Who did the wrong thing? The baby or the guy with the rocket?*

Child: *The guy with the rocket.*

Therapist: *Babies are innocent, that baby never did anything wrong.*

When George was choosing his stickers that day at the end of the session, he said, "*I left the blue sleeping bag in Seattle with my* (mumble) *and Travis* (the stepbrother)." George was distancing from his past due to his courage to face his fears and empower himself.

Therapist: *How does that feel? To know you didn't cause these things to happen to you?*

Child: *Like I want to play basketball. That's where I'm going now.*

STEPS IN SCANNING FOR REMAINING DISTRESS AND INSTALLING THE POSITIVE BELIEFS AND REEVALUATION

This process corresponds to saying the goodbye/termination phase in experiential play therapy.

Step 1: Clarify that therapy is going to end and validate the child's work. The therapist can also tickle the child's imagination about positive future possibilities.

> Therapist: *I think we are close to saying goodbye. Your mom feels you are doing very well and wants you to spend more time playing sports.*

Step 2: Check for remaining distress.

> Therapist: *Show me with your hands how scary it feels to think about the blue sleeping bag.*

George stopped his hands about 1 to 2 inches apart. "I'm just gonna play basketball from now on and maybe try soccer."

> Therapist: *Okay, great! How do you feel about going to your powerful place quickly and making sure that it's still filled up with the green light.*

As a part of the body scan, I asked how the green light feels in his body; I got a thumbs up. I asked how the light feels when he is playing basketball; thumbs up and a grin. There are no offensive colors or feelings at this moment in George's body. During his processing, a yukky brown feeling had morphed into a verdant green—indicating growth.

Step 3: As part of reevaluation, the therapist checks for neutrality, positive cognitions, and feelings.

At this point, George's behavior had shifted dramatically. He had chosen sports and diverted his attention to excelling in that arena. He also enjoyed drawing and, of course, video games. Academically, George caught up with reading and math; he made a few good friends and had a mending relationship with his mother. George was a forgiving type of person. He slept in his own room and slept well most of the time, and he was eating in a typical fashion.

George attended one more session and he played with Legos, symbolically demonstrating his ability to feel constructive and engage in typical play for a child his age. As he approached his seventh birthday, he was coping well—some of his scariest memories appeared to be erased although remnants of feeling trapped, exposed, and confused still seeped into the Lego play, but briefly. Legos are small; George experienced a great deal of mastery over his trauma at seven-years-old. He let me know that he could go to his safe place when he felt scared or needed to calm down. He was demonstrating emotional intelligence, and I was able to reflect that level of mastery to him.

Because George's behavior had changed drastically and his feelings of self-worth increased, I felt we had reached the end of the road for his therapy at this stage of his development. George's mother did not contact me and no-showed for a wrap-up session. I felt as satisfied as I could that we had accomplished many of the goals during previous sessions. The value of reevaluating George's feelings about himself as the therapy progresses in case the therapy process is interrupted prematurely is both necessary and helpful. George internalized the most important feeling of all, his own belief in his innocence and his own power to literally change his mind. I trust that George took his healing process as far as he could from where he stood on the developmental ladder. I envisioned him in the future with a basketball, a hoop, and friends to play with.

ON A PERSONAL NOTE

After playing with no less than 3,000 children and providing these services for almost 30 years in the playroom, I have learned from many people. As to the experiential play therapy, I relied mostly on Dr. Byron Norton (Norton & Norton 1997) and Dr. Garry Landreth (2012) and other leaders in the field of play therapy. Early on, I attended EMDR for children conferences and wrote a small book also listed in the references on the topic of EMDR and play therapy. I learned the adult protocol directly from Francine Shapiro in 1996.

REFERENCES

Landreth, G. (2012). *Child centered play therapy: A clinical session [DVD-ROM]*. New York, NY: Routledge.

Norton, B., & Norton, C. (Eds.) (1997). *Reaching children through play therapy: An experiential approach*. Denver, CO: The Publishing Cooperative.

Shapiro, F. (2018). *Eye movement desensitization and reprocessing: Basic principles, protocols and procedures* (3rd ed.). New York, NY: Guilford Press.

Tinker, R., & Wilson, S. (1999). *Through the eyes of a child: EMDR with children*. New York: W. W. Norton.

FOR FURTHER CASE EXAMPLES SEE OTHER PUBLICATIONS BY THIS AUTHOR

McGuinness, V. (1997). *Integrating play therapy and EMDR with children*. Author House.

McGuinness, V. (2011). Integrating play therapy and EMDR with children: A post-trauma intervention. In A. Drewes, S. Bratton, & C. Schaefer (Eds.), *Integrative play therapy* (Chapter 11). New York, NY: Wiley.

McGuinness, V. (2015). *We the children: The hidden language of children*. Carlsbad, CA: Balboa Press.

RECOMMENDED READING IN PLAY THERAPY

Axline, V. (1969). *Dibs in search of self.* New York, NY: Ballantine Books.
Gil, E. (1999). *The healing power of play: Working with abused children.* New York, NY: Guilford Press.
Sweeney, D. (2001). *Counseling children through the world of play.* Eugene, OR: Wipf & Stock.

20

Effectively Managing the Closure and Reevaluation Phase With Parents

ANNIE MONACO

INTRODUCTION

Popcorn Night is a term that was coined to assist caregivers in providing a calm and comfortable night for their child following a desensitization session. Following the reprocessing of a memory, the therapist works with the caregivers to manage the possible emerging behaviors and assist with a log to track any changes in symptomology. Communicating these changes during the reevaluation phase then allows the therapist to make a proper clinical determination for the next step in the child's treatment.

PHASES OF EMDR

Closure (Phase 7) and reevaluation (Phase 8)

MATERIALS

- Popcorn Night handout (see Appendix 20.1)

RATIONALE

In the preparation phase, the therapist's goal is to effectively equip the child to manage trauma memories in Phases 4 through 7. Afterward, children can still struggle to tolerate the beliefs, emotions, and body sensations that come with desensitization of these memories despite the best efforts of the therapist. Having productive closure in Phase 7 can help ensure successful in-between sessions and increase the likelihood that the child will participate in further reprocessing of memories (Adler-Tapia, 2008). Providing caregivers with a solid explanation of potential emerging disturbances and what to expect after the desensitization phase is critical for Phase 7. Reprocessing a traumatic event in counseling can be taxing to a child who will often continue to process the memory after the session, including through dreams or nightmares. Helping the child feel safe and have a positive soothing night can enhance the child's continued desensitization of the memory and the integration of the positive cognition. A disruptive and chaotic evening after a trauma-processing session can interrupt the continued processing and integration of adaptive material.

Because children are unable to completely manage their own in-between session disturbances, it is important that caregivers provide emotional safety and security during trauma reprocessing. There are many pieces to attend to while desensitizing children's memories, and it is important to warn parents about the effects of trauma reprocessing. One possible disturbance includes children having regressive behaviors after a therapist has processed a traumatic memory, including whining, sucking their thumbs, or clingy behavior. Parents are fearful that the child's behavior will stay permanent or that the therapist is causing harm to the child and therefore may be hesitant to allow their child to continue with eye movement desensitization and reprocessing (EMDR) therapy. Providing an in-depth debriefing of the possible outcomes that may arise in symptoms and behaviors is important for parents prior to the therapist starting Phases 3 through 7. With caregivers, which can include supports outside the home, providing the debriefing in the preparation phase and then again after the desensitization phase offers multiple opportunities to discuss what to expect, how to manage the potential disturbances, and how to track symptoms and behaviors. To emphasize these expectations, the Popcorn Night handout includes a description of possible symptoms or behaviors and a log to track behaviors. A discussion should include a list of both positive and negative behaviors and symptoms that may occur as well as pointing out that it may take more than one session of desensitization to effect positive changes in the child. It is of utmost importance to inform parents that it is impossible to predict the behaviors and that the most important task for a caregiver is to be supportive and observe changes in the symptoms, behaviors, emotions, moods, and statements following so that the therapist is well informed and can make a proper decision on how to move forward in treatment.

Despite therapists helping to stabilize children's home and school life, many of the families struggle to stay consistently stable. At some point, the therapist may decide that the family has made significant gains and that moving forward with Phases 3 through 7 is in the best interest of the child. If the child does regress or has increased acting-out behaviors, and the parents handle it ineffectively, the child may associate this negative consequence with the therapy session and be unwilling to do further processing work with the therapist. In working with at-risk families, parents who struggle with severe mental health issues, ineffective parenting, or caregivers with significant attachment issues, it is important to coach the parent on how to manage strong emotions and find success in the afternoon and evening after desensitization. Parents may not be able to provide emotional support consistently but can come through for one calm night. This is often *good enough* for their child to associate EMDR therapy with receiving care and support and the child can then be willing to continue with treatment. One night free of chaos is often doable with even the most challenging parents.

When the child and caregiver return for the next session, the therapist is in the reevaluation phase of EMDR therapy (Phase 8) with the goal of assessing the status of the memory worked on in the previous session(s) to determine if adequate integration and assimilation of maladaptive material have been made (Gomez, 2013). This reevaluation will allow the therapist to properly gauge the next steps in EMDR therapy by considering a number of questions, typically done with a conversation with the child and the caregivers. Has the desensitization of the memory been sustained from the previous session? If there was not a complete resolution in the last session, has the memory resolved in dreams or nightmares? Has any new material emerged? New developments may include insights such as *"It was not my fault,"* an additional detail of the memory, or an additional memory. The therapist attempts to determine if there are any decreases in symptoms, shifts in thinking, or if the positive cognition feels "more true" or has sustained since the last session. With children, we are also looking for behavioral change such as a decrease in temper tantrums, bed-wetting, or somatic symptoms, or a change in any of the problematic behaviors in the child's daily life.

This thorough approach is needed because caregivers who are frustrated with their child's problematic behaviors often do not adequately report the changes in the child's behavior or decrease in symptoms. They often respond by stating *"It's the same"* and then focus on the worst part of the week with the child's behavior. Often, there *are* behavior and symptoms changes, and a clinician has to pursue questioning to ensure a full picture of the child's symptoms is understood in reevaluation phase, including if the child has increased symptomology as this may be an indication that new material has emerged. However, a session may appear to have been negative, distressing, unproductive, or incomplete but may still lead to a reduction of symptoms (Gonzalez & Mosquera, 2012).

DESCRIPTION OF THE INTERVENTION

The first part of the Popcorn Night handout recommends an easy-going after-session experience for the child. It involves a night free of yelling, homework demands, critical comments, frustration, and most importantly should include a parent's tolerance for whatever comes from the memory work. The second part of the Popcorn Night document asks parents to monitor for noticeable differences in the child after desensitization. The handout includes a log (Royle & Kerr, 2010; Shapiro, 2001) presented in the closure phase to capture any new memories emerging or increases, decreases, or shifts in behavior experienced so that the clinician can determine next steps in the reevaluation phase. At the end of the desensitization session, the therapist, caregiver, and child review the log in the Popcorn Night document and practice by jotting down any disturbances during the previous week. I give caregivers a number of examples such as noticing any changes in their child's emotions like seeming happier, less angry, or more explosive, or noticing if the child is less upset about peer issues, handling teachers or academics more effectively. Possibly the child feels confident to handle the school bully or walked away from a sibling who was teasing. The child may have a change in thinking about a situation, such as understanding a parent's rule about being a good big brother/sister. I also ask caregivers to listen for unusual statements made by the child such as talking about a new memory, new fear, or new problem. I ask them to notice decreases in behaviors such as a bed-wetting or temper tantrums. Parents often say, *"He is still bed-wetting"* and neglect to tell me that this behavior has decreased in the past week. Providing thorough examples to parents (based on the child's presenting problems) ensures that the therapist can receive the best possible information for the reevaluation phase to make the next clinical steps. It is very important to let parents know that dramatic positive changes do not always occur immediately (although it is in this writer's experience that they often do) so that they do not become discouraged if significant changes are not made after one or two processing sessions.

This intervention focuses on informing caregivers of possible negative side effects of EMDR therapy that may cause additional problems for the child. It is an opportunity to inform parents of traumatic material being processed, how this affects the neural networks in the brain, and how the parents can assist the therapy process by ensuring an after-therapy session. This intervention also asks caregivers to monitor their child's behavior after the desensitization phase so that the following session can be a discussion of the behaviors of the week. During the reevaluation phase, the therapist initiates a conversation about the week(s) and is listening and inquiring about the increase, decrease, or elimination of symptoms and behaviors. This will allow the clinician to capture accurate data and determine next steps.

STEP-BY-STEP INSTRUCTIONS: CLOSURE PHASE

Step 1: Engage the parent as your cotherapist to help care for the child after the processing of a memory. I find it important to discuss this topic with parents at least several times before the processing of a memory occurs. Explain the importance of having a positive ending after a hard session and emphasize that you are in it together and can assist with additional resources.

Step 2: Explain the "side effects" of reprocessing memory. Typically, the child is very tired after reprocessing. Also, each child responds differently after reprocessing, and anything can happen after the session. I do explain that, typically, regressive behaviors are temporary and may indicate that more memories, feelings, body sensations, and thoughts are coming up for the child.

> *Positives:* Sometimes, the changes are positive and good for the child and for those who live with the client. These changes can be fewer nightmares, decrease in bed-wetting, fewer acting-out behaviors, fewer harmful behaviors toward others, more cooperation, or a decrease of tantrums.

Negatives: Sometimes, the changes are negative for a little while. These changes can be regressed behaviors, crying spells, refusal to cooperate, nightmares, requests to sleep in bed with the parent, refusal to go to school, or violent behaviors.

These behaviors can be frightening to a parent who already struggles with the child's behaviors so it is important to inform them that these difficult acting-out behaviors can occur. They fear that the child is forever harmed by your therapy when they see regressive behaviors. *"She is sucking her thumb!"* or *"She wants me to feed her and she is 8 years old."* If parents are triggered by a certain behavior that has increased due to the memory work, such as clingy or whiny behavior, it is important to work with parents on "tolerating" the behavior and managing their reactions as well.

Step 3: *Homework/chores:* Request homework or chores be done ahead of the session or not done at all—unless the child requests to do it (some children find it soothing to do homework or help out). The therapist can contact schools to explain that trauma therapy services are being provided and ask for an extension on homework.

Step 4: Suggest possible options for soothing. This is important for parents who are not effective at comforting or soothing their child. I give a significant number of examples for this option so parents can be successful. Parents can make their child a special meal, favorite meal, takeout, or allow a favorite dessert. Parents can allow the child to watch a special TV show or play video games on a school night. Playing a game together or visiting a park or favorite place reinforces to the child that although this is hard work, the parent wants the child to feel better. Encouraging affection between caregiver and child can be as simple as allowing the child to sit near the parent during the evening or rest on them (head in their lap). A good option is allowing whatever the parent can tolerate, even if it is small doses of physical touching or closeness. For extra comfort, I encourage allowing the child to sleep with the parent that night, if needed, and if not contraindicated in the treatment plan. I have also suggested that the parent not leave a child alone in a room unless the child is tired and wants to sleep. Checking on the child or providing comfort is important. Even the most challenging parents can typically provide good parenting for one night.

If the child is angry after EMDR, I encourage parents to acknowledge how hard it is, that they did good work, and how they can talk to me the next time about it. Sometimes allowing a child to text me their feelings or talking on the phone can help the child feel heard and supported. If appropriate, I will role-play with a parent to have them practice their part. Sometimes, parents witness extensive crying or overwhelmed feelings and want to soothe the child by telling them they do not need to continue working on their memories. I encourage parents to *not* say *"You don't need to do it again."* This can halt good processing work and discourage seeking treatment in the future.

Step 5: Document the behaviors. The chart is an opportunity for caregivers to take something tangible home and utilize it to monitor behaviors until their next appointment. I encourage them to see it as their role in assisting me with the next steps in the playroom. If caregivers are not good at following through, the document at least provides an idea of what changes I am looking for.

STEP-BY-STEP INSTRUCTIONS: REEVALUATION

1. **Step 1:** *Adequate preparation*: The therapist must have a clear understanding of all problematic behaviors prior to Phase 4. Having knowledge of the frequency and triggers for behaviors will help in knowing if there is an increase or decrease after desensitizing a memory.
2. **Step 2:** *At the reevaluation session*: If the parent did not fill out the log during the week, it can be given in the waiting room to fill out prior to the session or the therapist can fill out with the parent at the beginning of the session.
3. **Step 3:** *Ask additional questions if needed*: Discuss the log in detail to determine even minor increases or decreases in symptoms and changes in emotion, mood, or behaviors. The child might continue to have temper tantrums, but perhaps these have reduced in length of time or frequency since the previous session. Or a child is still oppositional but complies quicker. The child, who normally has problems at school, may have received a note during the week that indicates the child was more cooperative for several days.
4. **Step 4:** *Ask specifically about new behaviors*: It is important to ask if new behaviors have emerged such as a child now displaying a new positive coping behavior (i.e., utilizing Safe Place) or a negative coping behavior (i.e., picking at their skin). It is important to ask how long the child has engaged in a problematic behavior. This may include such examples as aggressive behaviors that ceased more quickly than normal or a child who is now remorseful after the behavior.

MODIFICATION: CAREGIVERS WHO ARE NOT AVAILABLE

All too often therapists do not have access to a caregiver during counseling treatment. The therapist may be providing services in school, and the parents not returning calls, or these may be parents who "drop off" the child for counseling services and do not readily join the session. Sometimes, another caregiver or relative is providing the transportation and does not have knowledge of the behaviors. Other times, the parent does not speak the same language as the clinician, which poses an additional barrier. In these circumstances, without access to a caregiver, the clinician will have to rely on the child to provide the entire picture of the past week.

Therapists also work with parents who are struggling to parent effectively due to many internal and external causes. If parents are not able to provide adequate information to the therapist about the changes, it is important to try and obtain that information from another source, by contacting extended family, school staff, in-home services, or other support systems that are in place. The Popcorn Night handout can be provided to multiple caregivers or supporters.

For children who live in group homes or residential settings, it is important to identify a positive staff person and attempt to ensure that the staff person is working in the evening shift to offer extra support. I contact the staff person to arrange for the child to be monitored or taken care of so that the child is safe and feels supported. Asking the staff to document their behaviors is key so that the therapist can determine the effects of treatment and discuss those changes prior to the reevaluation phase.

If the child's direct caregivers are not consistent or reliable, I search for someone in the child's life who can offer support. I have invited aunts, uncles, older cousins, and neighbors into my sessions (with consent) or engaged them in treatment over the phone. In one case, I had a long-distance aunt who was willing to call the child nightly after my desensitization sessions. The home was extremely chaotic, but each night the aunt and child would talk for 30 minutes. She then would leave me voicemail messages as to the interaction on the phone and any concerns or issues with the child.

CONSIDERATIONS

Overall, a very important consideration is to plan ahead. The therapist might have to contact the school or request the caregiver to inform appropriate school staff that you are doing EMDR therapy, especially to request that the school staff (e.g., teacher, counselor) be available for support and be understanding if the child has not completed their homework. Schools are often frustrated with a child's behavior, and it is important to attempt to get support from the child's school staff. Sometimes, this is futile and staff do not comply, but at other times it turns out to be the extra support needed for the child to succeed.

If parents do not come to session typically, it is important to try and meet with the caregivers several sessions before in case they do not show up on the days of Phase 4 through 7. If not, it is possible to send this document home with the transporter, follow up with a phone call, and reinforce the benefits of completing the document, addressing concerns, and reviewing requirements for the next session.

If the desensitization of the memory did not work or take effect, this strategy allows the therapist to try different options to increase the potential for success. This could include instances when the therapist determines safety is a concern, if feeder memories exist, or if a child is not reporting the difficulty of tolerating aspects of the memory and may need additional preparation. In this phase, the therapist also can ask the child about all the changes in symptoms and behaviors. Sometimes, the progress is not clear, as the child who has just gotten into trouble with the parent right before session or may be unable to report their changes in symptoms from the previous week.

CASE EXAMPLES

CASE EXAMPLE 1

Sturia* was a 6-year-old girl who had been returned to the custody of her mother who had three other children. The mother was overwhelmed with the care of the children and struggled to show any kindness, support, or loving gestures to her children. After the desensitization session with Sturia, I asked her mother to allow her to sit next to her on the couch while they watched TV. I asked her to fondly touch her hair once, fondly gaze at the child at least two times, and tell the child

---

*In order to protect client confidentiality, the information in this case example has been modified.

that she was proud of her for what she did in counseling. The girl fell asleep on the mother on the couch and had no acting-out behaviors for the entire night. The mother was instructed to allow Sturia to sleep in Mom's bed if she had a nightmare, which Sturia did and the mother complied. In the reevaluation phase, I provided the log in the waiting room a few minutes before I would meet with the mom. I asked her to fill it out while waiting for me. Mom was able to notice significant and positive changes in her daughter, never again missed an appointment, and always followed through with my requests between sessions! Sturia associated our hardwork in the playroom with having a positive impact and would ask when we were going to do EMDR again.

CASE EXAMPLE 2

An 8-year-old child, Rob*, was living with parents who were not consistent and reliable in many aspects of his life, which worried me in going forward in EMDR therapy, but I felt it was necessary to do so to provide some relief. Rob had significant nightmares that were disrupting everyone's sleep as well as his functioning in school. He was also bed-wetting, which caused punishments and arguments at home.

I contacted the school and Rob's favorite teacher who agreed to be his support for the week.

I did the processing of the memory on a Monday, then called the teacher on Tuesday morning to inform her of the session and what to expect. I provided her with the Popcorn Night handout and asked her to document any concerning behaviors. The teacher had all week to be supportive and check in with Rob. She provided hugs and encouragement for his work with me. The teacher agreed to write positive and encouraging notes and put in his bookbag, and Rob was instructed to read it right before bed. It was a model we used for all of the processing, and the school was amazing in their support. Rob's home life continued to be chaotic, but there was a noticeable difference in Rob's academics and friendships at school. Teachers stated that Rob was more cooperative with requests. His nightmares decreased and only on occasion did new memories surface. His bed-wetting only occurred after a difficult night with his family.

Rob's parents were able to provide me the information I needed in the reevaluation phase with behaviors at home; however, I had to ask more detailed questions than usual, such as *"Which night of the week did the nightmare occur?" "Did he bed-wet every night or just some nights? Which night of the week was that?"* and *"Was there one time he was nice to his siblings and didn't hit them?"* These detailed questions allowed me to see that Rob's behaviors were also improving at home every time I did a desensitization session of a memory.

A CREATIVE ALTERNATIVE TO THE POPCORN NIGHT

Laurie Belanger (*EMDR chicken soup analogy*, personal communication, 2019) offers "Homemade Chicken Soup" as a friendly analogy that explains how

---

*In order to protect client confidentiality, the information in this case example has been modified.

emotional content can be stirred up during processing and will just take time to settle. It normalizes and encourages increased patience for what would otherwise be seen as an increase in negative behaviors by caregivers. The soup picture can be drawn by the therapist, making the explanation more visual and appealing to younger children. The therapist can follow up with the analogy in the reevaluation session.

> *EMDR is a little like homemade chicken soup. Today, when we wanted to get at all the big things in our soup, we needed to stir it up a little bit. Once we stirred the soup, we spent time together sifting out those crunchy bits of celery (our EMDR target memory) that we don't want in there anymore. The flavor of the celery will stay (we don't erase our memory), but those pesky crunchy parts that were bothering us (those tough thoughts and feelings) get sifted out and do not get to bother us anymore. The thing is, once we've removed all those celery bits there may be many other sorts of vegetables (other possible EMDR memory targets) floating around in our soup that had been hanging out on the bottom before we stirred the soup. After getting that celery out, we might or might not notice a few of those other veggies. Not to worry, the soup tends to eventually settle back down and get clear on the top again. Our job is to be patient with this. Just notice this and be supportive of the person whose soup just got stirred. If the soup doesn't settle back down within the next couple of days, or if something totally unexpected and concerning pops up in the broth, you can call your EMDR chef and check in about what to do with that.*

CONCLUSION

Engaging caregivers and other outside support in EMDR therapy with kids leads to better outcomes as it provides additional support and additional information about the child's functioning. Popcorn Night is an instructional handout and log that helps guide caregivers in structuring a carefree and supportive evening after desensitization and track emerging symptoms or behaviors in the time between sessions. It is important to be transparent, flexible, and hopeful with this intervention as it can both inform treatment and encourage commitment to continued growth through EMDR.

REFERENCES

Adler-Tapia, R. (2008). *EMDR and the art of psychotherapy with children* (2nd ed.). New York, NY: Springer Publishing Company.

Gomez, A. (2013). *EMDR and other adjunct approaches with children*. New York, NY: Springer Publishing Company.

Royle, L., & Kerr, C. (2010). *Integrating EMDR into your practice*. New York, NY: Springer Publishing Company.

Shapiro, F. (2001). *Eye movement desensitization and reprocessing* (2nd ed.). New York, NY: Guilford Press.

APPENDIX 20.1: "POPCORN NIGHT" HANDOUT

> It is important that after a challenging therapy session, your child experiences an easy-going and relaxing evening. If possible: no homework, no fights, no room cleaning!

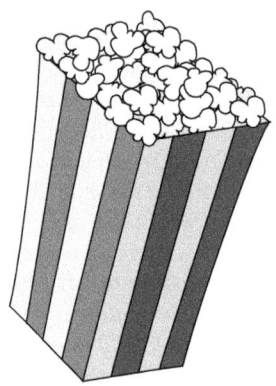

Following an EMDR session, your child may feel and experience different thoughts, emotions, or behaviors. Some children feel good, more relaxed, and calmer right away. Some children feel sensitive, overactive, or different. These are *all normal* feelings and reactions that usually last 1 to 2 days:

- Tired for the rest of the day
- More talkative than normal
- Physical reactions (e.g., headache, stomachache)
- Significant crying spells, temper tantrums, or agitation
- Might say, "I don't feel right" or "Something seems wrong or different"
- Might say, "I don't want to go back to therapy"
- May act younger than they are
- Lack of concentration: Cannot follow directions or seem confused
- May act spacey, like in a fog, or do not seem to hear you
- May have nightmares or more vivid dreams
- Other memories may come up
- Clingy, scared, or quieter than usual
- May feel like something bad is going to happen

WHAT YOU CAN DO . . .? MAKE POPCORN!

Caregivers should do everything possible to be soothing and attentive to the child. Expect and be prepared for different reactions and try your best not to get frustrated or angry. It might worry you to see your child regress, but my experience is that children are back to normal (and much better!) in a day or two.

SOME OPTIONS

- Prepare a favorite meal for your child, make popcorn, or a favorite snack.
- Hold them or let them sit close to you.
- Physical soothing: Hugs, rub their back, rub their feet, or touch their hair.
- Let them rest, watch TV, or play video games.
- Tell them they did a good job in therapy and that you are proud of them!

What do you think would help your child tonight or this week?

Over the next week, record in your phone or on this paper how your child is doing; specifically note any significant changes in the following areas. Please bring to next session.

Day	Feelings, Thoughts	Body Sensations/ Pains	Dreams/ Nightmares	Improved Behaviors	Regressed Behaviors	Interaction With others	Other Memories	Insights
M								
T								
W								
Th								
F								
Sa								
Su								

> **Reevaluation Phase: Next Session Questions**

After you left the session, how was your child that night?

During the week:
Any dreams or nightmares? Bed-wetting?

Were their behaviors better, about the same, or worse?

Even if negative behaviors are continuing, were there any moments of relief, cooperation, or improvement?

How have they been with others (family, siblings, peers, and others)?

What has school reported this week?

What physical symptoms did they have that night or during the week that were different from the usual? Were they more tired or more awake? Stomach issues? Headaches?

Any temper tantrums? Did the temper tantrums last as long as they normally do, less, or more?

Crying or unusual behavior? More clingy, anxious, or worried?

Did they have any new memories come up or talk about something that bothers them that you did not know about?

Have there been any new events in the family (moving, housing issues, canceled visitation, illness, or personal life of the parents)?

Adapted for children by Annie Monaco, LCSWR, www.anniemonaco.com
Source: Royle, L., & Kerr, C. (2010). *Integrating EMDR into your practice*. New York, NY: Springer Publishing Company, pp. 145–147

Index

acculturation levels, of Latinx children, 227–229
adaptive information processing (AIP) model, 3, 5, 6, 7, 10, 37, 110, 114, 115, 138, 153, 155, 302
    in family/play therapy context, 75–78
    and trauma, 146–147
adaptive memory networks, 125, 137–138, 139, 305, 321
Adolescent Dissociative Experience Scale, 260–261
Adult Attachment Interview, 25
adverse childhood events, 148, 155
affect avoidance theory, 258
affect dysregulation, and dissociation, 262
affect-regulation strategies, 57
AIP. *See* adaptive information processing model
All Tangled Up intervention, 57
AMAMECRISIS. *See* Mexican Association for Mental Health Support in Crisis
amnesia, and dissociation, 273–274
amygdala, 113, 312, 314
analogies, 124, 271
    Homemade Chicken Soup analogy, 420–421
    Latinx children, in EMDR therapy with, 231–232, 240
    pizza analogy, 231–232
    sore spot analogy, 263
anger volcano activity, 56, 57
apparently normal personality, 258
art expression, experience of, 184–187. *See also* expressive arts therapy
    gang age, 185, 186
    preschematic stage, 184–185
    scribble stage, 184
Art Therapy Relational Neuroscience, 188
Assessment and Treatment of Dissociative Symptoms in Children and Adolescents, 261
assessment phase, 17, 51–55, 56, 403–404
    CCPT/DPT, 171–176
    expressive arts therapy, 199

family-based play therapy, 99–101
    Latinx children, EMDR therapy with, 233, 242
    Lemon Squeezies intervention, 339–348
    Resource Wand intervention, 365–369
    Splatting Out the Trauma intervention, 379–391
    Theraplay, EMDR-infused, 349–363
Association for Play Therapy, 149
attachment, 162, 190
    building, CCPT/DPT, 170–171
    history, 155, 259
    new, interference of dissociation with, 261
    play, resourcing through, 158–160
    and trauma, 148–149
attachment theory, 34, 189, 258, 350
attunement, 170
    and expressive arts therapy, 196
    mentalization-based therapy, 195–196
    misattunement, 18, 122, 133
    of therapists, 124, 129, 133, 135, 303
    worksheet, family-based play therapy, 90–91
authenticity, therapist, 121–123
autonomic nervous system, 111
    activation, of therapists, 120, 121
    dysregulation, 113, 114, 115, 116, 118, 120
    regulation, 112, 116–119
Axline, Virginia, 4

back and forth games, 13, 15
Balancing Act intervention, 49, 50
BASK. *See* behavior, affect, sensation, knowledge model of dissociation
behavior, affect, sensation, knowledge (BASK) model of dissociation, 380
behavioral development, effect of trauma on, 147–148
belonging, sense of, 228
betrayal trauma, 259

bilateral stimulation (BLS), 6, 17, 27, 125, 153, 157, 158, 159, 247, 353, 380, 403, 404, 405
   CCPT/DPT, 160, 165, 168, 170, 171
   Color Hands intervention, 393–399
   expressive arts therapy, 215, 217
   family-based play therapy, 89, 97–98, 101, 102
   Fort Tent Calm/Safe Place intervention, 302, 304, 305, 306, 309
   Latinx children, EMDR therapy with, 230, 232, 233, 234, 237
   Lemon Squeezies intervention, 343, 348
   prop-based, playing EMDR with, 13–15
   resource wand prop, 365–369
   Splatting Out the Trauma intervention, 380, 391
   Superhero Shuffle intervention, 371–378
   synergetic play therapy, 128, 135, 136, 139, 140, 141, 142
   Theraplay, EMDR-infused, 356–357, 359–360, 361, 362
   trauma-sensitive yoga, 317, 320, 321, 322
   and TraumaPlay, 37, 42, 45, 47, 55, 61, 66, 69
bilingualism, 227, 228–229, 241
bingo game, 235
biopsychosocial model of art therapy, 189
BLS. *See* bilateral stimulation
body awareness, 158
body scan phase, 103, 395, 406–407, 409
   family-based play therapy, 101–102
   Latinx children, EMDR therapy with, 234, 245
   Theraplay, EMDR-infused, 349–363
booklets, 230, 231
boundaries, 212–214, 406
   Fort Tent Calm/Safe Place intervention, 303–304
   synergetic play therapy, 133
Bowl of Light story, 55, 294, 295, 297–299
brain–body connection, and trauma, 312–314
breathing exercise, 164, 165, 166, 315–320
Broca's area, 312
butterfly hug, 13, 27, 234, 246, 302, 304, 305, 308, 309, 359, 380

Calm Place exercise, 302. *See also* Safe Place exercise
caregivers, 24, 45, 46, 49, 129, 138. *See also* family-based play therapy in sand tray; parents
   access to, 418–419
   and affect dysregulation, 262
   assessment of, 86–91
   and attachment, 148, 350–351
   attachment history, 155
   betrayal by, 259
   and child, improvement of attachment between, 270
   debriefing to, 414
   educating on dissociation, 252–253
   explaining dissociation to, 271–272
   involvement

   in Playroom Parts-of-Self process, 283
   in therapeutic work, 24–28, 39, 76, 77
   and mentalization skills, 193
   Pocket Smock for, 335
   Popcorn Night intervention, 413–426
   preparation, CCPT/DPT, 160–162
   resourcing, 55, 166
   through attachment play, 158–160
   window of tolerance, 118
case conceptualization, 12, 39, 124, 155, 156
CCPT. *See* child-centered play therapy
chewing gum strategy, 296
Child and Adolescent Committee, ISSTD, 253, 261
child-centered play therapy (CCPT), 4–5, 6, 17, 40, 41, 145, 150–151, 156, 160, 299
   attachment building, 170–171
   for dissociation, 283–284
   EMDR assessment and reprocessing, 171–176
   history and preparation, caregiver, 160–162
   impromptu RDI, 167–170
   play objectives of, 157
   preparation, child, 162–167
   therapeutic alliance, 8–9, 10
Child Dissociation Checklist, 260
Child Dissociative Experience Scale and Traumatic Stress Inventory, 260
child–parent relationship therapy (CPRT), 4, 25
CIPOS. *See* Constant Installation of Present Orientation and Safety
closure phase, 395, 407
   family-based play therapy, 101–102
   Latinx children, EMDR therapy with, 239
   Popcorn Night intervention, 413–426
   synergetic play therapy, 125, 126
cognitive distortion, 65
cognitive interweaves, 22, 55, 176, 216, 243–244, 245, 367, 369, 382, 384
cognitive processing, and dissociation, 264–265
Color Hands intervention, 393
   case example, 397–399
   considerations, 396–397
   intervention, 394
   modifications, 396
   rationale, 394
   step-by-step instructions, 394–395
Color Your Heart intervention, 57
communication, 56, 78–79, 150
   among parts of self, 285
   with Latinx clients, 226, 228–229
Competency Surge, 45–46
complex posttraumatic stress disorder (CPTSD), 219
complex trauma, 149, 151, 157, 201, 219, 252, 312, 366
Conference Room Technique, 275
Constant Installation of Present Orientation and Safety (CIPOS), 28, 332, 368
container exercise, 157, 207, 208, 273, 348

Cool as a Cucumber intervention, 46
CopeCakes intervention, 48
coping, 113
  assessment/augmentation, TraumaPlay, 47–49
  skills, 124, 125, 158, 171
Coping Tree exercise, 48
Coping Umbrellas exercise, 48
covert traumas, 260
CPRT. *See* child–parent relationship therapy
CPTSD. *See* complex posttraumatic stress disorder
cradling exercise, 152–153, 170
crawl tunnel, 234
CREATE. *See* Creative embodiment, Relational resonating, Expressive communicating, Adaptive responding, Transformative integrating, and Empathizing and compassion
creative arts therapy. *See* expressive arts therapy
Creative embodiment, Relational resonating, Expressive communicating, Adaptive responding, Transformative integrating, and Empathizing and compassion (CREATE), 188, 189
Creative Meeting Place exercise, 208
Cuento therapy, 247
cultural competence, 224–227
culture, 224–227, 239–246

dart boards as TraumaPlay equipment, 51–54
deep breathing, 50, 315–320
depersonalization, 257
derealization, 257
desensitization phase, 22
  CCPT/DPT, 175–176
  Color Hands intervention, 393–399
  family-based play therapy, 101–102
  Latinx children, EMDR therapy with, 233–234, 244
  Lemon Squeezies intervention, 339–348
  Resource Wand intervention, 365–369
  Splatting Out the Trauma intervention, 379–391
  Superhero Shuffle intervention, 371–378
  Theraplay, EMDR-infused, 349–363
developmental play therapy (DPT), 5, 145, 151–153, 157, 160
  attachment building, 170–171
  EMDR assessment and reprocessing, 171–176
  history and preparation, caregiver, 160–162
  impromptu RDI, 167–170
  preparation, child, 162–167
developmental trauma disorder, 149
DID. *See* dissociative identity disorder
directive trauma narrative work, 62–63
discrete behavioral states model, 257
dissociation, 113, 199, 251–252, 256–257
  "aha moments" of therapists, 252–255
  BASK model of, 380
  categorization of, 256
  child-centered play therapy, 283–284
  clients, problems with, 254–255
  communication among parts, 285
  diagnosis of, 260–261
  directive play with parts, 284
  early life experiences leading to, 258–260
  educating parents on, 252–253
  extreme, 257, 267
  integration, 286–287
  mild, 256
  moderate, 257
  Playroom Parts-of-Self process, 272, 275–283
  potency of integrated models of treatment in, 28
  processing phase of EMDR, 285
    child parts, containing, 285
    playing, 286
  reason for knowing about, 253–254
  resources on, 253, 271
  screening measures, 260–261
  self-states
    in and out of therapy room, 265–268
    switching between, 268, 272
  symptoms of, 261
    affect dysregulation, 262
    behavioral control, 263–264
    biological, 261–262
    cognitive (information processing), 264–265
    emotional shifts, 262
    interference with new attachments, 261
  theories of, 257–258
  treatment, 268–269
    behavior, meaning of, 269
    caregiver and child, improvement of attachment between, 270
    evaluation, 269
    examples, 283–286
    future, building, 270
    harmful/destructive behaviors, children not remembering, 273–274
    as normal as possible, 270
    psychoeducation and working with parents to understand dissociation, 271–272
    reducing triggers to create safety, 270–271
dissociation doll, 275, 276, 277
dissociative identity disorder (DID), 272, 280
Dissociative Table Technique, 207–208
DPT. *See* developmental play therapy
dry-erase face activity, 57, 58
dual attention stimulation. *See* bilateral stimulation (BLS)
dual awareness, 116, 119–120, 129, 130, 313
dysregulation, autonomic nervous system, 113, 114, 115, 116, 118, 120
  nervous system symptoms of, 112

ETC. *See* expressive therapies continuum
educate model, for discovering self-states, 258

egg splat balls technique, 381
ego state resourcing, 158
El Espanto, 245
embodied play therapy, 311
  case example, 320–322
  interventions, 315–320
  materials, 311
  rationale, 312–315
EMDR. *See* eye movement desensitization and reprocessing
EMDR-IGTP. *See* EMDR integrative group treatment protocol
EMDR integrative group treatment protocol (EMDR-IGTP), 246
EMDRIA. *See* Eye Movement Desensitization and Reprocessing International Association
emotion ball games, 164
emotional development, effect of trauma on, 147–148
emotional flooding, 130–131, 135, 139, 162
  and boundaries, 133
  and involvement of parents, 134
  response of body to, 131
emotional literacy, 35, 36, 56–58, 158
emotional personalities, 258
emotional resources, development of, 137–138
emotional vocabulary, 164
enmeshment, 198
epistemic mistrust, 191, 192, 194, 212–213
epistemic trust, 191, 195, 196, 201, 203
epistemic vigilance, 191, 192
Erase the Place game, 66
experiential learning theory, 188, 192
experiential mastery play, 37, 59
experiential play therapy, 402
  exploratory stage, 402
  termination/friends saying goodbye, 402
  testing for protection, 402
  therapeutic growth, 402
  working stage, 402
explicit memory, 112
expressive arts therapy, 42, 150, 183–184, 197–198
  assessment phase, 199
  boundaries, 212–214
  collaborative approach, 200–201
  development of art expression and experience, 184–187
  directives, 205, 206, 210
  EMDR props, 211, 212
  enmeshment, 198
  feelings, expression of, 211–212, 213, 216, 217
  future template, 217–218
  history/treatment plan, 199, 201–203
  inside/outside self, 206
  as mentalization therapy, 194–197
  parts of self, exploration of, 207–209
  preparation phase, 211
  processing, 214–217
  psychoeducation, 203, 207
  resourcing, 207, 208
  self through time, 210–211
  skill building, 207, 214
  timeline, 201, 210–211
  use for healing, evidence, 187–190
  window of tolerance, 203–206, 207
expressive therapies continuum (ETC),189
external regulator, synergetic play therapy, 117–119, 141, 142
eye movement desensitization and reprocessing (EMDR), 3, 153–154, 403. *See also individual phases*
  and children, 154–155
  as clinical approach, 5–6
  effectiveness, limits for, 183
  informed consent language for, 86
  integration with play therapy. *See* play therapy and EMDR, integration of
  process, explaining to children, 124–125
  studies with children/adolescents, measures, 87–88
  therapists, training for, 76
Eye Movement Desensitization and Reprocessing International Association (EMDRIA), 268

face painting activity, 354–355, 359
Familismo, 239
family-based play therapy in sand tray, 84–85
  case example, 91–92, 93, 94–95, 96–99, 100–101, 102–104
  desensitization, body scan, installation, and closure, 101–102
  history and treatment planning, 85
    attunement worksheet, 90–91
    children, assessment of, 92–93
    families, assessment of, 93–94
    informed consent language, 85–86
    parents, assessment of, 86–91
  preparation, 95–96
    safe place practice, 97–98
    timeline, creation of, 98–99
  reevaluation and future template, 103–104
  target assessment, 99–100
  target setup, 100–101
  targeted memory, resolving, 102–103
Family Experience in Childhood Scale, 25
family therapy, 25, 92
  and AIP, 75–78
  play in, 77
fantasy play, 265
Fatalismo (Fatalism), 239–240
faulty neuroception, 312
  6Fs of, 313, 317–318, 321
fawn-or-fool around/fidget response, 312, 313
Feeling-State Addiction Protocol (FSAP), 360, 361, 362
felt safety, 28, 35, 42, 85, 95, 125

fight-or-flight response, 312, 313
filial therapy, 76, 151, 368
finger puppets as props, 350
first-generation Latinx children/teens, 227
flashforward procedure, 238–239
foam sword prop, 13, 14
folk stories, 247
Fort Tent Calm/Safe Place intervention, 301
  case example, 306–310
  considerations, 306
  intervention, 303
  materials, 301
  modifications, 306
  rationale, 301–302
  step-by-step instructions, 303–306
freeze-or-faint response, 312, 313
freeze response, 111
FSAP. *See* Feeling-State Addiction Protocol
Fuller, Buckminster, 109
Future Movies activity, 270

generational differences, and Latinx children, 227–229
genograms, 94
Gil, Eliana, 10, 12, 13, 29, 77, 380
gradual exposure, play-based, 58–59, 62, 279–280

hand model of the brain, 317, 321
HeartMath™, 272
history/treatment plan phase, 124, 129, 155–156, 366, 385
  CCPT/DPT, caregiver, 160–162
  dissociation, 269–272
  expressive arts therapy, 199, 201–203
  family-based play therapy, 85–95
  Latinx children, EMDR therapy with, 229–232, 234–235, 239–240, 245
  questions for immigrants, 235–237
  trauma history, play-based, 293–299
Homemade Chicken Soup analogy, 420–421
homeostasis, 114, 200
hot potato game, 227
hyperarousal, 34, 49, 95, 96, 380
hypoarousal, 34, 95, 96

ICE. *See* Immigration and Customs Enforcement
Immigration and Customs Enforcement (ICE), 227
immigration history, 227
implicit memory, 112, 115–116, 127, 146–147, 148, 259
infancy
  discrete behavioral states in, 259
  trauma in, 259
information processing, and dissociation, 264–265
informed consent
  language for EMDR, 86
  language for sandtray, 85–86

installation phase, 42, 157–158, 406–408, 409
  Color Hands intervention, 393–399
  family-based play therapy, 101–102
  Latinx children, EMDR therapy with, 234
  Lemon Squeezies intervention, 339–348
  Splatting Out the Trauma intervention, 379–391
  Superhero Shuffle intervention, 371–378
  Theraplay, EMDR-infused, 349–363
integration, 286–287
Integrative Attachment Trauma Protocol, 25
internal working model, 148
International Society for the Study of Trauma and Dissociation (ISSTD), 253, 261
interoception, 314
interpersonal neurobiology integration, impacts of play therapy on, 81, 82–83
interviewing a body part technique, 245
ISSTD. *See* International Society for the Study of Trauma and Dissociation

kindling process, 113

Landreth, Gary, 4
language
  informed consent, 85–86
  trauma language, 241
  use, during therapeutic process with Latinx children, 224, 227, 228–229, 240, 241
Latinx children, EMDR therapy with, 223
  background, 223–224
  communication, 226
  cultural/individual strengths, utilizing and emphasizing, 239–246
  culture and cultural competence, 224–227
  generational differences and acculturation levels, 227–229
  group protocol, 245
  integration of playful and cultural interventions, 229
    being curious, asking questions, and maintaining an open attitude, 234–239
    child's lead and interest, following, 229–234
  language, 228–229
  Latinx term clarification, 224
  legal status of family members, 228
  somatization, 245
  titration and pendulation, 237–238
  using story template and *Cuento*, 247
Lemon Squeezies intervention, 339
  case example, 344–348
  considerations, 344
  intervention, 340
  materials, 339
  modifications, 344
  paper slice template, 345
  rationale, 340
  step-by-step instructions, 340–344
limpia, 244

Lose the Bruise game, 66–67
loteria game, 240
Lowenfeld, Margaret, 78–79, 81

magic carpet swing, 59
magic eraser board, 233–234
Magical Realism. *See Realismo Magico* (Magical Realism) approach
Mal de Ojo (evil eye), 244
Marianismo, 245
Marschak interaction method (MIM) assessment, 39, 354
MBT. *See* mentalization-based therapy
medial prefrontal cortex, 312
mentalization, 25, 190–194, 197–198
  affect regulator, 192–193
  definition of, 191
  and reasoning, 192
  skills, and trauma/stress, 191, 193
  split self, 191–192
mentalization-based therapy (MBT), 190–194
  expressive arts therapy as, 194–197
metaphors, 10, 11–12, 17, 22, 28, 340, 362
  anger volcano, 56, 57
  CCPT/DPT, 175
  for coping, 48
  expressive arts therapy, 201, 206, 207
  Latinx children, in EMDR therapy with, 240
  Lemon Squeezies, 339–348
  props, 203
  story, 294–299
Mexican Association for Mental Health Support in Crisis (AMAMECRISIS), 246
MIM. *See* Marschak interaction method assessment
miniatures, sandtray therapy, 80
minority groups, self-descriptions of, 225
mirror neuron system, 120–121, 122–123, 128, 129, 142
Moments of Meeting, 330
Montessori, Maria, 188
Mood Music intervention, 57
music, 229–230
mutual regression, 120

NC. *See* negative cognition
negative cognition (NC), 66–67, 99, 100, 140, 242, 309, 314, 339–348, 382, 389, 397, 402, 403–404, 408
negative self-talk, 66, 384
nervous system, 115, 117
  autonomic, 111
  parasympathetic, 111, 312
  regulation activities from synergetic play therapy, 131–132
  sympathetic, 111, 312
  symptoms of regulation and dysregulation, 112
neuroception of safety, 116, 119, 130, 131, 135, 139

neuroesthetics, 187
neurosensitization, 113
neurosequential approach to play therapy, 16
NHDA. *See* Nurture House Dyadic Assessment
noticing, 332, 353, 354
Nurture House Dyadic Assessment (NHDA), 39, 45, 55, 63
Nurturing Narration, 62–63

open-ended questions, 235
origami, 231
Our Thermostat System, 327, 328, 329, 354–355
Our Three Channels poster, 330–331, 355–356
out of sight, out of mind, 200
oxytocin, 49

parasympathetic nervous system, 111, 312
parent–child dyad, 15, 25
  games, 45
  Nurture House Dyadic Assessment (NHDA), 39
  synergetic play therapy, 134–137
  Theraplay, 26–27, 55
parents, 273. *See also* family-based play therapy in sand tray
  assessment, family-based play therapy, 86–91
  attachment history, 155
  as cotherapists, 283, 416
  educating on dissociation, 252–253
  explaining dissociation to, 271–272
  involvement, 134, 151, 199
  in play therapy, 76, 77–78
  in Playroom Parts-of-Self process, 283
  throughout treatment, 24–28
  as partners, TraumaPlay, 34, 45–47, 55
  Popcorn Night intervention, 413–426
  presence, limiting, 26
  resourcing through attachment play, 158–160
  soothing of children, 417
Parts of Self exercise, 207–208
patty cakes game, 18–19, 152, 231
PC. *See* positive cognition
personalized board game journey activity, 54
PFS. *See* Positive Feeling Scale
physiology, soothing (TraumaPlay), 45–47, 49–50
pizza analogy, 231–232
play-based gradual exposure, 58–59, 62
play therapy, 3. *See also* family-based play therapy in sand tray
  and AIP, 75–78
  as clinical approach, 4–5
  definition of, 149
  impacts on interpersonal neurobiology integration, 81, 82–83
  models, 150
  for treatment of children, reasons, 149–150
play therapy and EMDR, integration of, 6–8, 154
  bridges from implicit to explicit trauma work, 20–23

INDEX 433

holding space for posttraumatic play, 10–13
involving parents throughout treatment, 24–28
memory targets
  expanding/addressing, 17–20
  ongoing reevaluation of, 24
prop-based BLS, playing EMDR with, 13–15
state change, expanding capacity for, 15–17
therapeutic alliance, 8–10
Play Therapy room, Pocket Smock for use in, 334
play therapy targets for EMDR processing
  body scan, installation, and reevaluation, 409–410
  case example, 405–410
  considerations, 404–405
  materials, 401–402
  rationale, 402–403
  reprocessing and installation phases, 406–408
  step-by-step instructions, 403
    assessment phase, 403–404
Playroom Parts-of-Self process, 272
  checking in with parts of self, 281
  dialogue/cooperation among parts, creating, 282
  gradual exposure, 279–280
  head honcho, engaging, 282
  hostile/perpetrator–imitator parts, 282
    checking for, 281
  investigating parts, 280
    questions to ask, 280–281
    types of parts of self, 280
  parent involvement, 283
  phobia of dissociated parts of self, 277
  preparation of therapist in accessing self-states, 275–276
  setup, 278
    imagining/creating space, 278–279
    thoughts of therapists, 279
  taking to the parts though the child, 281–282
  use of, 276–277
Pocket Smock intervention, 325
  blank template, 334
  brainstorm ideas, 330
  case example, 335–337
  considerations and modifications
    caregiver Pocket Smock, 335
    Play Therapy room Pocket Smock, 334
    voice and choice, 332–333
  draft
    assigning, 330
    designing, 330
    practice, 332
    structuring, 330–331
    wearing Pocket Smock, 331–332
  intervention, 327
  materials, 325–326
  Our Thermostat System, 327, 328, 329
  present examples, 329
  purpose, explanation of, 328

rationale
  lasting protective factors, 326–327
  responsibility, safety, and control/choice, 326
  step-by-step instructions, 327–332
polyvagal theory, 25, 56, 116, 256, 312
Poop Emoji props, 54–55
Popcorn Night intervention, 413
  alternative to, 420–421
  case examples, 419–420
  considerations, 419
  handout, 422–426
  intervention, 415–416
  materials, 413
  modification, 418–419
  rationale, 413–415
  step-by-step instructions
    closure phase, 416–417
    reevaluation phase, 418
positive cognition (PC), 66, 99, 100, 140, 234, 242, 314, 339–348, 372, 374, 381, 382, 389, 395, 397, 402, 403–404
Positive Feeling Scale (PFS), 361
posttraumatic growth, 69
posttraumatic play, 10, 29, 37
  dynamic, 10, 12, 19
  expanding/addressing memory targets in, 17–20
  holding space for, 10–13
  toxic, 12
  TraumaPlay, 53–54, 58–59
posttraumatic stress disorder (PTSD), 35, 62, 111, 113, 153, 258 259
  with dissociative symptoms, 261
  potency of integrated models of treatment in, 28
prefrontal cortex, 312
preparation phase, 15, 39, 55, 314, 365–367, 413, 414
  CCPT/DPT
    caregiver, 160–162
    child, 162–167
  dissociation, 272–274
  embodied play therapy, 311–322
  expressive arts therapy, 211
  family-based play therapy, 95–99
  Fort Tent Calm/Safe Place intervention, 301–310
  Latinx children, EMDR therapy with, 230, 232, 237, 240
  Pocket Smock intervention, 325–337
  self-management measures, 352
  stabilization measures, 352
  Superhero Shuffle intervention, 371–378
  synergetic play therapy, 124–125, 137–138
  Theraplay, EMDR-infused, 349–363
  trauma-sensitive yoga, 311–322
prescriptive play therapy, 3, 4–5, 7. *See also* play therapy

pretend mode states, 191, 192, 194, 199, 206, 208
prompts, sand tray therapy, 80
prop-based bilateral stimulation, playing EMDR with, 13–15
proprioception, 135, 234
psych equivalent states, 191–192, 199, 206
psychoeducation, 95, 203, 207, 247, 271–272, 317
PTSD. *See* posttraumatic stress disorder
Punching Holes in That Theory game, 66
puppets as props, 37, 38, 232, 308, 350

RDI. *See* resource development and installation
Real Deal Reel images, 362–363
Realismo Magico (Magical Realism) approach, 242
reasoning, and lack of mentalization, 192
reevaluation phase, 24, 103–104, 409–410
  family-based play therapy, 103–104
  Latinx children, EMDR therapy with, 239, 246
  Popcorn Night intervention, 413–426
  synergetic play therapy, 125–126, 127, 137
reflective functioning, 188, 205
regulation, autonomic nervous system
  external regulator, 117–119
  nervous system symptoms of, 112
  and SPT–EMDR integration, 116–117
  therapist as an instrument, 117
relational neurobiology, 189
relational resourcing, 37, 55–56
religious beliefs/figures, and Latinx children/families, 239
reprocessing phase, 22, 101, 406–408, 414
  CCPT/DPT, 171–176
  dissociation, 285–286
  expressive arts therapy, 214–217
  Latinx children, EMDR therapy with, 232–233, 233–234, 237–239, 240, 242–245
  side effects of, 416–417
  Splatting Out the Trauma intervention, 383
  Theraplay, EMDR-infused, 359
resource development, 125, 162, 166, 314, 371–378, 395
  emotional resources, 137–138
  expressive arts therapy, 207, 208
  Latinx children, EMDR therapy with, 229–231
resource development and installation (RDI), 157–158, 314
  CCPT/DPT, 167–170
Resource Wand intervention, 365
  case example, 368–369
  considerations, 368
  intervention, 366
  materials, 365
  modifications, 367–368
  rationale, 365–366
  step-by-step instructions, 366–367
resourcing through attachment play, 158–160
response to intervention model, 351

ribbon wand, 13, 14
rocking, 27, 117, 128, 167–169, 170, 171
role playing, 15, 274

Safe Place exercise, 157, 196, 314, 403, 404–405
  CCPT/DPT, 165–166
  child parts, containing, 285
  contamination of, 43–44, 97
  in family-based play therapy, 97–98
  Fort Tent Calm/Safe Place intervention, 301–310
  synergetic play therapy, 139
  in TraumaPlay, 42–44, 65
safety, sense of, 133, 159, 268, 302, 326
  and communication among parts of self, 285
  enhancing, TraumaPlay, 41–42
  family-based play therapy, 85, 89, 95, 97–98
  felt safety, 28, 35, 42, 85, 95, 125
  play-based trauma history, 296
  reduction of triggers, 270–271
  in synergetic play therapy, 130
  and therapist authenticity, 122
SAMHSA. *See* Substance Abuse and Mental Health Services America
sandtray, 5, 15, 84, 321, 348, 406. *See also* family-based play therapy in sand tray
  CCPT/DPT, 165, 172
  expressive arts therapy, 215–216
  informed consent language for, 85–86
  Latinx children, EMDR therapy with, 231
  as modality, 78–79
    cleanup, 83
    creation of tray, 80–81
    documentation of session, 83–84
    introduction of process to client, 80
    postcreation, 81, 83
    preparation of setting, 79–80
    shapes, 79
  TraumaPlay, 67, 70–72
    Safe Place, creation of, 42
Sands of Time intervention, 57
Scaer, Robert, 113
scaling, EMDR, 63–64. *See also individual scales*
school staff, 270, 419
second-generation Latinx children/teens, 227–228
secure attachment style, 332, 350–351, 352
security, 352
  enhancing, TraumaPlay, 41–42
  family-based play therapy, 89
self. *See also* Playroom Parts-of-Self process
  inside/outside, 206
  parts
    exploration of, 207–209
    types of, 280
  posttrauma, making positive meaning of, 69–72
  split, 191

use by play therapists, 41
self-states. *See* dissociation
Shapiro, Francine, 3, 5, 75, 110, 111, 153, 183, 302, 380
Skycurve Platform Swing equipment, 50
social development, effect of trauma on, 147–148
social engagement system, 312
somatization, 200
  and dissociation, 261–262
  of Latinx clients, 245
  somatic experiencing with trauma targets, 67–69
somatosensory activities, 272
sore spot analogy, 263
special words in Theraplay, 353
Splatting Out the Trauma intervention, 379
  case example, 384–391
  considerations, 384
  intervention, 381
  materials, 379
  modifications, 383
  rationale, 379–381
  step-by-step instructions, 381–383
SPT. *See* synergetic play therapy
Stages of Psychosocial Development, 332, 333
Star Theoretical Model, 258
state change
  expanding capacity for, 15–17
  playful activities for, 16
storytelling, 27, 247
  metaphorical story, 294–299
  story template, 247, 359
  Theraplay, EMDR-infused, 359–360
  in TraumaPlay, 45, 46–47, 61–62
strengths perspective approach, 224, 237
structural dissociation, 258
structural dissociation theory, 28
Subjective Units of Distress Scale (SUDS), 24, 63, 64, 100, 199, 202, 215, 216, 231, 233, 296, 343, 344, 346, 348, 353, 376, 381, 382, 383, 388, 389, 396, 399, 404, 406
Substance Abuse and Mental Health Services America (SAMHSA), 6
SUDS. *See* Subjective Units of Distress Scale
Superhero Shuffle intervention, 371
  case example, 376–378
  considerations, 375–576
  intervention, 372–373
  modifications, 374–375
  rationale, 371–372
  step-by-step instructions, 373–374
sympathetic nervous system, 111, 312
synergetic play therapy (SPT), 109
  assessment of child for EMDR readiness, 130–134
  bilateral stimulation, 128
  closure, 126, 137

coregulation, 109, 118, 124, 127, 129
dual awareness, 119–120, 129, 130
and EMDR, 109–111, 114–116
  regulation, 116–117
  synergy between, 123–130
emotional resources, development of, 137–138
empowerment, 130
external regulator, 117–119, 141, 142
foundational elements, 111–114
mirror neuron system, 120–121
nervous system regulation activities from, 131–132
parent–child dyad, 134–137
preparation phase, 124–125, 137–138
reevaluation phase, 125–126, 127, 137
reprocessing trauma, 138–142
therapist activation, 120
therapist as an instrument of regulation, 117
therapist authenticity, 121–123
synergetics, 109

teleological mode, 192, 196
Tell Me the Targets activity, 51
termination plans, 326–327
Terr, Lenore, 10
TF-CBT. *See* Trauma-Focused Cognitive Behavioral Therapy
Theory of Mind, 190
thera-tapper, 402, 404
therapeutic alliance, 8–10, 240, 303, 350
therapeutic powers of play, 40
therapeutic presence, 41
therapeutic relationship, 10, 124, 133, 151, 194, 293, 314, 375
  authenticity, 122
  with Latinx children, 235, 239, 240
  and play, 49
  and posttraumatic growth, 69
  and power, 225
  and sense of control of child, 394
  and therapeutic presence, 41
Theraplay, 5, 15, 17, 26–27, 55, 332–333, 336
Theraplay, EMDR-infused, 349
  case example, 361–362
  considerations
    Real Deal Reel, 362–363
    storytelling, 359–360
    Upside-Down Scale, 360–361
  intervention, 352
  materials, 349–350
  Our Thermostat System, 354–355
  predictability, 358–359
  preparation phase, 352
  rationale
    common foundation, 350–351
    fundamental therapeutic differences and professional training, 350

Theraplay, EMDR-infused (cont.)
   natural progression of therapeutic intervention, 351–352
   session sequence, 358
   step-by-step instructions
      adding BLS, 356–357
      cross-referencing client history sources, 353
      notes, 357–358
      noticing and complementing, 353–354
      VOC, assessing for, 357
      wonder, expressions of, 354–356
TheraTappers, 45
Thinking Caps game, 66
third-generation Latinx children/teens, 228
Thoughts Kit for Kids, 66
thought life, addressing during reprocessing, 65–67
time machine drawing, 238–239
time-orientation strategies, 201
timeline scroll metaphor, 201–202
titration, 51, 67, 68, 130, 140, 201
touch, 47, 135, 152, 153, 165–166, 170
toy brain prop, 37, 38
traditional games, 240, 246
translators, 226
Trauma-Focused Cognitive Behavioral Therapy (TF-CBT), 29, 58
trauma history, play-based, 293
   case example, 297–299
   identification of events, struggle in, 297
   intervention, 294
   materials, 293
   modifications, 296
   rationale, 293–294
   step-by-step directions
      distress level, rating, 296
      getting the history, 295
      safety, reestablishing, 296
trauma language, 241
trauma narrative work, 59–62
   Nurturing Narration, 62–63
trauma-sensitive yoga (TSY), 311
   case example, 320–322
   deep breathing for coregulation, 315–320
   interventions
      be spaghetti, 316–317, 322
      bubble piles, 316, 321
      fight-or-flight charades, 317–319
      lion-kitty, 315–316, 321
      noodle hug, 317, 322
      pass a breath, 316
      walk like a…, 319–320, 321–322
   materials, 311
   rationale, 312–315
TraumaPlay, 7, 33–35
   addressing thought life during reprocessing, 65–67
   assessment, 39–41
   assessment phase in EMDR, 51–55
   coping, assessment/augmentation of, 47–49
   and EMDR, integration of, 37–38
   emotional literacy, increasing, 56–58
   enhancing safety and security, 41–42
   experiential mastery play, 59
   flowchart, 34, 35
   goals of, 33, 34
   intake interview, 39
   making positive meaning of the posttrauma self, 69–72
   Mapping Tool, 35–36
   Nurturing Narration, 62–63
   ongoing assessment, 35–36
   parents as partners, 45–47, 55
   posttraumatic play and play-based gradual exposure, 58–59
   relational resourcing, 55–56
   Safe Place in TraumaPlay, 42–43, 65
      contamination of, 43–44
   scaling, 63–64
   somatic experiencing with trauma targets, 67–69
   soothing the physiology, 45–47, 49–50
   titration, 67, 68
   trauma narrative work, 59–62
TSY. *See* trauma-sensitive yoga
two hats game, 237–238

Upside-Down Scale tool, 360–361

vagus nerve, 116
Validity of Cognition (VoC) Scale, 100, 102, 172, 175, 233, 342, 344, 347, 348, 353, 374, 376, 381, 382, 383, 389, 395, 396, 399
ventral vagal response, 111, 116
Veo, Veo game, 238
VoC. *See* Validity of Cognition Scale

weighted blankets, use with body scan, 234
Why Wheel game, 66
window of tolerance (WOT), 16, 27, 35, 46, 54, 95, 96, 118–119, 130, 131, 132, 133, 135, 140, 203–206, 207, 237, 312–313, 355
Wisdom Feathers activity, 69, 70
World Technique, 78
worry dolls, 241–242, 243
WOT. *See* window of tolerance

yoga. *See* trauma-sensitive yoga (TSY)
young children, trauma in, 145
   adaptive information processing, 146–147
   attachment, 148–149
      building, 170–171
   child-centered play therapy, 150–151
   developmental play therapy, 151–153

EMDR, 153–155
  assessment and reprocessing, 171–176
  history and case conceptualization, 155–156
  integration of CCPT, DPT, and EMDR, 160
    history/preparation, caregiver, 160–162
    impromptu RDI, 167–170
    preparation, child, 162–167

play therapy, reasons for using, 149–150
resourcing through attachment play, 158–160
social, emotional, and behavioral development, 147–148

zone of proximal development (Vygotsky), 332, 333

www.ingramcontent.com/pod-product-compliance
Ingram Content Group UK Ltd.
Pitfield, Milton Keynes, MK11 3LW, UK
UKHW021837210426
5322IPUK00021B/343